THE EMOTION REGULATION SKILLS SYSTEM FOR CLIENTS WITH COGNITIVE CHALLENGES

The Emotion Regulation Skills System for Clients with Cognitive Challenges

A DBT-Informed Approach

SECOND EDITION

Julie F. Brown

THE GUILFORD PRESS
New York London

Published by The Guilford Press
A Division of Guilford Publications, Inc.
www.guilford.com

Printed in the United States of America

This book is printed on acid-free paper.

For product and safety concerns within the EU, please contact *GPSR@taylorandfrancis.com*, Taylor & Francis Verlag GmbH, Kaufingerstraße 24, 80331 München, Germany.

Last digit is print number: 9 8 7 6 5 4 3 2 1

Library of Congress Cataloging-in-Publication Data is available from the publisher.

ISBN 978-1-4625-5938-1 (paperback) — ISBN 978-1-4625-5939-8 (hardcover)

About the Author

Julie F. Brown, MSW, PhD, is the president of Skills System, LLC. She is an independent social worker who has practiced in the intellectual disabilities field since the 1990s. Dr. Brown has been a dialectical behavior therapy (DBT) trainer with Behavioral Tech Institute since 2005.

Preface

People sometimes ask me, "How did you come up with the Skills System?" It has been a journey that is difficult to sum up in a few words, so I often fumble. I sometimes say, "It was a gift," or "I created it with my clients." Both of these are accurate, although a bit esoteric and unclear. This Preface is an opportunity for me to share the story of the process.

DEVELOPING THE SKILLS SYSTEM

The Treasure Hunt

The development of the Skills System has been a 30-year journey. This adventure began shortly after I graduated from Boston University with my MSW. I was working as a clinician in a behaviorally based 25-bed residential school for intellectually disabled, emotionally disturbed adolescent males and females in New England. One day, a youth who had a significant history of committing sexual offenses, setting fires, treating animals cruelly, and assaulting others was sitting in my office. We were discussing his latest incident of aggression toward a staff member. I posed questions, trying to elicit alternatives to smashing a staff member in the head with a padlock. The young man was unable to generate useful options; thus, I suggested that he play the card game Uno instead.

In the midst of suggesting he play Uno, I experienced an epiphany. This boy had suffered numerous traumas and inflicted even more, and my solution was Uno! While pulling this suggestion out of my eclectic bag of therapeutic tricks, I suddenly became keenly aware that this isolated activity was a woefully inadequate intervention. The card game may have been a piece of a coping puzzle, yet the problem was that I did not have an adequate, synthesized framework or system to teach coping to this individual in a form that he could understand, apply, and generalize. If I did not have a comprehensive representation of a coping map, there was no way that this intellectually disabled adolescent was going to integrate my random teaching into a technically strong, yet flexible model that could help him manage the challenging internal and external factors he faced on a daily basis.

I possessed no vision about the path ahead, but the journey to find the Skills System had begun.

I spent the next 3 years immersed in treating this diverse and challenging youth population within the residential setting. I combed the literature for insights; I found more tiny puzzle pieces but still no map: no comprehensive tools to help youth with numerous mental health diagnoses integrate the necessary skills to reduce the need for supervision; no models complex enough yet simple enough to assist individuals who struggled with effects of neglect, violent behavior, physical abuse, sexual victimization, and/or social stigmatization. I could not find a program that could help these youth reduce the need for multiple antipsychotic medications, antidepressants, mood stabilizers, and other drugs to control behavior. Although the well-structured token economy within the facility was helpful, it was not sufficient to teach these children, who had complex needs, the necessary skills to regulate their reinforced patterns of dyscontrol in settings beyond residential care. Somewhere there had to be a better solution.

During a monthly consultation in 1997, a well-regarded trauma specialist recommended I find out more about dialectical behavior therapy (DBT; Linehan, 1993a, 1993b, 2025a, 2025b). Initially, I asked myself, "How could a treatment for women with borderline personality disorder [BPD] who demonstrated suicidal and parasuicidal behaviors apply to my clients?" During my initial phases of DBT training, I discovered that although few of my clients were formally diagnosed with BPD, many experienced the BPD behavioral patterns of emotional, cognitive, and behavioral dysregulation described by Linehan. I was cautiously optimistic that DBT would prove to be a piece of the treasure map.

By 1999, I was fortunate enough to have received intensive DBT training and started a small outpatient therapy clinic in New England. The program provided outpatient therapy services for adults with mild and moderate intellectual disabilities who experienced intense behavioral control problems. Standard DBT individual therapy, skills training groups, consultation team, and phone skills coaching were key ingredients of the program. The comprehensive DBT treatment model was designed to help people change highly reinforced, long-term patterns of behavior associated with impaired emotion regulation. While it was clear that the DBT technology was helpful in improving self-management capacities, accommodations were necessary to allow cognitively impaired individuals to learn and generalize new adaptive coping skills. Adherence to the DBT model was paramount; our challenge was to make DBT technology accessible to cognitively impaired clients without reducing the therapeutic viability of the empirically validated treatment.

Surprisingly, the individual therapy aspects of DBT (Linehan, 1993a) required minimal adaptation for this population. While learning to do DBT individual therapy and treating cognitively impaired people is intellectually demanding for the therapist, participation in the treatment as a client is relatively straightforward. Unfortunately, the skills component (Linehan, 1993b) was a more complex problem. During the first year, we followed the standard DBT skills manual, adjusting teaching strategies to help improve comprehension of the information. The concepts contained in the mindfulness, interpersonal effectiveness, emotion regulation, and distress tolerance modules (Linehan, 1993b) were vital, yet the language and format were barriers for the clients. Despite my enthusiasm, many participants struggled to pronounce, remember, and understand several standard DBT skills terms and were therefore unable to recall and utilize the concepts within the context of life when emotionally dysregulated.

The DBT skills curriculum did not provide individuals diagnosed with intellectual disabilities, who often experience executive functioning deficits, a framework that facilitated transitions from one skill to the next within complicated contexts that required multiple skills. I continually felt that my clients' reaction to the information in skills training group was like mine when I played the game 52 Pickup as a child. As a group leader, I felt as if I were my mean older sister, who would invite me to play cards and then scream, "Fifty-two pickup!" as she squeezed the deck, gleefully sending the 52 cards into the air and all over the floor for me to pick up. Just as I had been overwhelmed by the cards strewn all over the floor, the participants seemed to stare, dazed and confused, at the divergent information, without even knowing which skill (or card) to pick up first.

While I was driven to maintain adherence to the DBT model, I had a clear sense that I needed to present the DBT concepts in a more accessible way if my clients were going to grasp the essential principles. I began creating step-by-step progressions that the participants with intellectual disabilities could learn and utilize. I knew that I had to find a simple system that offered participants a template to use skills dynamically in a self-generated way that integrated information from both the internal and external experience within each moment. While it was critical that the concepts be uncomplicated, the function had to be highly complex to synthesize these elements. The system had to help the individual be mindful of the current moment, mobilize Wise Mind (Linehan, 1993b, 2025a, 2025b) in a consistent way, cultivate effective planning, and embody both the simplicity and the sophistication required to help the person handle life's most abstract and demanding events. I spent months working and reworking these concepts to piece together this intricate puzzle.

One day, as I was driving, merging into a high-speed lane at 60 miles per hour, I noticed the core idea of the Skills System passing through my mind. It was so simple and so complicated at the same time—how dialectical! The treasure had emerged, and I was lucky enough to have noticed it careening through my mind. Fortunately, I didn't know at that moment how exciting this gift was, because I probably would have driven off the road.

The Treasure

Since that day on Route 195, my clients, team, and I have grappled with DBT concepts and emotion regulation principles to develop this version of the Skills System. Over time and through years of collaboration, the Skills System has become a simple yet sophisticated emotion regulation road map for youth and adults. The nine skills and three System Tools provide a useful structure that helps the individual make effective choices in service of personal goals.

The Skills System Instructor's Guide: An Emotion-Regulation Skills Curriculum for All Learning Abilities was self-published in 2011. This platform allowed the material to be protected, disseminated, and improved. *The Emotion Regulation Skills System for Clients with Cognitive Challenges, Second Edition,* is the latest version, the culmination of over two decades of work.

Despite this long history, the empirical validation process is still in its infancy. In 2013, the pilot data were published in the *Journal of Mental Health Research in Intellectual Disabilities* (Brown, Brown, & Dibiasio, 2013). This single-group, longitudinal study examined reductions in negative behavioral outcomes of the 40 individuals with intellectual disabilities over a 4-year period who participated in DBT individual therapy and Skills System skills group. The findings indicated statistically significant reductions in low-, medium-, and high-risk challenging behaviors. Although this was not a randomized controlled trial, it is my hope that the findings encourage other professionals to explore use of the Skills System.

A DBT-INFORMED APPROACH

The Skills System is designed to be a set of skills for challenged learners. The skills are built from DBT concepts and in many places are direct adaptations of the standard DBT curriculum. DBT practitioners: Be prepared—the surgery to reconstruct and improve accessibility may seem radical. Upon reading this book, the naive DBT clinician may say, "Where are all of the DBT terms?", while the seasoned veteran will see how certain DBT skills are deconstructed and repackaged to meet the needs of vulnerable learners. Most adaptations for people with intellectual disabilities politely add clipart and simplify through elimination. I tried that; it was insufficient and failed to meet the needs of this population adequately.

The reconstruction of the DBT skills had to be done carefully and effectively. Three key elements were integral in this process: (1) the work of James Gross, PhD, in emotion regulation; (2) cognitive load theory (Sweller, 2010); and (3) ongoing collaboration with my clients. It was necessary to keep DBT concepts intact, while simultaneously ensuring that the alternatives offered effective emotion regulation strategies in a user-friendly format consistent with DBT principles.

More specifically, the standard DBT skills modules format was replaced by a Skills List and System Tools that are used in a type of skills algorithm or dynamic formula that guides the individual to create adaptive skills chains. The Skills System framework helps the individual know which skills to choose and how many to implement given his level of emotion in each diverse situation. Although the nondisabled learner may be able to pick and choose skills effectively from the vast skills menu presented in the standard DBT skills manual (Linehan, 2025a), the vulnerable learner, with memory and executive functioning impairments, becomes overwhelmed. Certain DBT terms were retained, while others required adaptation. The language had to maximize recognition and recall of DBT concepts to facilitate generalization. Additionally, key skills concepts such as mindfulness (Wise Mind, Participating, and Acting Effectively), Check the Facts, Pros and Cons, and Cope Ahead had to be integrated as the base of every skills chain (Clear Picture, On-Track Thinking, and On-Track Action). An adapted DBT skills curriculum must provide functional validation to this population by presenting a maximum number of DBT concepts in ways that are accessible.

From my 35-plus years serving this population, I believe that in order to teach an individual who has moderate/mild intellectual disabilities to regulate emotions using a dialectical perspective, the skills framework must offer a structure that provides cognitive support—scaffolding—to perform high-level tasks, given that the individual has impairment in those functioning areas. Complex needs require enhanced intervention. To treat these people with more intense needs, DBT practitioners working with this population need to be bilingual: able to speak the standard DBT skills and Skills System languages.

Today I may recommend playing Uno to a given client; however, I can be confident that the individual knows several other emotion regulation skills, when to use each skill, how many skills to utilize, and how to implement the skills as a result of Skills System training. For example, recently in a skills group, one client, who was diagnosed with an intellectual disability of moderate severity, recounted a stressful situation she had managed successfully during the previous day. She described first getting a Clear Picture of the situation. She stated she was mad at a Level 4. Her staff members were not listening to what she was saying. She reported having strong urges to scream at the staff. Immediately my client stopped and stepped back. She used On-Track Thinking to reflect on whether these urges were helpful in reaching her goal. Knowing that she wanted to increase her independence and improve her relationships, she determined that screaming was not helpful. Realizing that she was too upset to use Expressing Myself or Problem Solving at that time (although she had urges to!), my client decided to do a Safety Plan and go to her room. She then reported doing an On-Track Action by calmly informing the staff members that she was going to her bedroom. While in her room, she did a few New-Me Activities (listening to music and drawing) that helped her think clearly, feel better, and relax. My client stated that later during the shift, she did her Clear Picture skill again and determined that she was feeling much calmer. She used On-Track Thinking to make a Skills Plan to talk to the staff members about the problem. Because she was calm and focused, she was able to discuss and solve the problem with the staff members.

As I listen to my clients recount detailed and effective skills usage as a part of skills training group, I periodically think of that boy with the padlock so many years ago. I think about how grateful I am to him for showing me my inadequacies. It has been a privilege working with many dedicated people—both group members and co-therapists—to improve the Skills System over the years.

THE SECOND EDITION

It has been 10 years since I wrote the first edition of this book. During that time, people all over the world have been learning the Skills System. Although minimal changes have been made to the skills themselves, I have learned that support teams need more resources to teach skills to individuals within the complex environments where they live.

To address these needs, the second edition of the Skills System text includes this volume, which is an instructor's guide, and a companion volume, *The Emotion Regulation Skills System Workbook, Second Edition.* One subtle change to this edition is to refer to the person teaching skills as an "instructor" rather than a "skills trainer," as was used in the first edition. An instructor is anyone who will be teaching skills. Instructors may have differing levels of education and be from a wide variety of disciplines (e.g., therapist, direct support professional, parents). Instructors may teach individual and/or support providers in group and/or one-on-one settings. Since the range of people who are teaching skills has vastly expanded, adjustable resources are needed to fit those instructors and the individuals they teach.

The qualities of individuals receiving skills instruction has diversified as well. Children of all ages learn skills and geriatric populations learn skills; people with various mental health diagnoses learn skills; people with all different academic and intellectual abilities learn skills. A skills instructor learns how to adapt her teaching to address the learning needs of the person they are working with.

Instructor's Guide

This book provides a comprehensive set of materials to facilitate teaching the Skills System and to begin the process of implementing the model within various settings. The first eight chapters of this second edition have been updated with recent research and informed by 10 years of additional experience teaching instructors and working with support teams. Chapter 9, Targeted Instruction, is entirely new to this edition.

Chapter 1 offers a brief overview of the Skills System, while Chapter 2 presents detailed descriptions of each of the skills and the System Tools to fulfill this task. It is important to note that the descriptions in both of these chapters are intended to teach the instructor concepts and may not be in the form that individuals with intellectual deficits should learn.

Chapter 3 introduces the theoretical underpinning for the Skills System. It explores the literature related to emotion regulation, intellectual disabilities, DBT, and cognitive load theory that all impact Skills System design and instruction. This information teaches skills instructors about key underlying principles that help them use and teach the Skills System with diverse populations.

The Skills System's enhanced teaching strategies are an integral part of the model. Given that the concept of emotion regulation is abstract, creating fathomable learning experiences is a quintessential element of the process. Chapter 4 introduces different types of instruction that are used to address each individual's and setting's unique needs. Foundational teaching strategies that are used throughout skills training are presented in Chapter 5. Chapter 6 highlights teaching strategies that are utilized within specific phases of the E-Spiral framework.

A sample 12-week curriculum that offers a detailed, week-by-week breakdown and clear instructions is presented in Chapter 7. Depending on the group, the instructor may choose to follow the 12-week curriculum closely or adapt the format to meet the needs of the learners. The curriculum cites handouts, worked examples, and worksheets that are contained in the *Skills System Workbook.*

It is important for support providers to know how to use skills. Skills help the support person self-regulate effectively, reducing escalating transactions that lead to the individual becoming dysregulated. Additionally, when a support provider knows skills, he is better able to provide emotion regulation advice to the individual he is working with. In addition to knowing skills, it is important for the support person to know skills coaching strategies that create relationships and environments that foster co-regulation versus co-dysregulation. Chapter 8 outlines relevant information for being a skills coach.

Chapter 9 offers important information about how an instructor can work to help an individual develop skills competency. Pre-learning, learning skills, and reaching goals are strategies that are designed to help the individual fill specific skills gaps so she can reach her goals.

Skills System Workbook

The most obvious change from the first edition is that the teaching handouts and worksheets are all contained in *The Emotion Regulation Skills System Workbook, Second Edition.* The *Skills System Workbook* serves as a resource for the individuals learning skills. They can progress through the materials, explore their perspectives, and individualize their learning experience. In addition, support providers can complete the *Skills System Workbook.* Reading the handouts and worked examples teaches concepts; filling out worksheets offers the person an opportunity to apply the skills in a personal way. When a support provider knows skills, he can be an effective coach. The *Skills System Workbook* also includes 80 new pages of resources! For example, there are:

- 10 new Pre-Learning worked examples and worksheets
- 20 new Learning Skills handouts, worked examples, and worksheets
- 16 new Reaching Goals worked examples and worksheets

In addition, there are also new online resources available through The Guilford Press at the workbook's companion website to facilitate teaching skills to children and adolescents:

- 25 elementary school-age worked examples
- 25 high school-age worked examples

Instructors need diverse and flexible resources to be able to teach skills to the individuals, support staff, and families they serve. The new resources in this text and the *Skills System Workbook* greatly expand teaching tools for instructors and support providers.

THE COST OF NOT TEACHING SKILLS

Never has the need for the Skills System been greater. The Skills System creates a common language that helps individuals and the people who support them communicate. The Skills System gives both individuals and people in their environment tools to help them self-regulate and co-regulate. Those of us in the mental health and/or disabilities fields know the disastrous, vicious cycles that happen when co-dysregulation between people in support environments becomes the norm. Both individuals and their support systems need accessible and effective strategies; they need a shared toolbox that fosters connections and tangible ways for all involved to reach their goals.

Acknowledgments

As I reflect on my journey with the Skills System and how this second edition has evolved, I recall what seems like hundreds of small and large contributions people have made. At the top of the list are the individuals whom I had in skills groups, who partnered with me to create the Skills System skills. We all grappled with the dialectical behavior therapy (DBT) concepts, working to increase accessibility, reduce cognitive load, and facilitate generalization of skills. Developing the Skills System was a Partnership New-Me Activity!

My journey with The Guilford Press has been pivotal. After three painful rejections over several years, I finally was able to get the Skills System material in a form such that Kitty Moore, Publisher, was able to see the Skills System's potential. Her willingness to remain engaged though this 15-year-plus process has led to three books. I am also grateful to Katherine Sommer, who edited this book and the second edition of *The Emotion Regulation Skills System Workbook,* for her amazing focus and dedication to improving these resources.

The work of Marsha M. Linehan, PhD, the developer of DBT, provided important foundational information for the Skills System. I would like to extend a special acknowledgment to Cynthia Sanderson, PhD, for her mentoring and support. James J. Gross, PhD, editor of the *Handbook of Emotion Regulation* (2007, 2014b, 2024), offered valuable feedback that improved the model.

Finally, I would like to acknowledge the contribution of my family to this project. My husband, children, and grandchildren have informed my work in many important ways.

I am grateful to you all.

Contents

Purchasers of this book can photocopy the Appendix for personal use or use with clients (see copyright page for details).

THE EMOTION REGULATION SKILLS SYSTEM FOR CLIENTS WITH COGNITIVE CHALLENGES

CHAPTER 1

Introducing the Skills System

The Skills System is a set of nine skills and three system rules that helps the individual cope with life's challenges. This emotion regulation skills curriculum was developed to help the individual organize her internal and external experiences in ways that decrease discomfort and problematic behaviors, while increasing positive affect and goal-directed actions. This simple framework guides the person through the process of becoming aware of the current moment (mindfulness), directing attention, and activating behaviors that are in service of personal goals. The individual learns to follow steps that mobilize inner wisdom ("Wise Mind"; Linehan, 2025a) in each unique situation. As the skills and the System Tools (guidelines for assembling skills chains) are integrated into the context of the person's life, often effective coping behaviors increase. Each situation provides the individual with an opportunity for self-discovery and for active participation in events; she can move ahead effectively.

BENEFITS OF THE SKILLS SYSTEM

User-Friendly for Individuals with Learning Challenges

Learning new, more adaptive patterns of behavior is a challenging task for anyone. This is especially difficult when the individual must manage complicating factors such as mental health issues, intellectual impairment, physical problems, or other difficult life circumstances. These life challenges may increase stress and impact the individual's ability to learn new information. The Skills System, teaching strategies, and curriculum contained in this book are designed to help individuals who experience learning challenges. For example, an individual who experiences certain mental health challenges and/or an intellectual disability may have difficulty focusing attention, remembering information, and utilizing concepts within complex situations. The Skills System itself and the teaching strategies contained in this book and the accompanying *Emotion Regulation Skills System Workbook, Second Edition,* are constructed to maximize learning, integration, and ultimately generalization of the skills into life contexts. Even an individual who cannot read or write can learn to use the Skills System and participate in Skills System instruction.

DBT Skills for the Challenged Learner

The Skills System was developed as an accessible alternative for individuals with cognitive impairment who were participating in dialectical behavior therapy (DBT; Linehan, 1993a). DBT has two main delivery modes: individual therapy and skills training group. The skills curriculum (Linehan, 2025a) is broken down into four modules. The individual learns skills in the areas of mindfulness, emotion regulation, distress tolerance, and interpersonal effectiveness in the skills group and discusses implementation of the strategies in real-life settings during individual therapy.

The standard DBT skills (Linehan, 2025a) were not specifically designed for individuals with learning challenges. The multisyllabic terms, complex mnemonics, use of abstract language, modular teaching process, and lack of structure to facilitate integration of the divergent elements can create barriers for vulnerable learners (Kurban, 2024; Sweller, 2022; Sweller, van Merrienboer, & Pass, 2019; Kalyuga, 2011; Paas & Sweller, 2012; Sweller, 1988, 2010). Although the terms and format of the standard skills are challenging, the general concepts are vastly helpful for this population. The practitioner must make an informed clinical assessment and decide whether an individual with learning challenges can comprehend essential components of the standard DBT skills through enhanced teaching strategies or if key aspects of DBT will be lost. For certain individuals with significant learning deficits, merely modifying the teaching of the standard curriculum is not sufficient to capture the essence of DBT in a way that promotes generalization of the concepts. The current studies on DBT state that the skills curriculum requires adaptation (Patterson, Williams, & Jones, 2020; Brown, 2019; McNair, Woodrow, & Hare, 2017; Brown, Brown, & Dibiasio, 2013; Haq, 2013; Sakdalan & Collier, 2012).

This DBT-informed version may not look like DBT, because semantic sacrifices were necessary to enable this population access to the essence of DBT. The Skills System utilizes DBT principles, while the language and format are adjusted to address the needs of individuals who experience learning challenges. There may be cases when the Skills System is learned first and the standard DBT skills are added later in treatment.

As with the first edition, this book will be used by people who have DBT training and those who do not. Practitioners with various levels of training may be interested in the ways the Skills System concepts map on to DBT skills. Rather than attempting to duplicate Linehan's expert teaching, text boxes follow each description of the Skills System skills in Chapter 2. There and in the remaining chapters of this book, text boxes contain reference information for the foundational standard DBT concepts and teaching points in the *DBT Skills Training Manual, Revised Edition* (Linehan, 2025a) that are relevant to the Skills System skills and/or skills training procedure. These references help the DBT practitioner better understand how DBT concepts are integrated into each element of the Skills System. The text boxes allow DBT practitioners to know where to look for related DBT information, and non-DBT clinicians can skim the information if it detracts from the learning process. If a clinician is unfamiliar with DBT, it is recommended that he do self-study of the DBT skills manuals or attend DBT trainings to deepen his knowledge about the foundations of the Skills System.

APPLICATIONS OF THE SKILLS SYSTEM

Many people have experiences or physiology that complicate learning as well as their ability to demonstrate effective emotion regulation behaviors. Each person has unique clusters of strengths and deficits, abilities and disabilities. Any individual, with a diagnosed learning impairment or otherwise, may be prone to overwhelming emotions, unclear thinking, or unproductive actions. All people have the capacity to make impulsive decisions that hinder the accomplishment of personal goals. Even individuals who practice adaptive coping behaviors experience overwhelming circumstances that can stress such capacities. The Skills System materials are user-friendly concepts that are accessible to learners of all abilities.

The utilization of the Skills System is expanding, along with the resources to improve access. As mentioned in the Preface, the Skills System was originally designed for adults participating in DBT who experience cognitive impairment. Now, the model is integrated into many other treatments in addition to DBT, including cognitive-behavioral therapy, motivational interviewing, positive behavioral supports, applied behavior analysis, trauma-informed treatment, and person-centered supports. Practitioners treating clients with differing academic/intellectual abilities and mental health diagnoses teach the model. The Skills System is used with children and adolescents; there are handouts specifically designed for elementary and high school-age youth (some are provided in the online Appendices of the accompanying *Skills System Workbook*). In an effort to improve access, Skills System materials in the manuals and online resources are translated into languages other than English (see *https://skillssystem.com/do-you-want-to-translate-skills-system-materials-into-a-different-language*).

The Skills System model has been used in many different therapeutic settings. Hospitals as well as residential, day, vocational, corrections, and outpatient programs have implemented the Skills System concepts. In these types of settings, individuals receive skills instruction. Staff are trained to be skills coaches (Chapter 8). Clinicians use the Skills System as a therapeutic tool in individual therapy. The ancillary materials available on the Skills System website are useful for training staff, as well as family members or other people in the client's life.

OVERVIEW OF THE SKILLS SYSTEM

There are nine skills in the Skills System; these nine skills form the Skills List. There are also three System Tools that guide utilization of the skills and assembly of skills chains. An individual who tends to become overwhelmed by emotion, has difficulty focusing on thoughts that are in service of personal goals, and/or reacts impulsively to urges may benefit from learning step-by-step progressions to manage these factors. A person with these issues often has difficulty transitioning successfully from one strategy to the next in traditional coping skills education that provides individual elements without offering a system to guide implementation. The unified structure of the Skills System assists the person in remembering strategies and moving fluidly through a multistep coping progression, while experiencing intense emotional, cognitive, and behavioral regulation problems. As the individual learns the skills and the system, she integrates the capacity to successfully experience a full range of human emotions, practice self-determination, and acquire the means to navigate toward goals even in challenging circumstances.

The first three skills in the Skills System comprise a core progression that serves as the foundation for skills use. This sequence begins when an individual experiences a situation that prompts awareness; she begins by getting a Clear Picture (Skill 1) of the moment. Six steps lead the person to become aware of information within the current moment. This is crucial, because often individuals with self-regulation problems focus attention on the past or future rather than the present. Not only does focusing on the current moment give the person accurate information to use in making decisions, but it also allows for more in-depth processing of the experience. Mindfulness is a core DBT concept; Clear Picture leads the individual through steps of being mindfully aware in every situation.

Once the person gets a Clear Picture, he shifts to On-Track Thinking (Skill 2). In On-Track Thinking, the individual moves through a simple four-step sequence that leads her through the process of mapping out an effective coping plan. This cognitive framework serves to guide the individual's thinking patterns to promote emotion regulation and goal-directed behaviors. As the person learns the adaptive cognitive structure during instruction, practices it within his life context, and experiences positive reinforcement, the functional thinking patterns become increasingly sophisticated and automatic over time.

On-Track Thinking requires the individual to Make a Skills Plan. This component links the remaining skills together in a chain. Three simple rules (System Tools) determine which skills will be helpful and how many to use within the context of the present moment. Depending on the individual's self-reported level of emotional arousal (using the Feelings Rating Scale), she knows whether using more interactive skills (Skills 6–9) are options (using the Categories of Skills). The person learns that at high levels of emotional (and cognitive) arousal, it is necessary to choose more solitary skills (Skills 1–5) that function to reduce the sensations of uncomfortable feelings, to divert attention from problematic urges to effective actions, to minimize risks, and to improve focus. At all levels of escalation, the individual Makes a Plan to choose a sufficient number of skills (using the Recipe for Skills), targeting specifically the most effective skills according to the demands of the situation.

Next, the individual takes an On-Track Action (Skill 3). On-Track Actions are the behaviors the individual mobilizes to move in the direction of his goal. Therefore, the person gets a Clear Picture, does On-Track Thinking, and executes a series of On-Track Actions. If the individual is over a Level 3 emotion, he may engage in a Safety Plan (Skill 4) or New-Me Activities (Skill 5). If under a Level 3, the person can also use Calm-Only skills, which are Problem Solving (Skill 6), Expressing Myself (Skill 7), Getting It Right (Skill 8), and Relationship Care (Skill 9). Once a cluster of skills has been completed or the circumstances change, the individual returns to do Clear Picture again to become aware of the new situation that has evolved.

Initially, the individual conceptualizes the Skills System as a series of linear events; when a sequence of skills is finished, she returns to doing Clear Picture, On-Track Thinking, On-Track Action, and so on, repeating the process in each subsequent situation. As the individual integrates the Skills System, she is more able to utilize Clear Picture and On-Track Thinking throughout the coping process in a dynamic, transactional pattern to adjust On-Track Actions. Even individuals with significant cognitive impairment gradually improve the ability to make subtle adjustments; this flexibility can enhance the person's success in reaching goals and in maintaining On-Track Relationships. The Skills System is a structured yet malleable framework that can help an individual reduce reliance on avoidant behaviors, bear increased responsibilities, and fully engage in the human experience. Table 1.1 lists the skills on the Skills List and the System Tools.

THE SKILLS LIST

The following section includes brief descriptions of each of the skills and System Tools. This is intended as an initial exposure to the information. These concepts are presented in greater detail in Chapter 2. This introduction serves as a skeleton on which more information will be layered in the following chapters.

Getting Started with a Clear Picture

The first skill in the Skills System is Clear Picture; the metaphor of a television represents having a clear versus fuzzy vision of a situation. Clear Picture guides the individual through steps that bring focused attention to six aspects of her present experience to gain clarity. The first of the Clear Picture Do's prompts the individual to focus on her breath. Next, she shifts attention to notice what is happening around her. Once the individual has awareness of the environment, attention is then shifted to doing a Body Check; bringing attention to the body begins a series of self-reflections that help orient the person to her internal experience. The person then labels and rates her emotions and notices thoughts and urges.

There are two important facets of this skill: (1) gaining accurate information about these important internal and external experiences in the present moment, as they are, and (2)

TABLE 1.1. Skills List and System Tools

Skills List	System Tools
All-the-Time Skills	A. Feelings Rating Scale
1. Clear Picture	0- to 5-point scale for rating the intensity of emotions.
2. On-Track Thinking	
3. On-Track Action	B. Categories of Skills
4. Safety Plan	Skills 1–5 are All-The-Time skills.
5. New-Me Activities	Skills 6–9 are Calm-Only skills.
Calm-Only Skills	
6. Problem Solving	C. Recipe for Skills
7. Expressing Myself	Add one skill for every level of emotion (e.g., at a Level 2 emotion, use at least three skills).
8. Getting It Right	
9. Relationship Care	

effectively shifting attention. Some individuals who experience cognitive deficits and/or self-regulation problems have difficulty shifting attention in ways that effectively manage their level of arousal. The Clear Picture skill trains the person to see her moment as it is, creating a base from which to move in the direction of her goals.

Using On-Track Thinking

Once the individual has a Clear Picture of his internal and external circumstances in the moment, he strategically transfers attention to Skill 2, which is On-Track Thinking. The name "On-Track" uses the metaphor of a train to represent the concept of the individual moving incrementally toward a destination or goal. Thus, the image of "off-track" communicates circumstances that are not in service of the goal.

On-Track Thinking offers the person a series of four tasks to complete to create an effective thinking process. This sequence—(1) stop and Check It, (2) Turn It, (3) Cheerleading, (4) Make a Skills Plan—provides an adaptive cognitive structuring template for the individual to follow in each situation. This process helps the person reflect on desired outcomes, appraise whether taking action on the urge supports his goal, generate on-track thoughts to support adaptive behavior, and create a plan to reach his goal.

Taking an On-Track Action

Once the individual gets a Clear Picture and does On-Track Thinking, she uses Skill 3, which is On-Track Action. The reuse of the word "On-Track" is designed to reinforce the concept that the person transitions from On-Track Thinking to On-Track Action. It is challenging for any person to alter problematic patterns of behavior; On-Track Actions mobilize new, adaptive actions that are directly related to personal goals. It is useful to have On-Track Thoughts, but without On-Track Actions, the individual may revert to problematic behaviors. Using Clear Picture and On-Track Thinking, and taking On-Track Actions are ways to act in "Wise Mind" (Linehan, 2025a). The combined term "123 Wise Mind" communicates that to demonstrate wisdom consistently in context, it may be helpful to be mindful (Clear Picture), generate strategic thinking (On-Track Thinking), and engage in goal-directed actions (On-Track Action).

There are five different elements of the On-Track Action skill. First, this skill includes any action that the individual takes in the direction of his goal. An action is considered on-track if the person has taken time to be self-aware within the present moment (Clear Picture) and has made an effective decision (On-Track Thinking). The remaining functions of On-Track Actions include knowing when to Switch Tracks, make an On-Track Action Plan, Accept the Situation, and/or Turn the Page. Each of these concepts give the individual tools to proactively or reactively manage off-track urges and difficult situations.

Managing Risky Situations with Safety Plans

During the process of getting a Clear Picture and doing On-Track Thinking, the person may identify possible risks that may impede her progress toward goals. In a situation such as this, the individual may take the On-Track Action to create and execute a Safety Plan. Safety Plans,

Skill 4 in the Skills System, provide a framework that assists in evaluating the level of risk and in choosing the appropriate responses to manage the circumstances. It is important that the person be fully aware of risks, understand various options for managing the problems, and have the ability to implement actions that neither unnecessarily avoid situations nor recklessly engage in risky ones.

Doing New-Me Activities

New-Me Activities, Skill 5,[1] are activities that the person engages in throughout each day. The term "New-Me Activities" represents activities that position the person on-track to personal goals. Developing a broad array of preferred New-Me Activities can help an individual improve self-regulation and satisfaction.

New-Me Activities serve four basic functions. Focus New-Me Activities assist the individual in focusing attention, while other activities promote distraction. Some activities help the person feel good; others are intended to be fun. The individual does Solo New-Me Activities by herself, while Partnership New-Me Activities include other people. The individual learns to evaluate what his needs are in the moment and to choose a New-Me Activity that fits best.

Problem Solving

The individual may determine that she has a problem or the urge to take action impulsively to change a situation. Problem Solving helps the person strategically evaluate when and how to solve problems, so that she reaches personal goals. The individual may have previous experiences that involved rushed, ill-planned, or extreme responses that not only fail to repair difficulties but also augment problems. Learning when to solve problems is just as important as knowing how to do it.

The Quick Fix process is used to address small problems, while a more comprehensive, multistep Problem Solving is best to use when fixing medium and large problems. During Problem Solving, the individual takes time to gain clarity about the problem, reviews multiple options for solving it, and checks the fit of the choices. The person develops Plans A, B, and C to prepare for inevitable obstacles that occur.

Expressing Myself

Expressing Myself, Skill 7, involves the individual communicating what is on his mind or in his heart. Choosing from myriad communication methods and determining when to communicate are important decisions. A person may have a habit of expressing himself while at high levels of emotional arousal. Although this may serve to purge distress, provide distraction, or mobilize the individual in challenging situations, such impulsive expression often damages relationships or causes other problems. The Expressing Myself skill helps the individual strategically and

[1]The terms "Old-Me" and "New-Me" were used by Haaven, Little, and Petre-Miller in their book *Treating Intellectually Disabled Sex Offenders* (1989). Although the term "New-Me" is used in many other forums, a special acknowledgment of these authors' contribution to the field of disabilities is warranted. I thank James Haaven for his support.

effectively utilize communication to reach personal goals. The person learns to use other skills, such as New-Me Activities, to reduce emotions at times when he is experiencing discomfort, rather than venting on others.

Getting It Right

The person may be in a situation where she needs to get something from another person. Getting It Right, Skill 8, is used specifically for acquiring what the individual wants or needs. Getting needs met is a vital skill; unfortunately, skill deficits in this area have often contributed to cycles of ineffective behavior and high levels of dissatisfaction. When the person makes requests while at a high level of emotional arousal, she fails to elicit help and may reduce the likelihood that her needs will be met. It is essential to have the capacity to make requests, self-advocate, and negotiate to reach personal goals.

Getting It Right provides the individual with a simple framework to get what he wants from another person. The individual learns to be in the Right Mind, talk to the Right Person at the Right Time and Place, use the Right Tone, and say the Right Words. The Right Words include using Sugar (being polite), Explaining the Situation, Asking for What You Want, Listening, and Seal a Deal (SEALS).

Relationship Care

Our relationships with ourselves and others are primary parts of our lives that can cause us joy and suffering. Relationship Care helps us manage our relationship with ourselves and the world around us. Being human, each of us experiences countless urges each day that potentially harm our relationships.

Relationship Care, Skill 9, is designed to help the individual effectively assess relationship situations so that he can make personal decisions that improve his quality of life. Many life problems are fueled by ill-timed and impulsive relationship behaviors. While it is challenging to manage changing forces that are continually transacting as part of the human experience, the individual increases mastery within relationships when he gains the ability to use Relationship Care and the other skills effectively.

Relationship Care assists the person in improving her self-relationship and interactions with other people. Building On-Track Relationships, balancing On-Track Relationships, and changing off-track relationships are the essential components. As the individual becomes more aware of her personal needs and learns how various actions either enhance personal connections or lead to creating distance between people, she is better able to actively manage interactions with others.

SYSTEM TOOLS

A person who has coping skills deficits and self-regulation problems may have difficulty accurately evaluating internal and external experiences. Additionally, the person may not have the ability to monitor his levels of self-regulation strategically to choose behaviors that achieve desired outcomes. The Skills System is designed to help an individual develop coping tools and the ability to use the skills to create a life worth living. The System Tools are simple concepts that guide the individual's use of the nine skills on the Skills List. There are three System Tools: the Feelings Rating Scale, the Categories of Skills, and the Recipe for Skills.

Feelings Rating Scale

The Feelings Rating Scale is a simple 6-point (0–5) scale that the individual uses to rate the intensity of sensations she is feeling. It is an important tool to help the person be aware of and organize her current experiences. The scale concretizes the abstract experience of emotions, which is particularly important for an individual who has intellectual impairments.

Through the skills training experience, the individual learns to differentiate emotional experiences and categorize the feelings rating. A feeling rated 0 means that the person is not experiencing sensations related to the emotion. A feeling rated 1 means the person is experiencing a tiny amount of the sensation from the emotion. A feeling is rated 2 when the individual has a small amount of sensation. An emotion is rated 3 when a medium level of emotion is felt. Generally, the individual's ability to focus and control behavior is intact when emotions are rated between 0 and 3; above a 3, the person's cognitive and behavioral control abilities may be compromised. A feeling rated 4 is a strong emotion; often some kind of behavioral dyscontrol or urge to have off-track actions is present. A feeling is rated 5 when the individual becomes overwhelmed and exhibits behavior that harms self, others, or property.

The scale serves a dual purpose: (1) The Feelings Rating Scale helps the person get a Clear Picture of the current moment, and (2) the individual uses the rating to determine which skills (Categories of Skills) and how many skills to use in the situation (Recipe for Skills) in On-Track Thinking. The person learns that at lower levels of arousal, she has the capacity to think clearly and interact effectively; therefore, it is possible to use interactive skills at that time. Conversely, a higher rating communicates to the individual that she will have more difficulty thinking clearly and interacting effectively with other people. At high-rated levels of feelings, more skills are indicated to manage the experience, and the goal at that point is to reduce arousal. The Feelings Rating Scale helps the individual build the capacity to manage impulses and productively wait until she is in the proper mindset to utilize interactive skills.

Categories of Skills

Many behavioral problems result when an individual engages in interactive skills at high levels of emotion. While it is natural to experience strong urges to take action to fix situations, express feelings, address a demand that needs be met, and exert control over people, acting on these urges often fails to help the individual reach long-term personal goals. The Categories of Skills help the individual know which skills are effective at given levels of arousal.

There are two Categories of Skills. Skills 1–5 (Clear Picture, On-Track Thinking, On-Track Action, Safety Plan, and New-Me Activities) are called All-the-Time skills. All-the-Time skills can be used at any level of emotion, from 0 to 5. The other Category of Skills is called Calm-

Only skills. The person can use Skills 6–9 (Problem Solving, Expressing Myself, Getting It Right, and Relationship Care) only when he is at or below a Level 3 emotion. Therefore, the person can utilize all nine skills if he is at or below a Level 3 emotion and just Skills 1–5 if he is over a Level 3 emotion.

Recipe for Skills

Another common pitfall is when a person does not chain enough skills within a situation. When high levels of emotions trigger body sensations, the effects can be uncomfortable and long-lasting. It is essential that the person chain together multiple skills to use multiple strategies to span the extended duration of the feeling experience.

The Recipe for Skills calls for using at least one more skill than the level of emotion, including 0. For example, if an individual is at a Level 2 emotion, at least three skills must be used. If the individual is at a Level 5 emotion, at least six skills are needed. In this case, since the person is over a Level 3 emotion, it is necessary for the person to use an extra All-the-Time skill (e.g., using two On-Track Actions or two New-Me Activities), rather than having the sixth skill be from the Calm-Only category. The Recipe highlights the minimum number of skills; doing more skills than the Recipe dictates is often helpful.

The goal of the Recipe for Skills is to ensure that the person plans and executes enough skills. The number of skills changes relative to the severity of the situation; the intensity of the event is calibrated through the emotional impact the circumstance has on the individual. It is not uncommon for individuals with emotion regulation problems to rush through insufficient strategies that do not adequately address the multiple components of complex internal and external situations.

PUTTING IT ALL TOGETHER

When an individual begins learning the Skills System in a skills group or one-on-one instruction, her ability to recall all of the concepts and terms is expectedly inconsistent. Group teaching strategies continually expose individuals to the Skills List and the System Tools within the contexts of their lives. This revolving approach allows the individual to cobble together comprehension over time. Suggestions for structuring skills instruction, teaching strategies, and implementing a 12-week curriculum are presented in Chapters 4–7.

Relatively early in skills training, the individual learns to be increasingly mindful of the present moment. The individual becomes able to take a quick snapshot of internal and external factors using the Clear Picture Do's. With practice, the person increases his speed and accuracy in these tasks.

The information gathered during the Clear Picture Do's is used to help the individual generate On-Track Thinking. For example, the feelings rating score (e.g., Level 4, Angry) guides him to choose which Category of Skills will be helpful at his current level of emotion. The individual learns that All-the-Time skills (1–5) may be utilized at any level of emotion, while Calm-

Only skills (6–9) are only used when he is below a Level 3 emotion. In the previous example, at a Level 4 emotion, the individual would engage only in All-the-Time skills and not utilize Calm-Only skills. All-the-Time skills allow the individual to reregulate prior to engaging in the more interactive Calm-Only skills. Additionally, the individual learns to use ample skills for the situation. The Recipe for Skills sets guidelines for the minimum number of skills. Quickly the individual learns the adage: The more skills, the better.

On-Track Thinking is a relatively complex skill; mastery is slow and builds over time. The individual may initially have primitive self-dialogue. Often, as skills capacities develop, more sophistication evolves. For example, the person may initially self-reflect and think, "I feel angry at Level 4; I need to go to my room." As self-awareness continues to evolve, self-statements become more elaborated: "I am at Level 4 anger; I have to use my All-the-Time skills. I have the urge to use Expressing Myself skills, but I must wait until I am below a Level 3 emotion. If I do it now, I will yell. Instead, I will do a Safety Plan and New-Me Activities. I have to use my skills, because I want to reach my goals. I can do this."

Throughout the skills training experience, the individual often becomes aware of (and committed to) taking On-Track Actions versus off-track actions. The individual may have the ability to notice an urge and move away rather than being aggressive. Over time, with more group discussions and practice, the chains are elaborated. The mindfulness (Clear Picture) training paired with the cognitive structuring (On-Track Thinking) offers the individual a framework that guides him toward taking effective, self-determined On-Track Actions (123 Wise Mind). The individual may become increasingly able to strategically intertwine various combinations of skills to manage oscillating internal and external needs. The nine skills and three System Tools are repeated, practiced, and reinforced so that the adaptive coping patterns become default settings.

Integration within Living and Learning Environments

The Skills System may provide a therapeutic language base and adaptive coping skills model for many different environments. The Skills System can be helpful in inpatient, residential, outpatient, classroom, vocational, and/or home settings. Parents can partner with their children to learn and use the material together. The preliminary research is currently limited, yet the opportunities for future study and exploration are broad.

The visual nature of the Skills System can promote integration within environments. The visual aid materials can provide visual cues that prompt skill use for individuals and skills coaches. Programs mount skills posters and personalized decorations throughout the site. When the model becomes immersed in the Skills System, many creative programmatic, group, and individualized interventions are possible.

There are many benefits of integrating the Skills System into program settings. The Skills System provides common language and a framework of information related to managing emotions, thoughts, and actions. This shared framework and language facilitate learning. When individuals and support providers both actively engage in positive relating behaviors, opportunities for adaptive learning and relating increase. For example, there are multiple benefits for individuals and staff who take part in peer skills tutoring activities. Ideally, individuals and support providers learn how to cope effectively and are able to engage in positive social behaviors that are mutually beneficial and reciprocal.

TRANSITION TO CHAPTER 2

This chapter offered a brief overview of the Skills System concepts. Chapter 2 presents a more detailed explanation of the nine core skills and the subskills with those strategies. The chapter also explains the System Tools that help the individual use skills within the context of their lives.

CHAPTER 2

Learning the Skills System

Chapter 2 offers a detailed description of each of the nine skills and the System Tools that guide their utilization. It is important to understand that, while the Skills System is a structured model, it is not a prescriptive formula. Rather, it is a revolving process that shifts to respond to the dynamic perceptions and needs of each person within each changing moment. Knowing all of the elements of the Skills System helps instructors, coaches, and, ultimately, the individual make and execute self-determined Skills Plans that reflect their personal goals and values.

References to sections in the *DBT Skills Training Manual, Revised Edition* (Linehan, 2025a) citing relevant foundational DBT concepts and standard DBT teaching points are provided in boxes that follow each of the skills descriptions in this chapter.

THE SKILLS LIST

There are nine core skills on the Skills List:

1. Clear Picture
2. On-Track Thinking
3. On-Track Action
4. Safety Plan
5. New-Me Activities

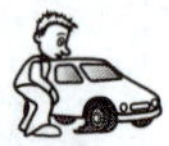
6 Problem Solving

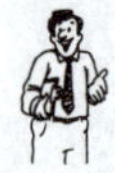
7. Expressing Myself

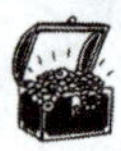
8. Getting It Right

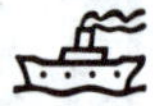
9. Relationship Care

Each of the nine skills have subskills that help elaborate for the individual how to execute the skill. The subskills help him design specific tactics within situations he faces. While some individuals may learn all of the skill and subskill names, this is not required. For example, one individual may learn the term "New-Me Activity" and the four types of New-Me Activities (focus, feel good, distraction, and fun); another individual may just know that making a puzzle or coloring helps him when he gets really upset. Every individual is different, and the Skills System model is designed to be tailored to each person's ability.

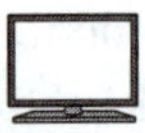

Clear Picture

Clear Picture is the first skill in the Skills System, and it is an All-the-Time skill. This means that Clear Picture can be used at any level of feeling, 0–5. There are six steps, which collectively are referred to as the Clear Picture Do's: Notice the Breath, Notice Surroundings, Do a Body Check, Label and Rate Feelings, Notice Thoughts, and Notice Urges. The purpose of Clear Picture is to help the individual become aware of and accept what is happening inside and outside herself in the current moment. This systematic progression leads her through steps to be mindful in each situation. The individual reviews the Clear Picture Do's when she notices a situation changing or when she is having a new reaction.

Clear Picture is an acceptance strategy versus a change strategy. The six Clear Picture Do's do not include changing anything about the moment, but rather focus on bringing awareness to the present moment and accepting it *as it is. Clear Picture helps the individual get a 360-degree view* and have an accurate perception of the *moment. This awareness* helps her know where she is, so she can take steps toward her goals.

The alternative is a fuzzy picture. A fuzzy picture occurs when an individual is experiencing cognitive dysregulation, is disoriented, or is not perceiving actualities within the situation. When the person has a fuzzy picture, she may be in emotional mind (Linehan, 2025a), when her emotions are in the driver's seat, off-track thinking prevails, and effective coping is impeded by the lack of clarity. Clear Picture is the first skill because being aware is the first step in the emotion regulation process.

The following steps help the individual become aware of internal and external factors that are currently happening. Although these Do's are presented in a particular order, the individual does not necessarily perform all of these processes or perform them in a specific order. The human experience is complex and fast moving and we cannot always stop to complete each step or control which of the Clear Picture Do's comes into awareness first. For example, if we stub our toe, we will become aware of physical pain in our feet first, therefore we will begin with Body Check. Similarly, if there is a knock on the door, we will Notice Surroundings before we Notice the Breath. Soon thereafter, it is helpful to Notice the Breath and do the other Clear Picture Do's to have skillful responses. The more Do's we perform, the clearer our picture will be.

Notice the Breath

The first step in Clear Picture is to Notice the Breath. In the moment, the individual brings her attention to the physical sensations of breathing. Noticing the air going in and out of her nose, feeling the chest expand, and observing the snugness of her waistband as she brings the air into her belly area are common focal points during breathing. The individual can also describe features of the breath or how it feels, such as rapid and shallow or slow and deep. It is important that in Clear Picture the individual notices the breath *as it is* versus needing to do a particular type of breathing (e.g., taking deep breaths). Accepting the breath *as it is* is an important step toward the individual seeing himself and the situation clearly.

Taking a breath begins the process of gaining intentional awareness that is free of distortions and avoidance. Being oriented helps him "Check the Facts" (Linehan, 2025a, p. 319) in the situation. Simultaneously, this concrete action of shifting attention from one Clear Picture Do offers the individual a concrete scaffolding to manage the intangible aspects of the current moment. Having clarity about the realities of the present, the individual is more capable of planning and executing impactful behaviors. Additionally, shifting attention from a stressor in the environment to the breath engages the emotion regulation strategy of "attentional deployment" (Gross, 2024, p. 8). When he brings 100% of his attention to the breath, attention shifts from the escalating emotions and cognitions, and only the breath is in awareness. Managing this one moment becomes more possible.

Teaching awareness of breath is a simple first step that triggers Skills System usage. Not only is the skill construct linked to this one simple step, but the individual also has the breath with him at all times, in all contexts. Learning, practicing, and reinforcing the linkages between taking a breath, completing the Clear Picture Do's, and executing other skills helps promote integration and automation of skills use in the person's life.

Notice Surroundings

It is important for the person to Notice Surroundings, the second step in Clear Picture. She must take a moment to look around to gain a clear understanding of what is happening outside of herself *right now*. The individual uses her senses to be aware of her surroundings, noticing what she sees, hears, smells, tastes, and touches around her in the moment.

This scan includes noticing aspects of the physical environment and of the relationships that are present. Awareness of surroundings may reflect immediate tangible experiences, as well as macrolevel realities (e.g., societal norms, legal ramifications). Seeing the situations, relationships, and environmental factors *as they are* is crucial. When the individual's emotions escalate, it is not uncommon for her to blur factors; inconsistencies between the realities of the situation and the perceptions of the individual can impede effective skills utilization. For example, focusing on what happened in the past, what might happen in the future, or what *should* be happening in the present hinders clarity in the present moment. Gathering accurate information, based on observations of the current situation, helps the individual handle the situation effectively. Notice Surroundings is a particularly important step if there are risks that must be managed.

As the person develops an understanding that it is easier to manage one clear moment in time, he is more likely to evaluate situations accurately. The individual learns that clarity, although potentially uncomfortable for the moment, allows effective coping and the accomplishment of personal goals. The individual may use fewer avoidant strategies as he experiences them as less effective and more problematic in the long term.

Again, shifting between senses engages attentional deployment. Individuals with histories of trauma, autism spectrum disorder, and/or other challenges may have difficulty shifting attention. Doing the Clear Picture Do's is one way to increase competency in shifting attention in a low-demand way. As the individual gains the ability to move from one Clear Picture Do to the next, the ability to strategically deploy attention is strengthened.

Body Check

Body Check is when the individual notices that sensations are happening inside *right now*. Noticing physical sensations such as heart rate, breathing, aches, and tension can help the individual understand emotional responses. Noticing body sensations can help the individual accurately label and rate feelings. In considering this step, it is important to note that an individual may have physical or mental health issues that affect the functioning of her mind and/or body. For example, an individual with autism spectrum disorder will have sensory experiences that can cause discomfort and affect processing and emotion regulation. Similarly, individuals with intellectual disabilities experience higher rates of medical challenges than the general population.

It is important that the individual get a Clear Picture of sensations that affect her mind and body in order to manage her internal and external environments. These realities also mean that when the individual does a Body Check, she may not receive "good news" with the awareness. This reiterates the need to have Skills Plans that incorporate Clear Picture and other skills, like On-Track Thinking and On-Track Action, to manage difficulties.

As the person monitors her physical being throughout the day, she also learns that sensations come and go through the natural course of each day. This mindful awareness helps her understand the concept of "this too shall pass." Understanding that painful experiences come and go naturally helps the individual tolerate being present in the moment. The awareness that painful feelings will abate in time helps the individual be present in, tolerate, and manage discomfort.

Label and Rate Feelings

The fourth step in Clear Picture is to Label and Rate Feelings. The person notices and describes emotions, such as fear, anger, disgust, envy, jealousy, love, sadness, shame, and guilt (Linehan, 2025a). Other sensations, such as hunger and fatigue, can be labeled and rated as well. Gross (2024, p. 4) explained that the term "affect" may be the best umbrella term to include emotions, stress responses, moods, and impulses. However, the term "feeling" (as opposed to "affect") is more familiar and accessible for individuals with cognitive challenges to describe the wide range of experiences that affect functioning.

Labeling a feeling is one part of the process to elaborate awareness and manage affective experiences (Vine, Bernstein, & Nolen-Hoeksema, 2019). It is optimal for individuals to develop language to describe a broad range of feelings. Some individuals have limited vocabularies and additional work is needed to learn and integrate terms to describe their feelings. Some individuals may have an emotion-processing deficit called alexithymia. Individuals with alexithymia tend to have difficulty identifying and describing feelings; these impairments often lead to emotion regulation difficulties and higher levels of negative affect (Preece & Sikka, 2024).

Once the person labels the feeling, it is important to rate its intensity using the Feelings Rating Scale (described more fully on pp. 50–53). For example, the individual could label and rate a feeling as a "Level 3 sad" or "3 sad" or "sad at a Level 3." The act of labeling and rating an emotion can serve to reduce ambiguity and improve emotion regulation (Lieberman, Inagaki, Tabibnia, & Crockett, 2011; Zaki & Williams, 2013).

In addition, the monitoring teaches the individual that emotions rise and fall, come and go. Feelings are like waves that go higher and then lower throughout each day. This awareness helps the person believe that painful states are transient and that emotions are survivable. As skills develop further, the individual begins to become aware that it is possible to decrease painful experiences while increasing pleasant ones. With practice, the individual can notice, accept, and allow challenging emotions to pass without taking impulsive action or retriggering more painful feelings.

Notice Thoughts

Notice Thoughts is when the individual pays attention to specific thoughts that pass through his mind *in a particular moment.* Although humans have automatic and generated thoughts throughout each day, Clear Picture tries to bring awareness to the thoughts that arise in the current situation. For example, an individual who is looking at a sunset might notice their thought, "That is beautiful"; when an individual is mistreated, she might find herself thinking, "He is a jerk." Situations can elicit thoughts, and thoughts, in turn, can elicit feelings and body sensations. Thinking about the beauty of a sunset may lead to feelings of peace; thinking a guy is a jerk may lead to feelings of anger. The process of noticing thoughts (like the breath, body sensation, and feelings), *as they are,* without change, creates the platform of acceptance that supports On-Track Thinking (generating thoughts that are in service of goals). Additionally, by noticing thoughts, the person learns that they continually come and go. Being aware of this flow helps the individual see that it is possible to not react automatically to thoughts.

Mental health disorders often affect the individual's thinking and are difficult to change. Some individuals experience involuntary intrusive thoughts that are violent or disturbing. Many individuals have worry thoughts that are disruptive and persistent. Some people have pervasive thinking that keeps them focused on one event and hinders them from shifting attention in an adaptive way. These types of thoughts can increase uncomfortable emotions and result in avoiding essential factors that would help the individual manage the situation effectively. Although challenging, the individual notices the thought in Clear Picture and engages strategies using the other skills to help her move in the direction of her goal. People who experience mental health disorders, such as psychotic disorders and autism spectrum disorder, may need to have specific Skills Plans to manage experiences when thoughts are causing discomfort and are overwhelming.

Thoughts may flood the individual in certain situations. Flooding may cause the individual to only Notice Thoughts and not complete the other Clear Picture Do's. Ideally the individual practices shifting attention to the six Clear Picture Do's to get a 360-degree view of the moment and then do On-Track Thinking to manage the situation. As the individual's abilities are developing, it may be helpful to immediately use On-Track Thinking Check It and Turn It to manage certain off-track thoughts before they hijack the individual's mind, body, and actions. It may be helpful to shift to a Safety Plan or New-Me Activity to interrupt patterns of cognitive overload.

Thoughts can be an abstract concept for some people. Using the metaphor of thoughts being like city buses can help some individuals have a tangible way to understand Clear Picture (noticing thoughts) and On-Track Thinking (checking and turning thoughts). Noticing thoughts is like watching as different buses (thoughts) go by. The individual watches each one and notices the sign on the front indicating where the bus is going. She does On-Track Thinking Check It to see if the bus will take her to her destination (goal). At that point the individual can choose to get on the bus that will take her where she wants to go. The preliminary step of Notice Thoughts (Clear Picture) is foundational to making goal-directed decisions.

Notice Urges

Notice Urges is when the individual becomes aware of action urges in the moment. Urges can come into awareness as a thought, such as "I'm tired, I want to rest," or "I'm bored, I want to go out." Fight and flight responses are examples of action urges of attacking or avoiding. Urges, much like sensations, emotions, and thoughts, naturally come and go.

Acting quickly on urges can be strategic in certain situations, but in others, reacting impulsively can diminish levels of effectiveness. In most nonemergency situations, taking a few seconds to notice the urge and other aspects of the moment (breath, surroundings, body sensations, feelings, and thoughts) can help the individual be grounded in awareness and avoid conditioned or default responses that do not serve them.

Urges can be an abstract concept for some individuals. For example, a person with autism spectrum disorder may have difficulty conceptualizing what an urge is. To help these individuals better understand what urges are, it can help to highlight common urges they may be familiar with, like the urge to go to the bathroom or the urge to eat.

Helpful Hints for Applying Clear Picture

- It can be helpful to initiate Clear Picture whenever there is an internal or external change. Clear Picture helps the individual know what is happening right here, right now.
- Even in challenging situations that the individual may want to change, it is helpful to see the situation as it is in the moment. Changing things before having clarity often reduces the individual's abilities to be effective.

- If an individual does not have the capacity to learn all six Clear Picture Do's, it is helpful to focus on a portion of the skill. The following are particularly important:
  - Notice the Breath: This is a simple task that enhances focus and shifts attention to using skills.
  - Label and Rate Feelings: This helps the individual know which Category of Skills to use (Calm-Only and/or All-the-Time) and the minimum number of skills that are needed in the situation (Recipe for Skills).
  - Notice Urges: This gives the individual an opportunity to stop and Check It and progress through the microtransitions in On-Track Thinking.

Clear Picture: Foundational DBT Concepts and Teaching Points (Linehan, 2025a)

- Mindfulness Skills (pp. 151–230)
- What Emotions Do for You (pp. 326–331)
- A Model of Emotions (pp. 334–345)
- Observing, Describing, and Naming Emotions (pp. 345–349)
- Check the Facts (pp. 350–359)
- Mindfulness of Current Emotions (pp. 403–406)
- Paired Muscle Relaxation (pp. 436–438)
- Self-Soothing with a Body Scan Meditation (pp. 444–445)
- Allowing the Mind: Mindfulness of Current Thoughts (pp. 472–476)

On-Track Thinking

On-Track Thinking, the second skill in the Skills System, is an All-the-Time skill, so it can be used at any level of emotion, 0–5. All skills chains begin with Clear Picture (1) and On-Track Thinking (2); this chain is represented in numbers as "12." The following four steps of On-Track Thinking help individuals appraise and navigate their internal and external experiences.

Stop and Check It

Check It is the first step in On-Track Thinking. When checking it, the individual pauses to reflect and evaluate the utility of the thought or urge in relation to his goal. Check It implicitly asks the person to step back and think about what he wants. The individual gives a thumbs up if acting on the urge will help him reach his goal. A thumbs down is given if the action would be off-track to the goal. For example, worrying about all the ways a situation could go wrong is likely to decrease, rather than increase peace, so if the individual's goal was to feel more peaceful, worrying about the situation would get a thumbs down. The urge to take a warm bath, however, can lead to his goal of feeling more peaceful, so that urge might get a thumbs up.

The thumbs-up and thumbs-down signs are useful visual aids that give tangible representations to intangible thoughts. Children as young as age 3 may understand the concept of thumbs up translating to something being helpful or positive. Individuals who have more cognitive deficits and less verbal abilities may not have the ability to describe elaborated Skills Plans, but they can communicate preference using the thumbs-up and thumbs-down hand signals.

In more complex situations, as the individual weighs various factors, costs, benefits, and potential outcomes, it is not uncommon to go from a thumbs up to a thumbs down and back to a thumbs up. Urges, wants, needs, short-term goals, long-term goals, and priorities can support each other or be in conflict. Potential outcomes of actions can be obvious at times and unclear at others, and sometimes people have trouble knowing exactly where they want to go.

Check It offers the individual an appraisal process through which he takes time to reflect on the internal and external factors happening in the moment; this opportunity is designed to help him make flexible and informed personal decisions. On-Track Thinking is a vehicle for the individual to bring her identity and wisdom to any situation, even as the context continually changes as life and the individual changes. In *The Emotion Regulation Skills System Workbook, Second Edition* (sold separately), there are updated Relationship Care worksheets that help the individual clarify goals, values, and priorities in order to help him do Check It.

Turn It

If the individual's thoughts and/or urges are assessed as off-track (the thought will lead the individual away from his goal), it is important to Check It and then Turn It. Turn It is reappraisal. It counteracts an appraisal and prompts the generation of on-track thoughts, often by highlighting the costs of taking the off-track action. For example, if the individual thinks, "I feel like hitting him," and gives it a thumbs down during Check It, he may Turn It by thinking, "If I hit him, I will get arrested." Turn It thoughts can also focus on the benefits of an On-Track Action alternative. For example, the individual may Turn It by telling himself, "I want to handle my anger in a good way."

Turn It is also used when an individual assesses that the feeling or feelings level is not aligning with their goals. For example, if the individual is at a Level 3 anxious, Checks It, and sees that her thoughts and/or urges are increasing the anxiety, she can Turn It to generate On-Track Thinking that supports her goal of reducing anxiety. Therefore, Turn It can support reaching situational and feelings rating goals.

Turn It thoughts can be very brief, like "No" or "I can't do that," or they can be more elaborate self-statements. If an individual is having strong off-track urges, more detailed, comprehensive Turn It thoughts may be needed. For example, if the person has a substance abuse problem and has the urge to use drugs, a Turn It thought of "no" will likely not be sufficient. A series of Turn It thoughts, one after the other, detailing (1) the costs of the action and (2) the benefits of not taking the action may be needed (e.g., "Drinking caused me to get divorced. I lost my job. If I drink, I am going to be broke again. I am finally in a good place. I am feeling healthy again").

It takes time and practice to manage urges effectively, especially strong ones that are continually provoked by the environment. As the individual is learning to use Turn It, he may need to avoid certain situations (Safety Plan) if cognitive load demands are too high to process information effectively. As the individual's skills get stronger, he will hopefully be able to manage more challenging situations and remain on-track.

Cheerleading

The word "cheer" as a verb means to encourage, offer comfort, and support. Cheering ourselves on, or cheerleading, is when the individual creates supportive self-statements. Cheers or cheerleading statements are thoughts that help strengthen the individual and invigorate him. When the person Checks It and finds that the urge is on-track or he successfully has turned it, he should then generate Cheerleading statements to support the process of making and executing a Skills Plan. A few specific types of cheers support skill use the following:

- *Skill-efficacy.* Generating thoughts that confirm that a skill will work, will increase the likelihood the individuals will use the skill. For example, "I *know* I can use my Safety Plan to deal with that situation," and "I *know* New-Me Activities make me feel better." Building skill efficacy is crucial; individuals need to use skills and develop trust that the skills will work for them (Gross, 2024).
- *Self-efficacy.* Generating positive thoughts that confirm the individual's capacity to manage the situation and/or to use skills increases the chances of her using sufficient adaptive strategies. For example, "I *know* I can do this" or "I *can* deal with this." Self-efficacy is essential, as well; if the individual believes she can prevail, she will be more likely take the necessary steps.
- *Hope.* Hopeful thoughts can help the individual stay and get back on-track during challenging experiences. Generating hopeful self-statements about the situation can help her endure waiting and times of limbo when situations remain difficult. For example, "I will be OK" and "This too shall pass" are hopeful cheers.

Cheerleading is necessary throughout the entire emotion regulation process. It can help the individual engage in the On-Track Thinking process that intertwines with the development and execution of each Skills Plan. Off-track thinking can divert an on-track plan at any point during the emotion regulation process.

People who experience chronic mental health issues, trauma, and strife often have beliefs that lead to low self-efficacy and hopelessness. They may not know how to cheerlead, requiring an overcorrection and high dose of Cheerleading. The individual may need to check, turn, and cheerlead frequently to avoid getting mired in off-track narratives. She may need to make lists of cheers and recite them proactively and reactively to create muscle memory. Inspiring visual aids and coaching support can help. As the individual develops more adaptive skills, integrates them into her life, and experiences the feeling of competency to manage emotions, more balanced dosages of Cheerleading may be possible. The new Blast It worksheet and worked example (Learning Skills, On-Track Thinking Worked Example 4 and Worksheet 5 in the *Skills System Workbook),* asks the individual to list ten cheers; this is intended to create new, more helpful self-talk.

Make a Skills Plan

Once the individual has gotten a Clear Picture and is oriented toward his goal by checking and turning thoughts and urges and doing Cheerleading, he makes a Skills Plan, choosing the strategies and tactics he will use to manage the situation. It is important the individual choose the best skills for the situation. The three System Tools—Feelings Rating Scale, Categories of Skills, and Recipe for Skills—help the individual know what skills to use (the System Tools are each explored in greater detail at the end of this chapter).

Rating Feelings

The individual's level of feeling affects her abilities to process information. At higher levels of arousal, she will have difficulty being strategic and effective. It is important that the individual use strategies in the moment that she can do successfully to manage her present state, so it is essential that the individual understand her level of feeling to develop a Skills Plans that will work.

During Clear Picture, the individual labels and rates her feelings on a 0–5 scale. Between 0 and 3, she can focus and talk and listen to others, at Level 4 feeling, she is unable to focus and has difficulty talking and listening to other people, and by Level 5, she is harming herself, others, or property. The feeling rating is important information that helps her choose which skills she can use effectively at her present level of feeling (Categories of Skills) and how many skills she will need to manage the situation (Recipe for Skills).

Choosing Category of Skills

Deciding whether the individual can use Calm-Only skills (Skills 6–9) is important. If the individual is over a Level 3 emotion, All-the-Time skills (Skills 1–5) should be used. Using Calm-Only skills when over a Level 3 often causes problems for the individual. It may be helpful to validate the individual's urge to solve the problem, express emotions, try to get needs met, or settle relationship conflicts immediately, but using the All-the-Time skills first to reduce arousal is generally more effective.

Recipe for Skills

The Recipe for Skills tells the person the minimum number of skills to use in the skills chain. It is necessary to use at least one skill for every level of feeling, including 0. Therefore, at Level 1, two skills are the minimum. At Level 2, at least three are needed. At Level 4, five skills are necessary. At Level 5 feeling, six skills are recommended. Since it is not possible to use Calm-Only skills over a Level 3, doubling up on one of the All-the-Time skills is necessary at a Level 5.

The Recipe helps teach about the basic construction of skills chains: Clear Picture (Skill 1) and On-Track Thinking (Skill 2) determine the On-Track Actions (Skill 3). This "123" chain of skills is a core progression of emotion regulation skills. For example, if a person's On-Track Action was to do a Safety Plan and move away from the risk, that skills chain would be a "1234." When the individual does a New-Me Activity after leaving the risky area, it turns into a "12345" chain. The "123" foundation becomes rote as the individual learns how to add on skills to better manage situations. The base of "123" helps the individual act with Wise Mind (Linehan, 2025a).

The Recipe for Skills conveys in simple terms the more complex idea of assembling skills into progressions to facilitate effective emotion regulation microtransitions through a situation. Cobbling together enough small steps to span an event effectively is like stretching a walking bridge across a ravine. Without knowing discrete steps to take in highly emotional situations, the person may have a polarized response and avoid the experience or fall off-track into the ravine. The Recipe for Skills guards against having insufficient links in the chain that will not bridge an intense emotional experience. Additionally, in skills coaching situations, coaches can ask the participant to calculate the Recipe for Skills to shift attention from off-track thoughts to On-Track Thinking and to improve focus.

Choosing the Best Skills for the Situation

Making a Skills Plan is a preliminary step toward charting a course of action to reach personal goals. There are *standard* and *a-la-carte* Skills Plans. A standard plan includes Clear Picture, Check It, Turn It, Categories of Skills, and Recipe for Skills. Standard plans address multiple processes that are involved in managing emotions and reaching personal goals. As an individual learns skills concepts and practices, she develops more elaborate, stronger Skills Plans that help navigate more challenging situations effectively.

Alternatively, an a-la-carte Skills Plan relies on one skill or tactic. A-la-carte plans may be necessary when an individual is experiencing high cognitive load and is unable to do 123 Wise Mind. Instructors may help shape the individual's abilities toward standard Skills Plans. For example, the individual's a-la-carte plan may consist of going to his bedroom to avoid risk (Safety Plan: Move Away). Over time, he can learn how to expand this into a standard plan to strengthen his abilities to manage more challenging situations. For example, he may notice when he wants to hit people (Clear Picture: Notice Urges) and then go to his bedroom to avoid doing that. This section will focus on the creation of a standard Skills Plan. Chapter 6 offers strategies to adjust instruction if necessary.

On-Track Thinking: Foundational DBT Concepts and Teaching Points (Linehan, 2025a)

- Cheerleading Strategies (p. 90)
- Mindfulness "How" Skills: Nonjudgmentally (pp. 199–208)
- Mindfulness "How" Skills: One-Mindfully (pp. 208–210)
- Mindfulness "How" Skills: Effectively (pp. 210–213)
- Skillful Means: Balancing Doing Mind and Being Mind (pp. 222–225)
- Wise Mind: Walking the Middle Path (pp. 225–227)
- Factors Reducing Interpersonal Effectiveness (pp. 237–241)
- Clarifying Goals in Interpersonal Situations (pp. 242–248)
- Evaluating Your Options: How Intensely to Ask or Say No (pp. 263–266)

- Troubleshooting Interpersonal Effectiveness Skills (pp. 266–270)
- Dialectics (pp. 285–293)
- Validation Skills (pp. 293–301)
- Recovering from Invalidation (pp. 301–306)
- Cope Ahead (pp. 393–395)
- Troubleshooting Emotion Regulation Skills (pp. 408–410)
- STOP Problematic Behavior Immediately (pp. 424–427)
- Pros and Cons as a Way to Make Behavioral Decisions (pp. 427–430)
- Improving the Moment (pp. 445–450)

On-Track Action

On-Track Action is the third skill in the Skills System. It is an All-the-Time skill; thus, it can be used at any level of emotion, 0–5. On-Track Actions are skillful actions the person takes. As a general rule, the individual is not advised to take an action unless it is an On-Track Action. Doing Clear Picture and On-Track Thinking before taking an action increases the chances that it will be on-track rather than off-track. There are five types of On-Track Actions in the Skills System.

First Step to My Goal

The first type of On-Track Action is when the individual takes a step toward his goal. For example, if the person is trying to lose weight, reaching for the bag of carrots when preparing lunch may be an On-Track Action. Reaching for a bag of chips may be an off-track action. An On-Track Action occurs when the individual does something that helps her reach a personal goal in a situation. Quickly reacting while hoping that an action is on-track may work, yet it may not incorporate the totality of available information and may not have maximum positive impact.

It is essential to understand that *only the individual, in that moment,* can decide whether an action is on-track or off-track. For example, perhaps an individual who has lost 10 pounds is at a holiday party. Perhaps having a few chips as a treat may still be an On-Track Action. The personal decision-making process is a vital opportunity for self-determination and activation of inner wisdom, or Wise Mind (Linehan, 2025a). The goal is to help the person engage in a skills process prior to taking actions versus leading him to particular choices.

It is important to note that when using the Recipe for Skills, often On-Track Actions involves doing other skills. For example, if the individual takes the On-Track Action of playing basketball, he gets double-credit in the Recipe for Skills. Playing basketball is an On-Track Action *and* a New-Me Activity. Getting a two-for-one communicates that the individual is generating a lot of adaptive actions, which bolsters self-efficacy and hope.

Switch Tracks

Switch Tracks is when the person does something to shift from off-track (or heading off-track) to on-track. For example, if a person is engaging in Getting It Right with his employer and he is met with resistance, his feelings may escalate above a Level 3, making it difficult to process information and communicate in an effective way. At that point, he may want to Switch Tracks to an All-the-Time skill, such as revisiting Clear Picture or On-Track Thinking to avoid taking off-track actions with his boss.

Being aware in situations helps the individual know when to Switch Tracks and when to keep moving ahead. Waiting too long to Switch Tracks can make it more difficult. For example, if I am sitting down watching a TV show during my normal exercise time, it might be helpful to Switch Tracks right away and go put on workout clothes. The longer I watch, the less likely I am to workout. Shifting behavior to do several On-Track Actions helps the individual be securely on the road to his goals. For example, changing into shorts, putting on running shoes, getting my music player, and filling my bottle of water would increase the likelihood that I would exercise.

There are times when the individual continues to trigger uncomfortable emotions and/or ruminates about certain thoughts and urges; these behaviors may serve to increase painful emotions and hinder movement toward goals. Jumping in with both feet to On-Track Actions is important. If one foot is on-track and one is off-track, the individual is still engaging in off-track patterns.

Taking an "Opposite Action" (Linehan, 2025a, p. 359), is another way to Switch Tracks. Doing the opposite of off-track urges can (1) initiate on-track behaviors and (2) reduce cues to avoid, because the individual approaches the task. Doing the Opposite Action of the off-track urges may decrease cues that perpetuate problematic patterns. For example, if the urge was to be rude, being polite would be its opposite. It is important that Opposite Action be done with 100% effort and focus. For example, being neutral to someone may not be rude, but it is not an Opposite Action. "Opposite" means that the individual goes all the way to the other end of the spectrum and is clearly polite. Clinicians should review pages 359–372 in the *DBT Skills Training Manual, Revised Edition* (Linehan, 2025a) to gain a complete understanding of Opposite Action.

On-Track Action Plans

On-Track Action Plans are activities that are part of the individual's daily routines that help balance his mind, body, and spirit. When the individual proactively manages his body, it helps him manage his mind. For example, the individual may have an exercise schedule, eat healthy food, take proper medications, get suitable amounts of sleep, and talk to friends as part of an On-Track Action Plan each day. Doing Written Safety Plans before medium- and high-risk events may be part of an On-Track Action Plan. When balancing various aspects of daily living, the person may be better prepared to mitigate and manage stressful situations that arise.

Accept the Situation

Certain situations are unfavorable and unchangeable—at least in the short-term. For example, an individual may want to have family visits, but his relatives refuse contact. Not accepting the realities of situations may lead to rumination and reeling against circumstances—both of which increase negative emotions. The individual calls the family multiple times per week and assaults peers who have family contact. Accept the Situation involves microtransitions of reappraising or thinking differently about the situation *and* pivoting to take On-Track Actions. Accept the Situation does not mean that the individual approves of the situation, but means that he demonstrates willingness to move ahead in an on-track way, despite a lack of comfort or agreement. The individual acknowledges his family's perspective and makes holiday plans with friends. Since merely thinking differently, without taking different actions, may not be sufficient to reach goals, Accept the Situation is an On-Track Action. If the individual only acknowledged the family's perspective and did not create an on-track Skills Plan for the holidays, the likelihood of the individual escalating to a Level 5 would increase.

It can be difficult to accept the situation when individuals have a high emotional connection to a situation. There may be strong feelings of hurt, loss, sadness, fear, and anger. It may be helpful to use other Skills Plans that include both All-the-Time and Calm-Only skills to help the individual manage feelings and improve situations. Pairing Accept the Situation with other types of On-Track Actions like Switch Tracks and/or Turn the Page can provide additional scaffolding for changing reinforced patterns of off-track behavior.

Individuals with intellectual disabilities, autism spectrum disorder, and other mental health challenges often experience heightened medical, psychiatric, and environmental challenges. Some aspects of the individual's life may elicit high levels of stress and may not be changeable. For example, the individual may have experienced a traumatic loss or have a medical condition or mental health disorder that is not fully curable; they may be on a plethora of medications that have side effects. Accept the Situation can help her accept certain realities, reduce the reactivity related to the difficulty, and focus on using skills to improve her quality of life.

Accept the Situation can also help the individual do things she doesn't want to do and accept not doing things she does want to do. For example, Accept the Situation may be helpful when she has to do chores, or when she feels like skipping work, but knows that action is off-track. Accept the Situation helps the individual manage short-term sacrifices for progress toward her long-term goals.

Turn the Page

Turn the Page is when the individual shifts from an action that is no longer effective to another, more goal-directed action. Turn the Page involves changing thoughts and actions. It isn't just thinking differently, it also includes doing differently. For example, if the individual wants to feel less angry (goal) but is continually talking about how her ex-partner betrayed her (plan), she may notice that her plan is not aligning with her goal. Talking about the betrayal is increasing her anger. What she is doing is making her feel worse not better. When the individual determines that she has invested enough time into something, when she decides "enough is enough," she may want to Turn the Page. The individual in this case might Turn the Page from talking about the ex-partner to new dating opportunities.

It can be difficult for the individual to Turn the Page from worries, memories, painful emotions, urges, or relationships that have gotten a lot of attention. Reinforced patterns and default settings are challenging to change. Former comfort zones that become dis-comfort zones can create strong holds that are difficult to move on from. Dealing with strong holds often requires a multifaceted approach to (1) address internal and external factors associated with managing connections to the former subject and (2) build new associations that support new actions. For example, the individual has to have ways to deal with reminders of the ex *and* has to have avenues to develop new relationships. If the individual has no way to move forward, she is not likely to leave patterns that have formerly offered comfort. In addition to several other skills, it may be helpful to combine Accept the Situation and Turn the Page to accept the old subject and move on to the new.

The individual must make the decision to Turn the Page herself. While people around the individual may be frustrated with apparently problematic patterns, the individual weighs the benefits and costs of the situation. When the cost outweighs the benefits, it may be time for Turn the Page.

On-Track Action: Foundational DBT Concepts and Teaching Points (Linehan, 2025a)

- Mindfulness "What" Skills: Participate (pp. 192–199)
- Mindfulness "How" Skills: Effectively (pp. 210–213)
- Build Mastery (pp. 392–393)
- Taking Care of Your Mind by Taking Care of Your Body (pp. 396–397)
- Sleep Hygiene Protocol (pp. 400–402)
- Radical Acceptance (pp. 451–465)
- Turning the Mind (pp. 465–467)
- Willingness (pp. 467–470)
- Half-Smiling and Willing Hands (pp. 470–472)

Safety Plan

Safety Plan, the fourth skill in the Skills System, is an All-the-Time skill. This means that Safety Plan can be used at any level of emotion, 0–5. If the individual determines, after doing Clear Picture and On-Track Thinking, that some kind of risk exists, a Safety Plan is often an On-Track Action. The person must decide what level the risk is, what kind of Safety Plan to use, and what actions are necessary to manage the current level of risk.

Levels of Risk

The first step in a Safety Plan is to get a Clear Picture of the risk. There are inside risks, such as off-track thoughts, urges, feelings, and fantasies (TUFFs). There are also outside risks (people, places, and things), including people who upset the individual, places that are dangerous, and objects that trigger off-track thoughts. The person handles inside risks and outside risks before larger problems develop.

There are three levels of risk: low, medium, and high. In a *low*-risk situation, the risk is far away and/or the contact may cause stress. For example, if the individual's neighbors are having a loud argument in their house, the danger is far away and there is little potential for her to be hurt. In a *medium*-risk situation, the danger is in the area and/or contact may cause problems. If the neighbor walked over to the individual's fence and started screaming at her, the risk is closer and the contact with the neighbor may increase problems. In *high*-risk situations, the danger is close and/or contact may cause serious damage. The irate neighbor might come over and start banging on the individual's door, threatening to break it down. This is high risk because the risk is close and the threat of harm is immediate.

It is important not to overrate or underrate risks. Overrating risk means that the individual rates the risk as high when it is low. This may cause the individual to avoid activities that are helpful. For example, if the person rates going to work on the first day as high risk because he is anxious, he may not go to work. In this case, it may be better to do an On-Track Action and jump in with both feet on the first day of a new job! Underrating risk is when the individual rates a risk that is high as being low. This can lead to danger and harm because his efforts to manage the risk are insufficient (e.g., if he drives a car after having four drinks and thinks it is fine). If the individual is not thinking clearly, it is important that he seeks support from someone to discuss options for managing the risk (Talking Safety Plan). Once the individual has a Clear Picture of the risk, it is necessary to choose the type of Safety Plan to use.

Types of Safety Plans

There are three types of Safety Plans: Thinking, Talking, and Written. In a Thinking Safety Plan, the person thinks about how to manage the risk safely. For example, if the individual hears the neighbors fighting, she may make the decision to watch through the window to see if the couple's fight escalates to a higher level of risk or turn up her TV so that they do not bother her as much. A Thinking Safety Plan is often used in low-risk situations.

In a Talking Safety Plan, the individual decides to tell someone about the risk to elicit support. It is generally helpful to use Talking Safety Plans in medium- and high-risk situations. For example, the individual may approach a skills coach and say, "I am having TUFFs right now. Could you help me make a good Safety Plan?" It is important to note that if the person's emotion level is over a 3, the focus of the communication during a Talking Safety Plan is strictly on tactics to manage the risk versus encouraging lengthy and detailed discussions about the content of the situation.

It is important that the individual understands the difference between a Talking Safety Plan and Expressing Myself. In a Talking Safety Plan, the discussion is related to the risk or strong emotions and how to manage the situation effectively. Expressing Myself, which is a Calm-Only skill, would communicate the individual's thoughts, concerns, needs, feeling, likes–dislikes, and hopes/dreams. Delving into Expressing Myself, especially related to the risk, increases levels of feelings (and in turn risk). It may be important for the individual to express feelings about the issues, but it is essential to choose the best time to do that.

In a Written Safety Plan, the individual, with or without assistance, writes down the possible risk and dangers prior to, during, or after risky events. Safety Plans need to be designed to help the individual. For example, if an individual can't read, the Safety Plan should include pictures of his safe places and images of New-Me Activities he may do when he is there.

The individual creates a personal Safety Plan that outlines tactics to manage risk, as well as strategies to deal with problems that may arise that impede the Safety Plan. Written Safety Plans are particularly important in high-risk situations. The individual may choose to share the written plan with a trusted friend who can assist him in following it.

Ways to Manage Risk

There are three ways to manage risks: focus on a New-Me Activity, move away, and leave the area. The first, least invasive way of managing risk is to focus on a New-Me Activity. New-Me Activities are various positive tasks that the individual does throughout the day. For example, if the person notices a low risk while at work (i.e., the risk is either far away or in the future), she may choose to remain at her position and focus on the work task she is doing—sweeping the floor, for instance. If she is not engaged in an activity, participating in one may help her remain safe, focused, and on-track. Focusing on a New-Me Activity prompts the individual to take a positive action versus merely ignoring the risk. It is important to give attention to the New-Me Activity and be alert to any changes in the environment and risk level of the situation.

For example, Jim is at work. He hears his coworker raising his voice in the next room. He decides to do a "1234" skills chain. When he thinks about what kind of Safety Plan to do, he knows that the coworker is merely venting and no significant danger exists. Jim also feels that he is at a safe distance from the trouble and therefore assesses the situation as low risk. He thinks about what he should do to handle the situation. Jim decides to stay where he is and focus on his work task.

The second way to manage risk is to move away. This means that the individual moves to a safer area and gets distance from the risk. Once the person has moved away, she may want to refocus on a New-Me Activity to stay on track. It is often necessary to move away in medium-risk situations when either the problem is nearby or there is the possibility that contact will cause problems. Continuing to have a Clear Picture and doing On-Track Thinking will help the person use other skills to manage the situation effectively. For example, Jim is in the break room at work. His coworker comes in complaining about the boss. Jim does a "1234" skills chain. He realizes that this situation could cause him problems, so he moves to the other end of the break room.

The third and most invasive way to manage risk is to leave the area completely. In high-risk situations where there is serious danger, it may be necessary to leave the area. Under these circumstances, the individual may need to go where she cannot hear, see, talk to, or touch the risk. Similarly, if the individual engages in self-injurious behaviors, it is important to remove all objects that may be used to inflict harm. Doing a Talking Safety Plan and letting another person know about the danger can help ensure that the individual remains a safe distance from perpetrators, potential victims, and possible weapons that are creating high levels of risk. If there is imminent danger, it is crucial to seek support. Additionally, after leaving the area, it may be helpful to refocus on a New-Me Activity. For example, Jim is in the break room. His coworker starts yelling and swearing about the company. The man starts trying to free the fire extinguisher to throw it. Jim quickly does a "1234" skills chain and leaves the area because of the high level of danger. He tells the security guard and returns to his work area on the other side of the building.

Safety Plan: Foundational DBT Concepts and Teaching Points (Linehan, 2025a)

- Cope Ahead (pp. 393–395)
- Taking Care of Your Mind by Taking Care of Your Body (pp. 396–397)

New-Me Activity

The New-Me Activity, the fifth skill in the Skills System, is generally an All-the-Time skill. This means that the individual can use New-Me Activities at any level of emotion, 0–5. It is possible to do New-Me Activities alone or with other people. While Solo New-Me Activities (activities the individual does by themselves) can be done at any level of emotion, Partnership New-Me Activities (activities an individual does with others) involve Relationship Care and are best done when all participants are below Level 3 feelings. Therefore, the individual chooses Solo New-Me Activities when over a Level 3, since Partnership New-Me Activities are a Calm-Only skill.

New-Me Activities are the on-track activities that the individual does during each day. New-Me Activities are a useful emotion regulation strategy to increase positive emotions and decrease negative ones. It is important to note that different New-Me Activities affect people in various ways, and situations require different tactics. There are four types: Focus, Feel Good, Distraction, and Fun New-Me Activities.

Focus New-Me Activities

Focus activities improve attention and focus in the moment. When the individual engages in activities that involve sorting, organizing, following step-by-step instructions, and/or counting, his mind becomes more focused. Examples of Focus New-Me Activities are sorting cards, playing solitaire, word searches, cooking with a recipe, counting money, folding clothes, cleaning, reading, and playing video games. Activities can be made into Focus New-Me Activities by adding counting or patterns. For example, counting a certain number of times while dribbling a basketball with the right hand and then switching to do the same number with the left would be adding counting and a pattern. Just playing basketball may be a Fun New-Me Activity instead.

When a person is highly emotional and not thinking clearly, it can be helpful to do a simple card-sorting activity. First, the individual separates the deck into two piles, with the red cards in one pile and the black ones in another. The person should try to keep the cards in organized, tidy piles rather than allow the cards to slide all over the table. Even this rudimentary task is challenging when a person is in an escalated state. Once that is complete, the person separates the deck by suits—hearts, diamonds, clubs, and spades—each in its own pile. Finally, the individual takes each pile containing one suit and puts it in order, either from the highest card down or the lowest card up. The goal is to perform a task that does not increase cognitive load demands and frustration significantly but rather helps the individual focus attention. If the person is unable to do one of the tasks, it may be useful to return to a simpler version of the sorting activity. Other sorting games can be created, such as separating the deck by the numbers on the cards (placing all four of the aces together, etc.).

Feel Good New-Me Activities

Feel Good New-Me Activities help the individual feel comfortable and soothed. It is important to note that everyone must have an opportunity to define what they find soothing. Each person's experience of activities and preferences vary. Engaging in activities that trigger memories, problematic thoughts, or painful emotions may not function to help the individual feel good. The following items are self-soothing activities that involve each of the senses.

- *Sight.* The individual may look at pleasant sights to increase positive feelings and experiences. For example, sitting and looking at a beautiful view, taking a walk in nature, and/or looking at attractive pictures may make the individual feel better.
- *Hearing.* The person may listen to things that increase joy. For example, putting on music, listening to birds sing, or hearing water in a stream can be soothing.
- *Smell.* Experiencing pleasant aromas can help a person feel good. Smelling cookies baking, burning scented candles, and using fragrant hand lotion are examples of Feel Good New-Me Activities.
- *Touch.* Various types of touch can soothe an individual. Putting on cozy slippers, taking a warm bath, and petting an animal are common ways to experience comfort through touch.
- *Taste.* Eating and drinking things that have a pleasant taste can provide pleasure and make people feel good. Having a nice meal, sipping hot tea, eating a piece of chocolate, or drinking ice-cold lemonade on a hot day are examples of some Feel Good New-Me Activities.

Distraction New-Me Activities

Distraction New-Me Activities help the individual Switch Tracks and focus on something different than the event that prompts challenging emotions or off-track behaviors. Distraction can not only avert emotional escalation, but it can also alter aspects of the emotional response (Linehan, 2025a). Some strategies are used to distract the mind, whereas others are used to distract the body. Distract-the-mind activities help the individual get his mind off one thing and onto something else that is more pleasant. Activities such as watching TV or movies, playing video games, reading, or helping other people can help the individual focus his mind on a positive alternative. For example, if the individual is waiting for a ride home from the doctor's office, staring at the clock may increase discomfort. Instead, the individual can look at a magazine.

Distract-the-body activities can help when an individual is experiencing uncomfortable sensations or circumstances that cannot be changed. For example, rigorous physical activity helps the individual Switch Tracks from focusing on factors that may increase emotions to focusing on his body. Although, this is a type of Focus New-Me Activity, it also functions to distract the person from factors that are driving affect up. Activities that get the individual's heart pumping, such as walking, jogging, yoga, and use of a workout video, distract through exercise. Using ice cubes/packs can distract with temperature. Spicy food, sour candies, and cinnamon gum are ways to distract through taste.

It is important to note that using Distraction New-Me Activities may be most helpful when the person has done everything possible to manage the situation and she just needs to relax or wait. For example, if the person needs to be picked up at the doctor's office, it is important to call to arrange a ride prior to reading a magazine.

Fun New-Me Activities

Fun New-Me Activities make the individual feel happiness and joy. Exploring new activities can help the person improve emotion regulation abilities by providing beneficial alternatives to experiences that tend to elicit problematic emotions and behaviors. Each person finds joy in different ways: Drawing, playing sports, video games, working, cooking, cleaning, reading, watching TV, listening to music, talking to friends, going out, and studying skills are just a few Fun New-Me Activities. Creating On-Track Action Plans that include a variety of these types of activities (that fit into his budget) can help a person maintain balance within his life.

Choosing the Best New-Me Activity

Each kind of New-Me Activity has a different function; choosing the proper New-Me Activity in a situation can help the individual reach personal goals. For example, if the person is becoming upset or confused, choosing a Focus New-Me Activity will help promote clear thinking. If she is feeling tense or stressed, a Feel Good New-Me Activity may increase relaxation and comfort. If the individual has to wait for something and does not want get frustrated, doing a Distraction New-Me Activity may be a beneficial choice. If the individual wants to feel good about life and experience connection with others, doing a Fun New-Me Activity would be helpful.

Some New-Me Activities serve more than one function. For example, video games may help the person focus, distract him from worries, and provide entertainment. Similarly, a phone call to a friend may make the individual feel better and be fun at the same time. The individual uses Clear Picture and On-Track Thinking to determine whether to do a Solo or Partnership New-Me-Activity and whether to choose a Focus, Feel Good, Distraction, and/or Fun New-Me Activity.

Individuals who experience mental health and/or learning challenges may avoid trying novel New-Me Activities that require them to stretch out of their comfort zone. It may be necessary for the individual to explore acting opposite to the urge to stretch herself and expand capacities.

New-Me Activities: Foundational DBT Concepts and Teaching Points (Linehan, 2025a)

- Pleasant Events List (pp. 382–386)
- TIP Skills for Managing Extreme Arousal (pp. 431–439)
- Distracting with Wise Mind Accepts (pp. 439–442)

- Self-Soothing (pp. 442–445)
- Improving the Moment (pp. 445–450)
- Acting Opposite to the Current Emotion (pp. 359–372)

Problem Solving

Problem Solving, the sixth skill in the Skills System, is a Calm-Only skill. This means that the individual can use Problem Solving *only* when below a Level 3 emotion. To attempt Problem Solving when over a Level 3 emotion generally creates more rather than fewer problems. Rushing through Problem Solving may lead the individual to miss effective options and choose alternatives that may feel good in the short term, yet not be helpful in the long term. Problem Solving when a person has over a Level 3 emotion tends to be impulsive and is therefore less likely to aid the individual in reaching personal goals. If the individual is interacting with other people during Problem Solving, it is important that all involved are below a Level 3 emotion. When anyone is escalated in the situation, it may hinder the Problem Solving effort; waiting may be beneficial.

Labeling the size of the problem helps the person appraise a commensurate emotional response and ample resources to fix it. A small problem can cause annoyance rather than serious issues; it usually leads to Level 2 or 3 emotions. Small problems can trigger higher level emotions, but often the individual can reappraise the situation (Check It and Turn It) to have a more regulated response. An example of a small problem would be losing a favorite hat. It makes her Level 2 sad, but it would not really cause other harm. Small problems usually get fixed with a few simple steps (e.g., she can buy another hat when she is at the mall). When the individual has an enhanced response to a small problem, it may mean there are other root issues amplifying the response that perhaps should be addressed. Medium-size problems generally cause higher emotions (Levels 3 to 4) and take more steps and time to fix. For example, if the individual loses his car keys, he then needs to call a taxi, be late for work, figure out how to get a new key, get a ride to get a new key, and pay $200 for a new digital key. Large or overwhelming problems are very serious; for example, if I lose my job or I get evicted. Large problems often cause me to have Level 4 or 5 feelings, may take much longer to fix, and change my life in serious ways.

Quick Fix

The Quick Fix worksheet (Learning Skills, Problem Solving Worksheet 1 in the *Skills System Workbook*) may help to solve small problems and clarify medium and large ones. Using the worksheet to examine the problem, the solutions, and barriers to the fix can help the individual make a simple problem-solving plan. A problem may seem small initially, but as the individual does the Quick Fix worksheet, it can become clear that the small issue is connected to other larger ones. Doing a Quick Fix worksheet can help the individual get a clearer picture of all sizes of problems.

In addition to walking the individual through steps to solve a problem, the Quick Fix worksheet highlights the different available options. He checks off whether he wants to follow through on fixing it, make lemonade (change how he thinks about the problem), Accept the Situation (as it is), or suffer (do nothing). If the problem is more complex and multifaceted, this worksheet will be inadequate.

Problem Solving

Solving medium-size and large problems is a more complicated, multistep progression. Gaining mastery in Problem Solving is a long-term learning process. The following steps find solutions to more serious or confusing situations:

1. *Getting a Clear Picture of the problem.* The individual has to determine what she wants in a situation, what the problem is, and what the barriers are to reaching the goal. Rating the size of the problem helps her gauge the amount of resources necessary to fix it.

2. *Checking all options.* During this step, the person brainstorms about many different options. She "fast-forwards" each option to see what the outcomes may be and weighs the "pros" (thumbs up) and "cons" (thumbs down) of each choice. Weighing the benefits and costs of options helps the individual understand and make decisions.

3. *Creating Plan A, Plan B, and Plan C.* The individual creates multiple plans to ensure some level of success. The individual creates a primary plan to address the problem that best fits her goal; this is Plan A. Life and people are unpredictable, so it can be helpful to have a Plan B in case Plan A doesn't work or takes more time than expected. Plan B may not get the individual exactly what she wants, when she wants it, but it helps her stay on-track to her goals. Plan C is a fallback position. If Plans A and B don't work, Plan C will help the individual stay on-track to her goal.

Getting a Clear Picture of the Problem

The first step in doing successful Problem Solving is for the individual to get a Clear Picture of what he wants and to clarify what is getting in the way of that goal. Clarifying goals and barriers may be simple or complex, depending on the situation. The person may need to take time to self-reflect or contact a skills coach to illuminate the issues. An example of a relatively simple situation would be Joseph finding out that he has a basketball game in 3 days. He wants to play in the game but realizes that he does not have sneakers that fit him. Wanting to play in the game is his goal, and not having the proper shoes is the problem. Once Joseph understands the problem, he can check all his options and make a Plan A, B, and C to get new sneakers.

There can be barriers that complicate Problem Solving. For example, sometimes the individual is unclear about personal goals; a situation can also be confusing or require multiple steps to solve the problem. There may be environmental challenges and/or power differentials that make it difficult for a person with mental health or learning challenges to solve problems within complex social systems. Dissatisfaction in relationships, family conflicts, and vocational problems are examples of multifaceted problems. It may be necessary for the person to address components of a problem as part of a larger Problem Solving effort. The individual may benefit from seeking consultation from skills coaches, professionals who support the individual, and trusted friends to get a Clear Picture of her goals and address complex problems. Feedback can be useful during the problem-solving process to assess what can be changed in a situation and what needs to be accepted.

Checking All Options

Once the person has clarified what she wants and what is in the way of these goals, it is time to check all options. The person begins by generating possible solutions to the problem. She then reviews the pros (positive outcomes) and cons (negative outcomes) for each option. The metaphor of fast-forwarding to see the end teaches the concept that reflecting on consequences of action can be helpful. The individual checks the fit of each option to determine whether the action would be on-track (thumbs up) or off-track (thumbs down) to the goal. As the individual weighs her options, she begins to develop a series of Problem Solving plans. Plans may be simple and have a single step or be more challenging, requiring multiple skills. It is often necessary to use Clear Picture, On-Track Thinking, On-Track Actions, Expressing Myself, Getting It Right, and Relationship Care to execute Problem Solving. Once multiple options are reviewed, the individual chooses the options that best fit her goal.

Making Plans A, B, and C

Plan A is the plan that the individual believes will work best to fix the problem. Plan A best fits the needs of the person and has the highest likelihood of solving the problem in an effective way. Consulting with skills coaches or supportive friends prior to taking action, thinking about what to say, and rehearsing tactics can strengthen a plan. It is sometimes necessary to negotiate with people while doing Problem Solving. It is therefore helpful to have other alternatives, including a Plan B, in mind when engaging in discussions with people. There are times when Plan A and Plan B are not possible. Rather than getting in an off-track situation that drives emotions up, the individual makes Plan C, or an "if all else fails" fallback position. Plan C usually is either a third, less desirable option that is acceptable or a plan to tolerate the distress of losing preferred options.

Not getting problems solved or solutions taking longer than expected can cause stress. Encountering resistance or barriers can lead to heightened emotional responses. The individual will need to get a Clear Picture, use On-Track Thinking, and implement On-Track Actions as he solves problems.

Problem Solving: Foundational DBT Concepts and Teaching Points (Linehan, 2025a)

- Options for Solving Any Problem (pp. 130–131)
- Preparing for Opposite Action and Problem Solving (pp. 359–361)
- Problem Solving (pp. 372–381)

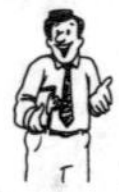

Expressing Myself

Expressing Myself, the seventh skill in the Skills System, is a Calm-Only skill. If the goal of expressing is to communicate, hear the other person's response, and create and maintain a Two-Way-Street relationship, expressing when both parties are below a Level 3 is likely best. When either person is over a Level 3, it can be more difficult to maintain balance in the relationship.

When we decide that Expressing Myself would be an On-Track Action, we give a thumbs up to communicate to ourselves or others. This section discusses what we communicate and why it may be helpful. We also explore many different ways of Expressing Myself and how it helps us reach our goals.

What Types of Things Are Expressed?

Expressing Myself is when the individual communicates what is On My Mind and In My Heart. Things On My Mind might be thoughts, concerns, and needs. For example, we might want to express our views on a social issue or opinions about sports, music, or movies. We may have a concern we want to share with someone to seek their advice or to get support. We might want to tell someone that we do or don't want to participate in an activity and why.

We express things that are In My Heart when we communicate our feelings, likes and dislikes, and hopes and dreams. For example, we may express love and gratitude to our friends and family. We may want to express our preferences so people around us can work with us. We may express our creativity though different activities, and we may want to share what is important to us, so other people know us more fully.

Why Express Myself?

Often, we express what is On My Mind and In My Heart to be connected with ourselves and the world around us. Expressing can help us get support from others, manage our emotions, clarify problems, communicate our needs, and improve our relationships.

Get Support from Other People

Expressing Myself can clarify aspects of our situation to ourselves and other people. For example, as we share our thoughts, needs, and concerns we organize our ideas, so we and the other person understand them better. When people know what is going on with us, it gives them important information about how they can support us in that situation. Unfortunately, when we express, we often don't know how people will react; they may or may not respond in ways that we like or expect. While Expressing Myself can make us feel vulnerable, that vulnerability may be an important first step to receiving emotional and physical support from others.

If we need things from people, we can begin by using Expressing Myself and shift to Getting It Right if the person does not respond to our initial expression. For example, if the individual says, "I hate broccoli" and the other person responds by not serving broccoli, the Expressing Myself worked. If the other person continues to serve broccoli, it may be time for the individual to use Getting It Right to get them to stop.

Manage Emotions

Sometimes people suppress expression, thinking that it will increase positive emotions and decrease negative ones. The research shows, though, that when we inhibit expression, it can reduce positive feelings (e.g., joy, happiness) and may not reduce negative emotions (e.g., fear, sadness; Rutherford & Joormann, 2024; Gross & Thompson, 2007). Therefore, inhibiting expression may not make us feel better, and may even make us feel worse. Overall, Gross and Thompson (2007) concluded that an individual appears to regulate emotions more effectively when he finds "ways of expressing them in adaptive rather than maladaptive ways" (p. 15). We use Clear Picture and On-Track Thinking to do Expressing Myself in ways that help us increase the emotions we want to be stronger and decrease emotions we would like to be weaker. The more we know about expressing, the better we are able to weigh the benefits and costs of Expressing Myself or choosing not to.

Solve Problems

There may be increased benefits to communication that promote "problem solving and interpersonal understanding" (Gross & Thompson, 2007, p. 15). As we express, we can clarify issues in complex situations; we can also get a clearer perspective of our goals, values, and priorities. There is a fine line between expressing to solve problems and venting out of frustration and aggravation. For example, if the individual has a difficult interaction with a coworker, it may be important to share the experience with someone to better understand what happened and how to address the situation. If that conversation continues for hours or days and is brought up again and again, it may become venting. Expressing Myself increases the level of emotions, so venting in this situation would make the employee even more frustrated and angry. When we have stopped clarifying issues in service of solving the problem and are instead "beating a dead horse," we may want to consider getting a Clear Picture, doing On-Track Thinking, and taking the On-Track Actions of Accept the Situation and Turn the Page.

Getting It Right

Getting It Right is the skill that helps the individual get what he needs and wants from other people (Getting It Right is explained in detail on pp. 41–44). Getting It Right includes using the right words: SEALS. SEALS stands for Sugar (being polite), Explaining (the context of the request), Asking (what he wants), Listening (to the response), and Sealing the Deal (pinning down the details). Using Sugar, Explaining, Asking, and Sealing the Deal involve integrating Expressing Myself. Choosing what to say, how to say it, and when to say it effectively (Expressing Myself), will improve the odds of Getting It Right. For example, the individual may want to express respect when he uses Sugar. He may want to express thoughts to Explain the situation and his feelings about why this is important. The individual may want to express his requests clearly when he Asks for what he wants.

Relationship Care

Expressing Myself is often used when people communicate with others to increase connections and/or create distance in relationships. For example, if the individual wants to have a two-way street with someone, expressing using On My Mind and In My Heart can create opportunities for connection. When both people express and listen, they may build an active dialogue. We can adjust how we use Expressing Myself to help us manage our different relationships.

How Do We Use Expressing Myself?

When the individual has something that she wants to express, she uses Clear Picture and On-Track Thinking to be sure the way she communicates is an On-Track Action that helps her reach her goals. Thankfully there are many different options for Expressing Myself.

Talking is one way to communicate. Some people talk by speaking verbally, while others use sign language and/or adaptive methods of communication. There are pros and cons with talking. Some of the pros are that talking can be a quick, easy, and clear way to make a point. The cons include miscommunication if the individual does not choose her words carefully. Speech and language difference between people can make it more difficult for them to understand each other.

Communicating through writing can be helpful. One pro is that when the individual writes, she can make her whole point without interruption. When writing, it is possible to communicate things that are hard to say face-to-face. A con for writing is the fact that the person may show it to other people. It is important to consider what the person may do with the communication when deciding what to write.

Social media is a common way that people communicate that also has pros and cons. Some people find social media platforms to be useful vehicles of communication that reach wide audiences and increase connections with people. Alternatively, the possible costs of hurtful comments being posted, provoking downward comparisons that make the individual feel worse, and overuse are reasons to thoughtfully consider the costs and benefits of using social media for Expressing Myself.

Expressing through body language is another option, but it can give a Fuzzy Picture. Utilizing body language can help us communicate our point, but it can also send messages that we may not intend. On one hand, body language can add nuance to communication, which increases engagement and understanding. For example, a smile, nodding, and a touch on the arm can communicate caring. On the other hand, using body language can communicate negative messages, intentionally and unintentionally. For example, if the individual rolls her eyes, crosses her arms, and looks down, this can communicate to the other person, "I don't care," "You are wrong," or "Whatever!" without a word being spoken. These types of expressions can lead to one or multiple people in interactions increasing levels of feeling to over a Level 3 and derail communication. When the individual chooses not to communicate via verbal or written means, and solely relies on body language, the likelihood of miscommunication increases.

When Do We Use Expressing Myself?

It is important to use 123 Wise Mind to know when Expressing Myself will help the individual reach his goals and live aligned with his values and when it will not. As the individual makes a 1237 Skills Plan, he chooses how he wants to communicate. The following factors help us make decisions about when (and when not) to use Expressing Myself.

Start at Lower Levels of Feeling

As previously discussed, Expressing Myself can increase the feeling of the emotion being expressed (Gross & Thompson, 2007). When the individual is considering whether or not to express herself, she should consider whether or not she wants the emotions she is currently experiencing to increase. It may be helpful to use Expressing Myself at emotion Levels 0–2, because the process of expression may naturally bring the individual to a Level 3 or higher. In addition, she may not hear what she is hoping to. Starting to use Expressing Myself at a Level 2 allows the individual opportunities to Switch Tracks, rather than ending up in her emotional mind.

Notice When Expressing Myself Turns Into Venting

The individual may start Expressing Myself and feel on-track. When she feels like she has fully expressed, the individual may Switch Tracks and Turn the Page. Other times, though, she may get stuck, ruminate, and find her uncomfortable feelings increase. Instead of helping herself clarify the problem, she is getting bogged down in the muck. While it may "feel good" being on a venting rampage, it may actually make the individual more miserable and give her a fuzzier picture. It is helpful to reflect, as she is stuck, "Do I want to feel better or worse in this situation?" If she wants her feelings level to go down, she should consider using Switch Tracks.

Expressing Myself In the Level 3 Sweet Spot

The Level 3 sweet spot is when the individual can use Expressing Myself while experiencing strong feelings *and* remain able to talk and listen. Once the individual stops being able to talk and listen, he is at a Level 4. For example, if a couple is discussing important relationship issues in a way that keeps the two-way street open without letting their emotions intensify, they are in the Level 3 sweet spot; this is when there may be optimal expression and mutual respect for each other's boundaries. Important information can be expressed in ways that build understanding between them. Additionally, by communicating effectively during times of rising emotions, both people get a sense of what is important to the other person. In order to stay in the Level 3 sweet spot, the individual must maintain focus and the ability to talk and listen without lashing out or shutting down. This requires being attentive to keeping a Clear Picture, using On-Track Thinking, and taking many, many On-Track Actions, such as creating a Safety Plan when necessary.

When the individual is over a Level 3 emotion, urges to express emotions are often strong. Over a Level 3 emotion, it may be more likely that communication can morph from effective Expressing Myself to venting, blaming, ranting, demanding, yelling, and swearing. Unfortunately, in situations where the individual is trying to gain cooperation, these tactics cause the other party to recoil, disengage, and even retaliate. We use Clear Picture and On-Track Thinking to help us Switch Tracks to a Safety Plan when we need to.

Expressing Myself Over Level 3

There are occasionally times when it may be effective to use Expressing Myself when an individual is over a Level 3 emotion. If the individual's football team wins a huge game, screaming with joy is warranted. Seeing his favorite band in concert may be a perfect time to scream support and dance like a fool. This kind of expression can be freeing. It is also a bit risky, as it may not lead him in the direction of his long-term goals. The likelihood of doing things the individual regrets, creating conflict, or needing to repair relationships is higher when Expressing Myself over a Level 3.

There may be times when we make a conscious decision to use Expressing Myself at a Level 4. If communicating in an escalated way is on-track for the situation, it may be helpful to do so. For example, if a family member is engaging in dangerous behaviors and does not respond to verbal or written communication, it may be helpful to try Expressing Myself at a Level 4 to communicate concern and urgency. It will be difficult to process information and do Problem Solving while either person is over a Level 3, so waiting to further address issues until both are below a Level 3 is recommended.

There are times when the individual does Clear Picture and On-Track Thinking, and decides that expressing *to himself* when over a Level 3 is on-track. The individual may decide to do this if he is on a walk and is talking to himself with no other people present. Alternatively, he may go to a private area to express feelings verbally where it isn't going to affect another person; maybe he chooses to write down what is on his mind or in his heart in a diary/journal. Similarly, a person may pray to a higher power and decide that this is still on-track when she is above a Level 3. This may be an On-Track Action because those types of spiritual relationships are built to support Levels 0–5 expression without damaging the relationship. Individuals create their own toolboxes that fit their goals and values.

The individual can also express through New-Me Activities such as singing, dancing, playing a musical instrument, drawing, and acting. There are times when the individual is over a Level 3 and feels the urge to express through New-Me Activities. If it is a Solo New-Me Activity, we can express at any level of feelings. For example, dancing and singing by ourselves may be good ways to express Level 4 feelings. If other people are negatively affected by the New-Me Activity (e.g., the music is too loud for the neighbors), the individual may experience conflict that increases stress. We use 123 Wide Mind to adjust our Skills Plans as needed.

Getting It Right and Finding Middle Ground

Finding Middle Ground is used to resolve relationship conflicts. Within Finding Middle Ground, Getting It Right is used to ask for a situation or person to change. Getting It Right ensures that the individual is in the Right Mind, communicates with the Right Person, at the Right Time and Place using the Right Tone and Right Words. Expressing Myself is used during Finding Middle Ground (as it is integrated into Getting It Right) to help the individual decide what, how, and when to communicate when resolving a relationship conflict.

For example, Expressing Myself is useful for communicating general statements about preferences, like "I don't like having to put the toilet seat down," or "I think men should put toilet seats down after they go." This allows anyone in the area to hear an individual's preferences and respond as he wishes. If the individual wants the person to put the seat down, Getting It Right is a better bet. When using Getting It Right, she might remark about how thoughtful her partner is (Sugar), Explaining her discomfort when she falls in the toilet at night when the seat is up, Asking him to put the seat down, and Sealing the Deal with hugs and kisses. This strategy has tactics built in that support making requests. Using Expressing Myself to "confront" people is likely to perpetuate or worsen relationship problems. For example, if the individual expresses only "the ask," without being in the Right Mind, Tone, and Words ("You need to put the seat down or else . . . !"), relationship strife may increase. Both Getting It Right and Finding Middle Ground are discussed in greater detail in the next sections of this chapter.

Expressing Myself: Foundational DBT Concepts and Teaching Points (Linehan, 2025a)

- Objectives Effectiveness Skills: DEAR MAN (pp. 248–255)
- Relationship Effectiveness Skills: GIVE (pp. 255–260)
- Self-Respect Effectiveness Skills: FAST (pp. 260–262)
- Evaluating Your Options: How Intensely to Ask or Say No (pp. 263–266)
- Validation Skills (pp. 293–301)

Getting It Right

Getting It Right, Skill 8, is a series of tactics that the individual considers when attempting to get something that he wants from another person. This eighth skill in the Skills System is a Calm-Only skill, which means that the individual can use Getting It Right *only* when below a Level 3 emotion. It is important to note that the other person also needs to be below a Level 3. If either person in the interaction is above a Level 3, it may be best to wait until a later time, when both individuals' emotions are less escalated.

To acquire things successfully, the person must be in the Right Mind and talk to the Right Person at the Right Time and Place, using the Right Tone and the Right Words. The word "right" refers to effectiveness of the strategies to help the individual reach her personal goals and live aligned with her values. The term "right" does not reflect an external judgment about social or moral correctness.

Right Mind

Being in the Right Mind to use Getting It Right means that the person has a Clear Picture and has used On-Track Thinking to make a plan related to the best tactics to get what is desired. The individual must be acting in Wise Mind; she should be prepared, focused, below a Level 3 on the Feelings Rating Scale, and be ready to do what works. It is helpful if the individual has a clear sense of what she is asking for before Getting It Right. Asking for one, clearly defined thing can increase the individual's chances of receiving it. Being vague and/or adding multiple requests can confuse the situation and decrease positive outcomes. As with Expressing Myself, it is common for emotions to rise prior to and during use of Getting It Right. It is important for the individual to self-monitor her emotional status. To become demanding, to act as though she is right and the other person is incorrect, or to use intimidation are signs that the person is starting to go off-track.

Approaching another person to make requests can increase emotional responses. It is vital that the individual continue to use all necessary skills to manage the situation. Creating a Getting It Right Plan (see Learning Skills, Getting It Right—Worked Example 1 in the *Skills System Workbook*) can help the individual be organized; rehearsing and practicing can increase effectiveness as well. Planning ahead can help the individual remain effective even if he unexpectedly experiences cognitive overload in the moment. If the person has a fuzzy picture or engages in off-track thinking, Getting It Right will quickly turn into getting it wrong. Therefore, if either person's emotions begin to escalate to the Level 4 or 5 range, it is best to retreat, returning to Clear Picture and On-Track Thinking to make another Skills Plan.

Right Person

When making a Getting It Right Plan, it is important to talk to the Right Person. This is the person who can and will help the individual get his needs met. For example, the individual may want to discuss a raise with his employer rather than with his coworker. In complex situations, it may be challenging to know who is best. For example, if the person lives in a residential program, he may talk to either a supervisor, a program manager, or a psychologist regarding a clarification about his individual service plan. Seeking consultation from skills coaches to make these choices may be beneficial. Additionally, if the Right Person is not readily available, it may be necessary to set up a specific time to talk. There may be delays that are frustrating. It is important to use other skills while waiting to talk to the Right Person. Getting a Clear Picture, using On-Track Thinking, and doing On-Track Actions, such as New-Me Activities, may help him wait and remain in the Right Mind.

Right Time and Place

Choosing the Right Time and Place is important. The individual will want to choose an opportunity when the Right Person is able to give full attention to the interaction. The circumstances have to be conducive to the Right Person helping the individual. The individual may want to rush to use Getting It Right at a time that is not convenient for the Right Person. It is often more effective to adjust the Getting It Right plan and wait, rather than have emotions dictate the timing of this process.

Right Tone

Using the Right Tone is critically important. The individual must get a Clear Picture and do On-Track Thinking to gauge what tone will work best. Usually being too passive or wimpy makes the Right Person not take the individual seriously. Often, being demanding makes the Right Person pull away, stop listening, and think that the individual is not able to handle the situation. When the individual utilizes an aggressive tone, it may stress the relationship so much that the Right Person will not want to help again, and it may make the circumstances more difficult.

Right Words

SEALS represents the Right Words or tasks in Getting It Right. Sugar, Explaining the Situation, Asking for What I Want, Listening, and Sealing a Deal are the Right Words in Getting It Right.

Sugar

Using Sugar represents adding sweetness to the situation. This means that the individual is respectful and polite to the Right Person to create a positive relationship environment—for example, "Excuse me, Ms. Smith, may I speak to you for a moment?" Sugar is an ingredient that makes the Right Person want to help the individual get what she needs. Throughout the interaction, the individual responds to the Right Person's needs (showing strong Relationship Care) while advocating for her own agenda: "Ms. Smith, I know you run a business that helps many people. I would really appreciate your help at this time." If the individual remains positive, the Right Person may want to return the favor.

Explaining the Situation

Next, the individual explains the situation. The individual highlights why it is important that the Right Person help him: "Ms. Smith, as you know, there was a huge flood in Nepal last year. The homes of over 60,000 villagers were destroyed. Many people are still homeless there." Explaining the Situation helps the Right Person become motivated to do whatever it takes to help the individual. The individual wants the Right Person to feel good about contributing. Rushing to make the request before using ample Sugar and fully Explaining the Situation can fail to mobilize the Right Person's motivation to help.

Asking for What You Want

After using Sugar and Explaining the Situation, the individual asks for what she wants: "Ms. Smith, my organization is collecting donations of money and supplies to send to Nepal to help build homes for families whose houses were destroyed in the flood." It is helpful to be specific, so that the Right Person clearly understands the request. "If you could either donate $100 or send tools to our organization to ship there, it would benefit many people. A donation of $300 builds one temporary home for a family." Asking for What You Want in a clear and direct way helps the Right Person reflect on her ability to help and make a decision about how to proceed.

Listening

Throughout the entire process of Getting It Right, it is important to listen to the Right Person's opinions and feedback. For example, the answer from the Right Person may be "no." In this case the individual listens to the reasons and tries to negotiate; perhaps only a portion of the request can be fulfilled. Right Person might say, "I'm sorry, Julie, but our company already made donations to the flood survivors." The individual may say, "Ms. Smith, is there any way your company could donate used tools to our efforts?" or he may thank the Right Person for her time.

The Right Person may say "maybe" or "I will need to check." It is important to check and turn urges to assume these responses mean "no." Listening and using skills to keep two-way-street communication can give the Right Person the opportunity to help. Throughout Getting It Right, the individual uses Clear Picture and On-Track Thinking to be assertive enough to maximize the likelihood of success while being respectful and maintaining the relationship. Sprinkling Sugar throughout the interaction can help the individual reach the goal and facilitate future success.

Sealing a Deal

Finally, the individual works on Sealing a Deal with the Right Person—for example, the Right Person says, "Julie, I am going to give $500 and send three toolboxes to your organization." The individual then seals the deal by saying, "Thank you, Ms. Smith, for your generosity. The check is made out to Helping Homes. The check and tools can be sent to 22 Main Street in Harrisville. I really appreciate this. Do you have a sense of when you will be able to make this donation?" It is very important to pin down the details as part of Sealing a Deal. It is great when the Right Person agrees to help, but it is vital to ensure the execution of the plan.

Getting It Right: Foundational DBT Concepts and Teaching Points (Linehan, 2025a)

- Objectives Effectiveness Skills: DEAR MAN (pp. 248–255)
- Relationship Effectiveness Skills: GIVE (pp. 255–260)

Relationship Care

Relationship Care, the ninth skill in the Skills System, is a Calm-Only skill. Managing relationships is a complex task that may require using other Calm-Only skills, such as Problem Solving, Expressing Myself, and Getting It Right. Just as with the other Calm-Only skills, it is helpful to use Relationship Care when all involved are below a Level 3. If the individual is in a conversation with someone who shifts to over a Level 3, he needs to get a Clear Picture and do On-Track Thinking to plan how to handle the situation. Similarly, if the individual is over a Level 3, it may not be the time to self-reflect and evaluate her life; the assessment might not be as accurate over a Level 3.

There are multiple elements of Relationship Care. Building On-Track Relationships, balancing On-Track Relationships, and changing off-track relationships are a few aspects of the skill. Healthy, balanced, fulfillment of On-Track Relationships with the self and other people can significantly add to the individual's quality of life.

Building an On-Track Relationship with Myself

The concept of the core self helps the individual understand what it means to have a strong self-relationship. There are four elements of the core self: self-awareness, self-acceptance, self-value, and self-trust.

Self-Awareness

Clear Picture teaches the individual steps that foster self-awareness. In addition, On-Track Thinking prompts the individual to reflect on goals and values. When the individual is clear about goals, it is much more likely that she will implement effective strategies to reach her goal in a situation. When he knows his values, it is easier for him to make choices that align with them. A positive recursive process happens: As the individual learns skills, his ability to be self-aware increases, and as he becomes more self-aware, his ability to apply skills improves. Both factors help the individual manage more challenging situations and be on-track with himself and his goals.

Self-Acceptance

When the individual can be present in the moment, he begins the process of self-acceptance. Seeing himself *as is,* is more possible when he has the capacities to manage the awareness and realities of the situation. Unfortunately, seeing the self *as is* may generate painful emotions. Factors such as medical issues, physical disabilities, mental health problems, trauma, and chronic behavioral dysregulation are a few examples of challenges that can significantly complicate the person's self-acceptance efforts.

Self-Value

The process of strengthening the core self often continues as the person improves self-awareness and self-acceptance to include increased self-value. Practicing Clear Picture, demonstrating On-Track Thinking, and taking On-Track Actions helps the person accomplish mastery. Experiencing success in more challenging situations leads the person to have a positive self-experience versus self-avoidance. The Skills System is built to continually mobilize the person's inner wisdom and guide him to engage actively in adaptive behaviors. Over time, the person discovers self-capacities and in turn develops the ability to self-value.

Self-Trust

Each of the previous elements of the core self serves to improve the individual's self-trust. The person sees situations clearly, accepts the realities, remains positive in the face of challenges, and makes skillful decisions that help her move toward personal goals. Experiencing these abilities gives the person the knowledge that she can not only survive but also get what she needs. Previous patterns of overdoing and underdoing are replaced by skillful self-management and, ultimately, improved self-trust. As the individual's core self strengthens, self-efficacy builds; self-efficacy is an important ingredient for using effective self-regulation strategies.

Building Relationships with Others

Developing capacities of self-awareness, self-acceptance, self-value, and self-trust may positively impact the individual's abilities to self-regulate *and* to have functioning relationships with others. For example, the individual's ability to be aware of other people may allow him to be more aware of what other people are experiencing. Being more aware of the other person can help the individual be more responsive and empathetic. Similarly, as the individual self-accepts, he may become more accepting of other people. Likewise, valuing and trusting other people may offer the individual opportunities for richer relationships. Having the ability to be aware of, accept, value, and trust other people potentially improves relationships and enhances the individual's ability to reach personal goals.

Balancing On-Track Relationships with Others

It is the right and responsibility of each individual to make personal decisions related to her level of participation in relationships on an ongoing basis. The person uses Clear Picture and On-Track Thinking to balance her changing needs and the needs of other people. For example, if a housemate has a brain injury, the person may choose to accept that her housemate repeats statements frequently. Conversely, there may be a situation in which the individual seeks to move from the home because the housemate's behavior is unacceptable. Thus, Relationship Care is not prescriptive but is a process of using skills to make adjustments within each moment that reflect her Wise Mind. Balancing relationships is a dynamic process that requires the individual to use many tools throughout each day.

Types of Relationships

Each individual has many different types of relationships in his life, and these relationships may change through time. For example, the person who has an intellectual disability may need to relate with residential agencies, employers, job coaches, support staff, housemates, friends, organization members, state social workers, family, and significant others. It is important that the individual learn about the socially effective ways to manage each different type of relationship. As the person ages, his individual role and the roles of other people may transform. Developing and maintaining effective relationships with all the different people in the individual's life requires utilization of all of the skills in the Skills System on an ongoing basis.

Relationship Behaviors

The individual uses Clear Picture and On-Track Thinking to make decisions about on-track relationship behaviors. The person continually assesses and balances actions that reflect her personal preferences, values, and goals within the moment. It is vital to use Clear Picture, On-Track Thinking, and On-Track Actions with Relationship Care to manage the multiple changing internal and external factors that transact in relationships. The process of caring for relationships is dynamic. It is necessary to enact a sequence of actions that serve to maintain self-respect and respect for other people as the individual changes, as other people change, and as life changes. Because there are no Relationship Care prescriptions, it is important to use various relationship tools to make adjustments in each moment.

To manage the variability within relationship environments, it is helpful to understand what factors tend to affect relationships so that the individual can make adjustments within the current moment. For example, certain Relationship Care behaviors tend to increase positive feelings between people: acting like the person is important, responding with thoughtful comments, calling the person and making plans, using appropriate touch, giving gifts, paying compliments, doing activities together, being flexible, and so on.

The individual may have important people and relationships in his life. It may be helpful for him to incorporate Relationship Care behaviors into On-Track Action plans that proactively maintain relationships. Using tools that enhance connection, communication, and support from him to those significant friends, family members, or support providers can help the relationships stay on track.

Conversely, certain behaviors tend to increase distance between people in relationships. Keeping conversations short, avoiding disclosing personal information, avoiding making plans, and setting clear personal limits are examples of how to create distance in relationships. Awareness of these tools can help the individual understand the impact of such actions, so that relationship behaviors can be strategically utilized to meet personal goals. For example, if the individual has gone out on a date with someone she is not interested in seeing again, she may discuss her lack of interest directly or she may use tactics that add distance. As she becomes more mindful of these diverse tools, increased self-determination and active Relationship Care can improve the quality of her life.

Two-Way-Street Relationships

One goal of the Skills System is to give the individual proper tools to participate in Two-Way-Street relationships. A Two-Way-Street relationship is a reciprocal relationship in which there is mutual respect and communication. Although the individual cannot control the behavior of the other person, Relationship Care teaches him to act in a way that allows a Two-Way-Street relationship to happen. The individual must learn to participate actively, both as a giver and receiver, in a Two-Way-Street relationship. For example, the individual must talk and listen to the other person. He clarifies his points of view and prompts the other person to use Expressing Myself. Within a Two-Way-Street relationship, participants are able to be present, discuss, negotiate, and collaborate. Working together creates a synthesis and a heightened development of each person and the relationship.

One-Way-Street Relationships

One-Way-Street relationships occur (1) when the individual does relationship behaviors that add distance in the relationship or (2) when she experiences the other person not reciprocating. There are times when the person may evaluate a One-Way-Street relationship as out of balance and do Problem Solving to make a plan to address the relationship problem. In this case, the receiver is dissatisfied. To rectify the problem, she may decide to increase Relationship Care behaviors that improve connections or use Finding Middle Ground to assess and change the off-track relationship. If the one-way street is "as good as it gets," using Safety Plans and Accept the Situation may be skill options.

At other times, the individual may want to create a One-Way-Street relationship. Restricting her participation as a giver may be effective to maintain alignment to her goals. For example, if there is an unwanted advance by a coworker, the individual may want to restrict involvement to communicate her boundaries.

Changing Off-Track Relationships

When the individual's self-relationship becomes off-track, it can impede reaching personal goals. For example, off-track thinking that is self-devaluing may undermine an individual's abilities to function to his potential. Another common problem is when he has a fuzzy picture about goals and is therefore unable to make and execute effective Skills Plans. Additionally, certain behavior patterns may be hindering him from reaching goals. Changing off-track habits, such as smoking, alcoholism, drug use, overeating, undereating, and medication inconsistency, may improve the individual's self-relationship and help him be on-track. It is challenging to change any kind of off-track habit. Therefore, it is necessary to use all of the skills in the Skills System to manage off-track urges and create new behavior patterns.

Changing Relationships with Others: Finding Middle Ground

Addressing relationship problems often requires using all of the Calm-Only skills. For example, the first step to change an off-track relationship may be to do Problem Solving to get a clear picture of the relationship problem. If the individual determines that meeting and discussing the issue with the other person is Plan A, she then chooses the best means of Expressing Myself. She decides whether talking face-to-face, on the phone, or writing a letter or email is the best tactic. If she wants the other person to change his behavior, she will have to use Getting It Right. She will have to be in the Right Mind, choose the Right Time and Place, and use the Right Tone and the Right Words.

Finding Middle Ground expands Getting It Right to be a collaborative process in which both the individuals talk and listen to hear both sides. Through this Two-Way-Street process there is a give and take and search for a win–win solution to the relationship problem. When they can negotiate a resolution that benefits both, the pair uses Finding Middle Ground to create a new level of balance in the relationship.

There are times when the individual's best efforts at Finding Middle Ground do not fix the relationship problems. If the other person is not responsive, chooses not to engage in the collaboration, and does not make accommodations for the individual, then ending the relationship may need to be considered. Revisiting Clear Picture, On-Track Thinking, and Problem Solving may be necessary to determine the next On-Track Action.

To learn the processes of Finding Middle Ground, it may be helpful to engage in negotiations and compromises related to low-intensity situations. For example, discussing where to order takeout from with a friend is a form of Finding Middle Ground. The individual explains her preference for pizza. The friend articulates his desire to have burgers. The pair discusses the alternatives and finds a win–win. Perhaps it is pizza today and burgers tomorrow. Practicing Finding Middle Ground in situations that do not generate high levels of feelings allows the individual to employ the strategies in a low-demand situation.

Steps of Responsibility

When the individual feels that he has created a relationship problem, it may be helpful to repair the relationship by doing the Steps of Responsibility. This process involves (1) clearly admitting the problem and the impact the behaviors had on the other person, (2) apologizing for what the individual regrets, (3) committing to change his behavior, and (4) taking an On-Track Action. It is not easy to take responsibility, because the individual may feel shame, have the urge to be stubborn, blame the other person, or insist that he is right. Although doing the Steps of Responsibility may cause discomfort, the process can ultimately strengthen the individual's self-relationship and his relationship with the other person.

Ending Relationships with Others

There may be instances when the individual has made efforts to repair the relationship, but relationship problems still exist. The individual may determine that a relationship is off-track. For example, if the other person is continually demonstrating poor Relationship Care behaviors or encouraging the individual to make off-track choices, perhaps the relationship needs to be ended. The individual can begin to use One-Way-Street behaviors that increase the distance in the relationship, or she can formally end the relationship. The individual uses Clear Picture, On-Track Thinking, On-Track Action, and Problem Solving to determine how best to stop an off-track relationship. Living with problematic relationships can lead her to be off-track, out of balance, and miserable.

Individuals must also learn to deal with relationships changing or ending through no actions of their own. For example, staff leaving, romantic partners breaking up, people moving away, and people dying are common reasons for disruptions in relationships. It may be necessary for the individual to use many skills to cope effectively with relationships that are ending. Although these are often painful experiences, the individual can remain on track toward her goals while managing loss and grief.

Relationship Care: Foundational DBT Concepts and Teaching Points (Linehan, 2025a)

- Mindfulness Practice: A Spiritual Perspective (pp. 214–218)
- Wise Mind: A Spiritual Perspective (pp. 218–219)

- Practicing Loving Kindness (pp. 219–222)
- Walking the Middle Path (pp. 233–234)
- Factors Reducing Interpersonal Effectiveness (pp. 237–241)
- Skills for Finding Potential Friends (pp. 270–275)
- Mindfulness of Others (pp. 275–280)
- How to End Relationships (pp. 280–284)
- Validation Skills (pp. 293–301)

SYSTEM TOOLS

There are three System Tools within the Skills System. The Feelings Rating Scale, Categories of Skills, and Recipe for Skills help the individual organize his current experiences and execute a series of behaviors intended to reach personal goals. The System Tools are designed to help the individual create effective skills chains.

Feelings Rating Scale

The Feelings Rating Scale is a self-report scale, from Level 0 to Level 5, used to rate the intensity of emotions, feelings, and/or sensory experiences that are happening during a situation in the moment. The more intense the sensations and impact on thinking, the higher the rating. The term "feeling" is generally used in the Skills System because it is the broadest term and the simplest to pronounce. The Feelings Rating Scale is used to rate both uncomfortable and more pleasurable experiences.

Emotions impact the individual's capacity to focus. The Feelings Rating Scale can also be conceptualized as a focus rating scale. At the lower levels of emotion, focus is often sharper. At higher levels of feeling, focus is more variable, fuzzier. The individual learns to do more interacting at lower levels of feeling when focus is intact. In addition, the Feelings Rating Scale assesses the individual's level of relationship ability in the moment. Often her capacity to relate effectively is lower as feelings are higher.

The Feelings Rating Scale serves a dual purpose in the Skills System. First, the individual learns to continually rate her feelings as part of getting a Clear Picture. The scale is a tool that provides a simple framework that promotes self-awareness and internal organization. Second, the Feelings Rating Scale is utilized during On-Track Thinking. She uses the Feelings Rating Scale to determine which skills and how many skills would be helpful in a particular situation (Categories of Skills). If the individual is below a Level 3 emotion, it is possible to use all nine skills in the Skills System. If the rating is over a Level 3 emotion, only the All-the-Time skills are used.

Each person experiences and expresses feelings differently. The same situation may elicit a Level 1 emotion from one person and a Level 3 from someone else. Similarly, different people may express the same emotion in different ways. Individuals can label and rate their own feelings, while the labels and ratings of others are only estimates.

Discussions about ratings and the similarities and differences in peoples' perspectives in skills group can help individuals become aware of how their ratings align with others. For example, if an individual becomes aware that he has high-level reactions in a situation in which others consistently have low-level reactions, then he has an opportunity to explore different, enhanced skills options to address the strong responses.

Feelings ratings adjust as a person gains emotion regulation capacities. The individual is able to experience stronger emotions, enact skills chains, and remain emotionally, cognitively, and behaviorally regulated in increasingly challenging situations. For example, a situation that would have previously elicited a Level 4 emotion may only produce a Level 3 emotion as more effective skills chains are used earlier in the escalation process. When this shift happens, the individual is more able to handle stressful, demanding, and increasingly tenuous interactions in on-track ways. For example, the individual may gain the ability to do on-track Finding Middle Ground, talking and listening in situations that would have previously elicited a Level 4 feeling, precluding the use of a Calm-Only skill.

A *Level 0 feelings rating* means that a feeling is not being experienced. For example, Level 0 anger means that the individual is not experiencing anger at that moment. She may be a Level 2 sad at that time, but not angry (0 angry). While awake, unless in a meditative state, it is difficult for humans not to have some type or level of feelings. Disorders like alexithymia and states of dissociation can affect the individual's awareness of feelings.

If an individual consistently reports feelings at Level 0, this pattern may mean that he may be repressing feelings or relying on affect suppression to manage emotions. If the individual can't manage the feeling, he may block awareness of it or choose not to communicate it. Although those strategies may be effective in specific circumstances, globalizing them can lead to difficulties with escalating emotions and challenges making goal-directed choices. As the individual develops the capacity to use skills and manage emotions, the accuracy of rating will likely improve.

A *Level 1 feelings rating* is a tiny reaction to something that is just noticeable, a twinge. For example, if the individual sees a nice car driving by, he may feel Level 1 envy. He may notice a twinge of the emotion and fleeting thoughts about how nice that car is and how he would like to have one like that. If he allows the emotions and thoughts to pass, the feeling dissipates; if he perseverates about what a piece of junk his own car is, the feeling increases.

A Level 1 feelings rating may be as high as the emotion goes, or a stronger feeling might be forming. Conversely, the individual might have reduced arousal from a stronger emotion. It is crucial that the individual learn to become aware of Level 1 feelings, because it can help him maintain awareness and effective coping throughout the situation.

At a Level 1 feeling, the person is likely able to think clearly; thus, he can use any of the nine skills on the Skills List. Because of the individual's capacity to cognitively regulate, he can use Calm-Only skills. The slight sensations and minimal cognitive disruption contribute to the relative ease of managing urges, impulses, and actions at a Level 1 emotion.

A *Level 2 feelings rating* is a small feeling. The sensations of a Level 2 feeling are noticeable, yet they do not generally cause disruptions that negatively impact the individual's capacities to be on-track. For example, at Level 2 anger she may feel her heart beating faster and notice her muscles tightening. Although there may be discomfort at Level 2, she is able to use all nine of the skills on the Skills List. This may be a good time to use skills that involve Expressing Myself, rather than at a Level 3 or above feeling. Optimally, the individual can experience the situation and move strategically toward personal goals.

A *Level 3 feelings rating* is a medium-size feeling. This level of emotion will cause noticeable and possibly multiple body sensations. Sweaty hands, stomachache, racing heart rate, and pacing are a few examples. At Level 3, "negative" feelings such as sadness, fear, anger, guilt, or jealousy may be uncomfortable for the individual. Although he may notice more off-track thoughts and urges at Level 3, he is able to focus attention and be on-track relative to his goals. He can talk and listen in ways that preserve his relationship to himself and the other person. If the individual is crying but is still able to talk and listen, he may be at a Level 3; when those abilities diminish, he is at a Level 4.

At Level 3, the individual can use Calm-Only skills; careful self-monitoring through Clear Picture and On-Track Thinking are necessary to ensure that he engages in on-track versus off-track actions. The Level 3 sweet spot is when the individual is able to balance experiencing medium-strong feelings (positive or negative) and interacting in ways that are aligned with her goals and/or values. For example, situations in healthy, intimate relationships may contain Level 3 sweet spot interactions that include communication of strong emotions while maintaining the safety of the partners. A Level 3 sweet spot may not be comfortable but may lead to deeper levels of connection and intimacy.

If the person begins to use the more interactive Calm-Only skills (Problem Solving, Expressing Myself, Getting It Right, and Relationship Care) and notices that emotions are increasing or the strategies are not working effectively, it is best to Switch Tracks to use the All-the-Time skills (Clear Picture, On-Track Thinking, On-Track Action, Safety Plan, and New-Me Activities) until he is more regulated. If the individual rates the feeling as 3.5, it is over a Level 3, and Calm-Only skills are not recommended.

A *Level 4 feelings rating* is a strong feeling. At a Level 4 feeling, it is likely that the individual is experiencing sustained, intense emotions and body sensations. For example, she may cry uncontrollably, tremble, breathe quickly, sweat profusely, or feel nauseated. Thought processes are disrupted. For example, her thoughts may be racing, disorganized, or nonexistent (blank).

At a Level 4 feelings rating, the individual may be having strong off-track urges to say or do things that will harm his relationship with himself or with another person. He is unable to talk and listen effectively at a Level 4. Using Calm-Only skills, such as Problem Solving and Expressing Myself, can be a desperate attempt to reduce emotional discomfort that unfortunately leaves goals unmet and creates collateral damage that makes situations worse. Interactive, Calm-Only skills are not recommended at a Level 4 feeling because of the high level of emotional, cognitive, and behavioral instability. At a Level 4, the individual is not harming himself, others, or property.

A *Level 5 feelings rating* is when the individual harms himself, others, or property. Often, either a Level 5 is an overwhelming event, or it is a Level 4 situation that escalates to Level 5 due to a lack of skills use. In the latter case, the actual sensations of a Level 5 may or may not be different than a Level 4, but the individual is overwhelmed and unable to manage his behaviors.

Each individual's appraisal of what out-of-control behaviors or what harming self, others, or property means may be different. One person may rate her anger at Level 5 when she yells at someone (hurting the person emotionally and injuring the relationship), while someone else may view behaviors such as slamming doors, storming around, and/or yelling as not directly causing harm, and may therefore rate them at Level 4. Just as each person's perceptions of what is on-track and off-track are individualized, feelings rating is a personal process.

At Level 5, All-the-Time skills are necessary. Clear Picture, On-Track Thinking, On-Track Action, Safety Plan, and multiple New-Me Activities generally are necessary to help the individual reduce high-level feelings. These skills help the individual regain the control and capacity to function safely. The situation may require Problem Solving, Expressing Myself, Getting It Right, and/or Relationship Care at a later point, but the individual must utilize other skills to reduce the level of escalation prior to engaging in these interactive skills.

Categories of Skills

There are two Categories of Skills. The first five skills (Clear Picture, On-Track Thinking, On-Track Action, Safety Plan, and New-Me Activities) are All-the-Time skills that can be used at any level of emotion, 0–5. When the individual is over a Level 3, All-the-Time skills are used. All-the-Time skills are designed to help the person self-regulate internal factors. Knowing how and when to step back and self-regulate emotions through All-the-Time skills is crucial to reaching personal goals. Table 2.1 lists the All-the-Time and Calm-Only skills.

The second Category of Skills is Calm-Only skills. The last four skills (Problem Solving, Expressing Myself, Getting It Right, and Relationship Care) often require interaction with other people and should therefore be used *only* when an individual is calm. If a person is even a tiny bit higher than a Level 3 feeling, All-the-Time skills should be used first.

Calm-Only skills are essential in helping the individual manage social relationships. Interacting with others and getting personal needs met is a challenging, ever-changing, ongoing process. Calm-Only skills are more complex, multistep, and take longer to complete than All-the-Time skills. The individual must continually use skills chains (e.g., "1236," "1237," "1238," "1239") to remain on track during these experiences. When doing Problem Solving, Expressing Myself, Getting It Right, and Relationship Care, there are more variables and more opportunities for the environment to drive the individual's feelings up.

Despite the increased risks, it is essential that the individual engage in Calm-Only skills to manage her life. A key factor is knowing when she can do them effectively given her level of

TABLE 2.1. Categories of Skills

All-the-Time Skills (Level 0–5 emotions)	Calm-Only Skills (Level 0–3 emotions)
1. Clear Picture	6. Problem Solving
2. On-Track Thinking	7. Expressing Myself
3. On-Track Action	8. Getting It Right
4. Safety Plan	9. Relationship Care
5. New-Me Activities	

feeling. Avoidance of Calm-Only skills can be associated with patterns of off-track behavior. For example, if the individual avoids Problem Solving, problems grow, become overwhelming, and lead to off-track actions.

The Category of Skills is used during Make a Skills Plan. At that point, the person reflects on his current level of emotion (via Clear Picture) and determines which skills can be used. If the level is over a 3, All-the-Time skills are the only option for the moment. If 0–3, then both All-the-Time and Calm-Only skills can be used.

Not all individuals can recall all nine skills and understand the specifics of the Categories of Skills. The concept of Categories of Skills remains important and instruction and coaching strategies need to integrate it in accessible ways. More conceptually, the messages of the categories are:

- When we have strong emotions, it is hard to be focused and on-track.
- When we are upset, it isn't the best time to solve problems because doing so at that time can make things worse instead of better.
- It can help to do Safety Plans and New-Me Activities when we are upset.

Recipe for Skills

The Recipe for Skills is a System Tool that helps calculate the minimum number of skills necessary in any situation. The Recipe recommends that the individual use *at least* one skill for every level of feeling, including Level 0. Therefore, at a Level 1, at least two skills are needed. At a Level 5, six are necessary and they need to be All-the-Time skills. The Recipe for Skills is intended generally to guide the individual to use more skills at higher levels of feeling. Medium, strong, and overwhelming feelings have higher intensity and last longer. Spanning a skills chain across those events increases the likelihood of getting through it successfully.

The Recipe for Skills is a conceptual framework that offers guiding principles about assembling skills chains. It is not a prescription about the number of skills that must be linked; it highlights minimum requirements. Executing longer chains of All-the-Time and Calm-Only skills at low levels of emotion (0–3) is more effective than following the Recipe for Skills minimum recommendations. For example, doing a 12369 chain at a Level 2 feeling far surpasses the Recipe for Skills and likely addressed important issues.

The Recipe for Skills is useful during the skills planning process. For example, "I am at a Level 3 mad, so I need to use at least four skills." The Recipe for Skills is also helpful when looking back on experiences to see whether ample skills were used. For example, if an individual is reflecting on an off-track incident, he may be able to see that he used no skills at a Level 4, when at least five skills were needed.

Each individual may use the Recipe for Skills differently. During the initial skills learning phases the Recipe for Skills may be used more consciously. As building adequate skills chains becomes more automatic, checking the Recipe for Skills is less necessary.

The cognitive demands of the Recipe for Skills may impact individuals differently at different times. For example, if the individual has difficulty with math concepts, the Recipe for Skills could trigger emotional reactions that reduce cognitive functioning rather than improve focus. Conversely, for other people, reflecting on what skills have been used and doing the simple math computation can improve focus in the moment. The Recipe for Skills is a general guideline rather than a complex math equation or strict rules to overengineer skills plans.

If the instructor or coach decides it is best to communicate the Recipe for Skills in a more conceptual way, these are a few helpful messages:

- Skills help us manage emotions.
- The bigger the feeling, the more skills we need.
- If we don't do enough skills, we can feel worse or go off-track.

Skills chains are when the individual makes and executes a series of skills in a situation. Standard skills chains include the foundational skills of Clear Picture, On-Track Thinking, and On-Track Actions. The bullets below offer some helpful hints about assembling skills chains at ascending levels of feeling.

- At Level 0, it may be helpful for the individual to do Clear Picture to be aware of the moment as it evolves.

- At Level 1, using Clear Picture (1) and On-Track Thinking (2), a "12" skills chain, can be advantageous. This puts the individual in the position to take various On-Track Actions that will help him reach his goals.

- At Level 2, at least three skills are necessary. Doing Clear Picture (1), On-Track Thinking (2), and an On-Track Action (3)—a "123" skills chain—are helpful. Given the On-Track Actions likely utilize other skills, the individual is probably going to use more skills than the recipe recommends.

- At Level 3, at least four skills are needed. Any number of skills chains can be created at this level (e.g., "1234," "1235," "1236," "1237," "1238," "1239"). If there is risk, a "1234" (Safety Plan, 4) may be best, or if the individual is bored, a "1235" (New-Me Activity, 5). If the individual has a problem to be solved, "1236" may work well. If he wants to express something, "1237" may be a good option. If he needs something from someone, "1238" may be useful. If he wants to sort out a Relationship Care issue, a "1239" may work. Longer chains that combine multiple All-the-Time and/or Calm-Only skills may be even more effective (e.g., "12345," "123455," "12367," "12378," "12379").

- At Level 4, at least five skills are needed. Because the individual is over a Level 3, the five skills must be All-the-Time skills. A common skills chain for when the individual is at Level 4 is "12345." At Level 4, when there may be off-track urges and off-track actions, doing a Safety Plan helps the individual manage the risk, and engaging in New-Me Activities can focus attention.

- At Level 5, at least six skills are needed. Since there are only five All-the-Time skills, it is necessary to double up on one of the All-the-Time skills. For example, the individual may use multiple New-Me Activities. In that case, he would get a Clear Picture, use On-Track Thinking, take an On-Track Action, do a Safety Plan, and engage in two New-Me Activities (e.g., playing a video game and listening to music in his room), resulting in a "123455" skills chain. The individual could choose to double up on On-Track Actions such as Accept the Situation or Turn the Page.

TRANSITION TO CHAPTER 3

Chapter 3 introduces the multiple models that create the theoretical foundation for the Skills System. This information teaches the skills instructor about emotion regulation, cognitive load theory, and the design of the Skills System. The information helps the instructor understand emotion regulation skills deficits and how to support individuals to fill skill gaps.

CHAPTER 3

Theoretical Underpinning of the Skills System

This chapter presents information about the theoretical underpinning of the Skills System that includes DBT, emotion regulation research, and cognitive load theory (CLT). A full explanation of DBT is beyond the scope of this text, but emotional vulnerability and biosocial theory will be highlighted. While there are multiple theories about emotion generation and regulation, the Skills System is built upon the process model and the extended process model of emotion regulation (Gross, 2024). Both of these are explained in this chapter. This information influences the design of the Skills System and underpins the Targeting Strategy that is presented in Chapter 5. CLT influences Skills System design, coaching strategies, and instruction techniques, so this chapter will offer an overview of CLT that will be foundational for the Quick Step Assessment strategy that is also presented in Chapter 5.

DBT

The Skills System is a "DBT-Informed" model, so exploring DBT's biosocial theory is a useful place to start. Linehan's (1993a) biosocial theory proposes that people who experience biological vulnerabilities and live in invalidating environments may develop patterns of emotional dysregulation. An individual who experienced this type of emotional vulnerability is described as being highly sensitive and responsive to emotional stimuli. Additionally, the person returns to an emotional baseline slowly and may experience re-escalations during the de-escalation process. From a DBT perspective, learned behaviors coupled with emotion regulation skills deficits lead to emotional, cognitive, behavioral, relationship, and self-dysregulation.

The Skills System integrates many DBT principles. For example, the Skills System is a transactional model that conceptualizes relationships between people as bidirectionally influencing each other. Coaching and instruction relationships can be positive transactions that involve co-regulation between partners. Conversely, these relationships can include negative transactions that involve bidirectional patterns of co-dysregulation where both people are adversely affected. The Skills System is designed to support positive transactions. The nine core skills, System Tools, and coaching strategies are built to help individuals, coaches, and instructors to self- and co-regulate.

Some DBT strategies are also incorporated implicitly into the Skills System due to their high cognitive load demands. Chapter 2 provided lists of DBT concepts that are implicitly integrated into the Skills System. Conversely, validation strategies are explicitly part of the Skills System A + B = C skills coaching framework and behavioral strategies are a foundational teaching strategy presented in Chapter 4.

The goal of DBT is to help people who experience emotional dysregulation create and maintain lives worth living. People who experience patterns of emotional dysregulation and deficits in the areas of executive functioning, attentional control, memory, and impulse control often have difficulty learning and generalizing DBT skills. The Skills System is designed as an accessible tool set that increases emotion regulation capabilities, so the individual can manage her emotions and reach her personal goals. The emotion regulation research in this chapter provides information to help practitioners better understand emotion regulation processes, barriers, necessary competencies, and Skills System concepts that address areas of need.

The biosocial theory, the theoretical underpinning of DBT, is presented as it relates to skills training in Chapter 1 (pp. 5–11) and later in the Teaching Notes (pp. 138–143) of the *DBT Skills Training Manual, Revised Edition* (Linehan, 2025a).

WHAT IS EMOTION REGULATION?

Emotion regulation includes using strategies to change the trajectory of an emotion (e.g., duration and intensity) and to reach desired goals (Gross, 2024). The goals may be to change an emotion and/or to achieve a specific outcome. The Skills System is constructed to help an individual modulate emotions, cognitions, and actions. These foundational competencies are essential for improving quality of life, reaching personal goals, and living aligned with one's values.

This chapter provides information about emotions and emotion regulation processes. This information can be used by practitioners to target emotion regulation skills instruction interventions for individuals with complex learning and behavioral challenges. Fortunately, adaptive emotion regulation strategies are implicitly built into the Skills System model, which eliminates the practitioner's and individual's need to understand these theoretical concepts.

Research related to emotion regulation has expanded rapidly, yet much is still unknown about how people choose and apply emotion regulation strategies in different contexts (Hartmann, Pruessner, & Barnow, 2024; Denny, 2020), as well as how practitioners can systematically target (e.g., reducing maladaptive and increasing adaptive) emotion regulation skills competency (Southward, Sauer-Zavala, and Cheavens, 2021).

Model-Based and Model-Free Emotion Regulation

Etkin, Bushel, and Gross (2015) described two types of emotion regulation approaches: "model-based" and "model-free" emotion regulation. A model-based regulation is when "frontoparietal regions are recruited for implementation of an internal model to guide behavior" and involves a "rule-based decision-making and dynamic computation of optimal actions" (Etkin et al., 2015, p. 694). Model-based emotion regulation allows the individual to respond to the demands of their environment in flexible ways while still maintaining orientation to goals. When the individual does model-free emotion regulation, he reacts to the environment with a limited range of "environment-dependent" responses as opposed to reflecting on an internal model (Etkin et al., 2015, p. 693). Model-free emotion regulation employs fewer cognitive resources and is therefore quicker but less flexible and less useful in helping the individual reach their personal goals.

The Skills System is designed to provide the individual with knowledge that serves as a foundation for model-based emotion regulation. The skills and System Tools provide scaffolding for myriad emotion regulation processes. Adding Skills System strategies to the individual's repertoire of emotion regulation skills (e.g., All-the-Time and Calm-Only skills) is intended to increase adaptive and reduce maladaptive strategies.

Iterative Cycles of Emotion Generation

In order to optimize skills instruction, it is helpful for practitioners to understand how emotions function. As we experience the world, emotions are generated. Having an emotion is not a single event; they have different phases. Gross (2024) explained that emotion generation as a four-part sequence: situation–attention–appraisal–response. The individual first experiences a *situation.* He brings *attention* to the situation because it is relevant to his goals. The relevance or meaning of the situation elicits the emotion. The individual then makes an *appraisal* or assessment about the situation or the emotion that leads to an emotional *response.* Emotional responses involve experiential, behavioral, and neurobiological systems.

The Process Model of Emotion Regulation

The process model (Gross, 2024) has four phases (identification–selection–implementation–monitoring). In the identification phase, the individual decides if action is needed when she experiences an emotion. If managing or changing the emotion is deemed necessary, she decides to change the emotional experience in the selection phase. Gross describes five "families" of strategies that help regulate emotions. The strategies offer tactics to manage each step of the emotion-generative sequence (situation–attention–appraisal–response). These emotion regulation response categories are "situation selection, situation modification, attentional deployment, cognitive change, and response modulation" (Gross, 2024, 2014a, p. 7; see also Gross 2013; Gross & Thompson, 2007). Table 3.1 defines each of the five families of strategies and how Skills System concepts support the emotion regulation processes.

The third phase is implementation, when the individual chooses which tactics to use to regulate the emotion. This sounds easy, but the human experience is complex; emotion regu-

TABLE 3.1. Emotion Regulation Response Categories and the Skills System Concepts That Support Them

Definitions	Skills System concepts
Situation selection occurs when one seeks "to alter emotion by selecting which situations are encountered" (Gross 2024, p. 7).	The Skills System's first three skills (Clear Picture, On-Track Thinking, and On-Track Action) lead the individual to make a goal-directed choice about whether to approach or avoid situations in their lives. Safety Plans help the individual managing risky situations.
Situation modification is an effort to "directly modify the situation so as to alter its emotional impact" (Gross, 2014a, p. 9).	The Calm-Only skills—Problem Solving, Expressing Myself, Getting It Right, and Relationship Care—are designed to help individuals modify situations. The System Tools assist individuals to know whether they can use Calm-Only skills at that time.
Attentional deployment is how the individual seeks "to alter emotion by changing which what aspects of the situation are attended to" (Gross, 2024, p. 7).	Completing the Clear Picture Do's helps the individual recognize aspects of the current moment, as it is. Check It guides the person to assess whether acting on the thought or urge will lead the person to the person's goals.
Cognitive change is when the individual "appraises a situation so as to alter its emotional significance, either by changing how one thinks about the situation or about one's capacities to manage the demands it poses" (Gross, 2014a, p. 10).	If the individual's thoughts/urges align with the individual's goals (i.e., are thumbs up), they progress to take On-Track Actions to manage the emotion and/or to create a desired outcome. If the individual's thoughts/urges will lead the individual off-track, the individual does Turn It to stay on-track to the goals.
Response modulation strategies "alter emotions by directly modifying emotion-related experiential, behavioral, or physiological responses" (Gross, 2024, p. 7).	New-Me Activities (Focus, Feel Good, Distract, and Fun) are commonly used as response modulation strategies.

lation strategies are difficult to prescribe. Stanoi and Ochsner (2024) explained that emotion regulation processes are currently viewed as a "dynamic open-ended process" and acknowledge that strategies and outcomes are affected by the individual and their context, rather than the assumption of uniform responses and outcomes. For example, cognitive modulation (reappraisal) is often considered an adaptive response and may be more effective in low-intensity situations and less effective in high-intensity situations. Attentional deployment (distraction) may be better in high-intensity than in low-intensity situations. It is important for the individual to have strategies to help them navigate a wide spectrum of situations in ways that help the individual's up- and down-regulation feelings in ways that align with her goals.

Certain strategies tend to elicit different outcomes. For example, affective suppression has been shown to decrease positive emotional experiences, but it does not reduce negative ones. While affective suppression may help the individual endure an unavoidable, difficult situation, over-relying on this strategy may increase symptoms of depression. The current research on polyregulation explores how individuals rely on multiple strategies simultaneously and consecutively to manage emotions (Hartmann et al., 2024; Ford, Gross, & Gruber, 2019). Having a broad range of tactics like the Skills System skills, helps the individual respond to each moment in a flexible way depending on her needs.

The process of identifying, selecting, and implementing is an "iterative process" (Gross, 2024, p. 9) that is ongoing. The individual engages in the fourth phase of monitoring as she notices the need to change tactics and updates strategies to fit her goals. The construction of the Skills System skills of Clear Picture, On-Track Thinking, and On-Track Action are repeated to scaffold and facilitate identification, selection, implementation, and monitoring processes.

The Extended Process Model

The extended process model elaborates valuation or how we weigh what aligns with our goals, choose general strategies, and elaborate tactics to reach our goals. The extended process model also shows us that emotions have many microprocesses and microtransitions. Practitioners can see skill gaps and target specific processes to improve the individual's functioning. The Skills System builds these processes into the mechanisms of the model, so the instructor does not have to explicitly teach these concepts.

The extended process model elaborates how valuation cycles happen throughout the three stages of the process model of emotion regulation (Gross, 2015, p. 12). The first stage of the process model is the "identification stage," when the person decides whether to regulate an emotion. The second, "selection stage," is when the person chooses a general strategy (i.e., one of the "five families" of emotion regulation strategies). Finally, the "implementation stage" is when the person initiates a specific tactic.

Within each of these three stages are substeps. The same four substeps happen within each stage: world–perception–valuation–action (Gross, 2015). The first is the world, which represents the internal and external stimuli that becomes the focus of the four-part valuation cycle. Second is perception, when the person brings attention to relevant aspects of the stimuli. Third is valuation. During valuation the person reflects on her goals and appraises whether the perception is neutral, positive/favorable, or negative/unfavorable for her. The valuation leads to the fourth substep, action. Action urge responses are generated to "bridge the gap between the perceived state of the world and the desired state of the world" (Gross, 2015). Table 3.2 explains the stage, substep, and function of the substep of the extended process model.

In each of the stages (identification, selection, and implementation) there are world–perception–value–action cycles of substeps. Emotion regulation is a dynamic process. Each world–perception–valuation–action cycle affects aspects of the world, leading to a new cycle of the substeps. There are several points during this process when the individual can either successfully or unsuccessfully regulate the emotion and/or take action to reach his desired goal. People

TABLE 3.2. Stages of the Extended Process Model, Substeps, and Functions of the Substeps

Stage	Substep	Function of the substep
Identification		
Decision point: Deciding whether to regulate	World	There is an internal or external stimuli (e.g., "I noticed my housemate stole my video game").
	Perception	Detect the emotion (e.g., "I feel angry").
	Valuation	Weigh cost–benefit of regulating the emotion (e.g., "I can lose my temper or use my skills. If I lose my temper, I will be off-track from my goals").
	Action	If there are benefits of regulating, the individual generates an emotion regulation goal (e.g., "I want to be on-track to my goals").
Selection		
Decision point: What strategy to use?	World	The goal to regulate the emotion becomes the focus (e.g., "I want to use my skills to stay on-track").
	Perception	Think about potential emotion regulation strategies (e.g., "I could yell at the person. I could do Clear Picture").
	Valuation	Weigh cost–benefit of using potential emotion regulation strategies (e.g., "Clear Picture would help me be on-track more than yelling would").
	Action	Choose the most promising emotion regulation strategies for the context (e.g., "Clear Picture is best for me right now").
Implementation		
Decision point: Implementing a tactic for the situation.	World	The goal to execute an optimal strategy for the context and level of feeling becomes the focus (e.g., "I will do Clear Picture").
	Perception	Translate the strategy (Clear Picture) into a series of tactics (e.g., "I will do the Clear Picture Do's").
	Valuation	Weigh cost–benefit of potential tactics (e.g., "Notice My Breath will help me slow down").
	Action	Take actions on the tactics (e.g., "I notice my breath").

may have ability gaps in one or more of the substeps. If the individual increases competencies at each stage and substep, his overall ability to regulate emotions effectively is likely to improve. General instruction and targeted instruction aimed to fill ability gaps may increase adaptive strategies and reduce reliance on maladaptive behaviors. Table 3.3 explains the function of each substep, barriers, and tasks to help the individual develop competency within each stage of the emotion regulation process.

The extended process model offers useful information to help skills instructors better understand emotion regulation processes, necessary competencies, barriers, and how the Skills System model can improve functioning. It is important to note that people make decisions about their actions by integrating many factors, rather than progressing through a linear set of processes that result in the objectively highest-value outcome (Suri, Gross, & McClelland, 2020). We don't always do things that appear to be in our "best interest," and subjective factors influence our decisions.

An individual may rely on reinforced "default" responses rather than activating a novel behavior chain. For example, a person who relies predominantly on distraction to manage emotions, might stay at a dead-end job rather than choosing strategies and tactics that require managing conflicts. Additionally, our temperament or personality affect how we value options. If a person tends to be more passive, options that offer an outcome of needing to demonstrate leadership to be effective, may tend to be weighed as less favorable. These types of "hidden" processes affect how options are weighed (Suri et al., 2020, p. 158).

For individuals with cognitive and/or mental health challenges, smooth navigation through the numerous elements of the extended process model may be affected. For example, if the individual has autism spectrum disorder, she may have difficulty with perspective taking, which affects how the individual experiences the "world" around her. If the individual has executive functioning deficits (e.g., difficulty weighing factors and sequencing), processes involving valuation and implementation may be difficult. If a practitioner's goal is to help an individual gain the competency to manage emotions in ways that align with her goal, on a consistent basis, targeting competency gaps, shaping abilities, and scaffolding will likely be necessary. CLT is integrated into the Skills System model to help the practitioner understand how to adjust instruction to maximize engagement and generalization of skills.

Cognitive Load Theory

CLT is a learning and instruction theory that is used to design instruction of complex tasks to maximize cognitive functioning capacities and learning (Sweller, 1988, 2010, 2022; Sweller, van Merrienboer, & Paas, 1998, 2019). Cognitive processing (like that involved in regulating emotions effectively) is limited by the capacity of humans' working memory and ability to manage complex, interactive situations. Given the complex nature of emotion regulation, the cognitive challenges vulnerable learners experience, low self-efficacy, and the complexity of the world in which people live and use skills, it is essential to actively manage cognitive load demands during instruction and coaching. CLT works to design interventions in ways that utilize the large resources of long-term memory and limited capacities of working memory to maximize learning and generalization of adaptive skills (Kalyuga, 2011). The term "cognitive load" represents

TABLE 3.3. Extended Process Model and Skills System Supports

Identification stage

Identification substep: World

Function	*Barriers*
The individual experiences an internal and/or external stimuli.	• Cognitive and sensory vulnerabilities • Executive functioning deficits • High environmental stress

Tasks to improve world functioning during identification stage:

Help the individual get a Clear Picture to increase awareness of internal and external cues.

Identification substep: Perception

Function	*Barriers*
Detect the emotion	• Low emotional awareness • Low body awareness

Tasks to improve perception during identification stage:

Help the individual learn to label and rate feelings by doing Label and Rate Feelings.

Identification substep: Valuation

Function	*Barriers*
Weigh cost–benefit of regulating the emotion	• Undervaluing emotion regulation (ER) goal • Low ER self-efficacy—executive functioning deficits

Tasks to improve valuation during identification stage:

Help the individual use On-Track Thinking to reflect on the benefits of using skills and costs of not using skills in their lives.

Identification substep: Action

Function	*Barriers*
If there are benefits to regulating the emotion, the individual generates an emotion regulation goal.	• Staying with "default" strategies and continuing to act the same way regardless of the emotion, even if it does not reach the goal • Thinking that emotions cannot be changed by using strategies

Tasks to improve action during identification stage:

Help the individual clarify their goals and values (Pre-Learning Worksheet 1 on p. 6 and the related worked examples and worksheets on pp. 11–14 of the *Skills System Workbook*)

(*cont.*)

TABLE 3.3 (*cont.*)

Selection stage

Selection substep: World

Function	*Barriers*
The goal to regulate becomes the focus.	Emotional, cognitive, and behavioral dysregulation makes it difficult to focus on a goal.

Tasks to improve world functioning during selection stage:

Help the individual focus their attention on their emotion regulation goals and use Check It to assess whether the individual wants the feeling to increase or decrease.

Selection substep: Perception

Function	*Barriers*
Think about potential ER strategies	• Does not know enough strategies • Only uses "default" strategies • Forgets strategies in context

Tasks to improve perception during selection stage:

Help the individual develop a wide range of ER strategies to choose from by learning the nine core skills (and their subskills) on the Skills List.

Selection substep: Valuation

Function	*Barriers*
Weigh cost–benefit of using potential ER strategies	• Undervaluing the cost of an ER strategy • Undervaluing the benefit of an ER strategy • Overvaluing the cost of an ER strategy • Overvaluing the benefit of an ER strategy • Low ER self-efficacy

Tasks to improve valuation during selection stage:

Help the individual understand how skills can be used in their lives by using the System Tools: Feelings Rating Scale, Categories of Skills, and Recipe for Skills.

Selection substep: Action

Function	*Barriers*
Choose the most promising ER strategies for the context	• Not choosing enough strategies • Low self-efficacy related to the strategies

Tasks to improve action during selection stage:

Help the individual develop skills plans in diverse settings by using

Make a Skills Plan that integrates All-the-Time skills (0–5) and Calm-Only skills (0–3).

(*cont.*)

TABLE 3.3 *(cont.)*

Implementation stage

Implementation substep: World

Function	*Barriers*
To execute an optimal strategy for the context and levels of feeling	• Lack of practice creating and executing Skills Plans • Lack of adequate scaffolding to promote generalization in context • High-intensity relationships and environments that complicate the process of using skills

Tasks to improve world functioning during implementation stage:

Help the individual practice component elements and complete skills plans.

Implementation substep: Perception

Function	*Barriers*
Translate the nine core skills, subskills, and System Tools into tactics.	• Cannot think of adequate strategies • Cannot elaborate the strategies into tactics • Cannot recall tactics

Tasks to improve perception during implementation stage:

Help the individual develop skills plans to manage real life by reviewing worked examples, brainstorming hypothetical situations, and strategizing to how to manage current/future real-life situations.

Implementation substep: Valuation

Function	*Barriers*
Weigh cost–benefit of potential tactics.	• Under- and/or overvaluing the cost and benefits of tactics • Low self- and/or situation awareness • Low self-efficacy related to the strategy

Tasks to improve valuation during implementation stage:

Help the individual discuss the pros and cons of using various skills options in contexts relative to the individual's personal goals, values, and ER goals.

Implementation substep: Action

Function	*Barriers*
Take actions on the tactics.	Not executing the tactics effectively

Tasks to improve action during implementation stage:

Help the individual use skills in real-life situations, reflect on how elements of skills plans worked, and create adjusted skills plans to improve future functioning.

the amount of mental resources a particular thinking or reasoning task demands (American Psychological Association, 2007, p. 189). There are three types of cognitive loads in CLT: intrinsic, extraneous, and germane.

Intrinsic Cognitive Load

Intrinsic cognitive load is the fixed "natural complexity" of information that must be understood (separate from instructional issues); this internal complexity can only be changed by altering the nature of the information or by changing the knowledge level of the learner (Sweller et al., 2019). High element interactivity increases cognitive load demands, and low interactivity reduces it. Low interactivity means that information is presented in discrete components (Sweller, 2010). For example, dividing Clear Picture into six parts that are learned one at a time requires lower cognitive load than a broader concept of mindfulness. Breaking complex, multistep emotion regulation tasks into component parts decreases cognitive load demands. On-Track Thinking schemata consolidate adaptive, goal-directed thinking into four steps (Check It, Turn It Up, Cheerleading, Make a Skills Plan). As these schemata are stored and elaborated in long-term memory, demands on working memory are reduced. Conversely, the standard DBT skills do not describe an explicit thinking process or schemata but instead rely on the learner's ability to consolidate information effectively (while under duress) from the four separate modules.

Connectivity that links discrete bits of information facilitates recall (Kalyuga, 2011). Without an organizing system of parts, retrieval of divergent, unlinked chunks creates high cognitive demand. To address this function, the System Tools (Feelings Rating Scale, Categories of Skills, and Recipe for Skills) guide the assembly of the component skills into skills chains. The DBT skills (Linehan, 1993b, 2025a, 2025b) do not have instructions integrated into the modules to guide skills usage. This type of "search-and-match" design creates cognitive load demands (Kalyuga, 2011, p. 2).

Extraneous Cognitive Load

Sweller (2010) explained that extraneous cognitive load is associated with "nonoptimal instructional procedures" that impede learning. CLT is primarily concerned with techniques designed to reduce extraneous cognitive load (Sweller et al., 2019). Cognitive overload impairs schema acquisition, which results in a lower performance (Sweller, 1988). The threat of cognitive overload derailing skills acquisition and retrieval is a concern for individuals with complex learning challenges.

Instruction design can increase cognitive load. For example, simultaneous process increases cognitive load demands. If information is introduced at different times or in different areas, it increases demand on working memory. The Skills System instruction strategies introduce the basic elements (nine skills and System Tools) early in the curriculum to begin the process of storing information in long-term memory. Conversely, the standard DBT skills are broken down into four modules that are taught over a series of months; this deconstruction impedes retrieval of skills concepts. When the individual with cognitive challenges is in her natural environment, cognitive load demands are higher and the impact of extraneous cognitive load is more pronounced.

It is important to use terms that do not waste cognitive load resources. Terms that are intrinsic to the task create lower cognitive load demands than does unassociated jargon. For example, the term "On-Track Thinking" contains the concept of being oriented to a goal through the use of the term "on-track"; it is also linked to the term "thinking," which communicates the concepts of goal-directed thinking. This schema draws on existing knowledge stored in long-term memory and creates a relatively low cognitive load demand in relation to the complexity of the concepts that are being retrieved.

Germane Cognitive Load

"Germane cognitive load" refers to the working memory resources the learner devotes to the process (Sweller, 2010). If the extraneous cognitive load is high, germane cognitive load is reduced, because there is more demand on the working memory. If the design of interventions is thoughtful, it is possible to maximize germane cognitive load. Individuals diagnosed with an intellectual disability have cognitive impairments that impact germane cognitive load levels. Consequently, interventions need to be efficiently designed to minimize cognitive load and maximize cognitive functioning and learning. CLT brings attention to extraneous processing that impedes efficient integration of information. The Quick Step Assessment (described in detail in Chapter 5) is a Skills System foundational strategy that helps coaches and instructors actively manage cognitive load demands during interactions to enhance learning.

TRANSITION TO CHAPTER 4

Chapter 4 presents ways to structure Skills System instruction. Five different types of instruction are discussed to help guide coaches and instructors in teaching skills. The chapter also explains the E-Spiral framework that is used during instruction sessions to enhance generalization.

CHAPTER 4

Structuring Skills System Instruction

People with differing psychiatric, psychological, and developmental profiles experience emotion regulation challenges. The Skills System is used with people of all ages and abilities, who are supported in many different settings. The Skills System is a user-friendly tool that can be adjusted for these people within the contexts of their lives.

In this chapter we explore. Then we review five different formats for instruction that can be used together or separately to maximize skills different types of instruction that are used to address each individual's and setting's unique needs. The first part of this chapter describes explicit and implicit learning strategies generalization. The last part of the chapter introduces the E-Spiral framework that is used to structure one-on-one and/or group instruction sessions.

EXPLICIT AND IMPLICIT INSTRUCTION

Given the heterogeneity of Skills System learners and the settings where instruction and skills application happen, it is necessary to have the ability to use different types of instruction to address the abilities and readiness of the individual. Explicit instruction is direct teaching that transfers information about the nine core skills, the subskills, and the System Tools. For example, during Week 3 in the 12-week curriculum (Chapter 7), individuals learn the six Clear Picture Do's. While specificity of explicit learning increases cognitive load, the benefits of learning the skills and System Tools helps the individual have a power-packed toolbox of strategies. Having the ability to use 123 Wise Mind increases the individual's capacities to generalize skills into a myriad of human experiences. Explicit instruction can be used in any of the different instruction formats explored later in this chapter.

Implicit strategies teach Skills System principles and concepts in informal ways; learning that happens in an incidental or indirect manner. As compared to explicit strategies, implicit ones generally create lower cognitive load. Implicit strategies can therefore create accessible learning experiences for individuals of differing abilities and levels of motivation. There are three important strategies that are commonly part of implicit instruction: experiential, environmental, and conceptual approaches.

Experiential implicit instruction involves the instructor engaging to do skills with the individual during interactions. For example, perhaps an individual is new in treatment and is not able/ready to learn the elements of Safety Plan (type of risk, levels of risk, types of safety plan, and ways to handle risk), but needs to move away from a hostile housemate. Instead of explicitly teaching the concepts of Safety Plan, the coach may engage the individual to take a walk when the housemate raises his voice. This strategy implicitly teaches Move Away. Taking a walk will help manage risk in the moment and the individual may know that moving away in that situation in the future could be an effective strategy. The coach can positively reinforce adaptive behaviors, fading supports, to shape more autonomous functioning to help the individual improve how and when to Move Away. The instructor can shift to add explicit teaching as the individual gains competency and readiness.

The instructor or coach can lead the individual through a conversation that implicitly does 123 Wise Mind. For example, asking questions like "How are you feeling?", "What do you notice about your breath right now?", and "What sensation do you notice in your body?" This does not explicitly teach the Clear Picture Do's, but it experientially leads the individual through the process of getting a Clear Picture. While not as transferable as having a framework for systematically and consistently being aware of the moment, an implicit Clear Picture can be helpful.

In environmental implicit instruction, the environment itself is infused with skills-based concepts. When skills are integrated into the normal operating procedures, cognitive load demands for the learner are often low. For example, it can be helpful to designate areas that the individual uses on a regular basis as Safety Plan areas (e.g., bedroom, sensory room, den, porch, or yard). This teaches her that when she is experiencing risk, moving to these areas is doing a Safety Plan. Similarly, programs or homes can have closets or bins that contain different New-Me Activities that are used each day. Schedules can include Skills System language, such as "New-Me Activity Time." Visual aids throughout the environment, such as laminated sheets that highlight various skills hung on the wall or on lanyards, can expose the individual to skills concepts in organic ways that demand a low cognitive load. Interactive and environmental implicit strategies can be used in all five types of instruction.

When an individual is not ready to learn Skills System terms, it can be useful to teach elements of the model using a conceptual approach. This means that the instructor describes a concept in general terms, rather than using specific Skills System language. For example, "When we have high emotions, it can be difficult to think clearly and solve our problems." This implicit instruction describes several skills concepts (Feelings Rating Scale, Categories of Skills, and Problem Solving) without using unfamiliar terms. Shifting to a conceptual approach can be useful when the individual verbalizes skepticism about explicit learning formats. If she has low self-efficacy and/or learning barriers, using a conceptual approach can reduce cognitive load and assist the individual to experience growth. While conceptual strategies are often an important gateway, the goal is usually to shift from a conceptual approach to other explicit and implicit strategies that help the individual build a more comprehensive and generalizable skills set.

FIVE TYPES OF INSTRUCTION

It is important to understand that the form of instruction needs to accommodate the needs of the individual as well as the setting within which the instruction is happening: Form follows function. An essential element of the Skills System model is the ability to adjust the instruction format and teaching strategies as needed. There is a dialectical tension that exists within the model: The instructor needs to maintain the fidelity to the Skills System concepts while simultaneously adjusting instruction to maximize learning and generalization for each unique learner. Table 4.1 lists five different types of instruction that can be used separately or in conjunction with each other to maximize learning. Each of these are explored in more detail in this section.

Standard Instruction

Standard instruction is when the instructor teaches the Skills System concepts following the 12-week curriculum format. The goal is to teach the individual the necessary component capacities to regulate emotions (Table 4.2). The individual learns to get a Clear Picture, do On-Track

TABLE 4.1. Types of Skills System Instruction

- Standard instruction
- Targeted instruction
- A-la-carte instruction
- Instruction during coaching (A + B = C +)
- Environmentally based instruction

TABLE 4.2. Standard Instruction

Type of instruction	Instruction objectives	Instruction format	Primary teaching resources	Focus of instruction
Standard instruction	Instructors teach all skills concepts: • Nine core skills • Subskills • System tools	Format options: • Skills groups • One-on-one instruction • Individual therapy Possible group/one-on-one titles: • Reaching My Goals • Managing Emotions • Improving Relationships • Learning to Be Safe	• 12-week-cycle curriculum • Repeat cycles though the curriculum	• Learn the nine core skills and subskills. • Broaden and deepen skills knowledge. • Develop the ability to use 123 Wise Mind. • Practice skills concepts and skills plans.

Thinking, and take On-Track Actions that help her reach her goals. Table 4.3 presents the progression of topics that comprise a standard teaching approach.

Standard instruction can happen in one-on-one or group sessions, in-person, or online. Chapter 6 offers many helpful hints to help you prepare to do a group or one-on-one standard instruction. The 12-week curriculum (presented in Chapter 7) is a detailed description of activities that instructors may choose to use. Standard instruction can follow the 12-week curriculum closely or use other materials to address the progression of topics.

Although the progression of topics (see Table 4.3) is followed in standard instruction, it is often useful to focus the instruction on a subject that is relevant to the learner. For example, instead of using the term "skills group," consider a more focused subject, like "improving my relationships," "managing my emotions," or "reaching my goals." Focusing the instruction on something relevant can (1) increase the learner's motivation and (2) target instruction in ways that increase skills application and generalization.

Targeted Instruction

Targeted instruction focuses on improving how the individual applies skills in their life (Table 4.4). Structured targeted instruction that systematically addresses targets and fills skills gaps most commonly happens in individual therapy settings. For example, during structured targeted instruction, the individual meets with the therapist on a weekly, ongoing basis to explore the individual's goals and life contexts, create skills plans, and review progress on skills plans. This type of targeted instruction elaborates the learning process and is a vital step toward generalizing skills. Informal targeted instruction can happen in diverse settings when coaches and support providers examine the individual's pattern of escalation and create instruction that helps the individual learn new skills to regulate her feelings and her goals. Both types of targeted instruction are important to help the individual improve her ER capacities.

Targeted instruction integrates information gleaned during pre-instruction activities that are presented in Chapter 6. During pre-instruction, the individual explores his goals and the

TABLE 4.3. Standard Instruction Topics

- Skills List
- System Tools: Feelings Rating Scale, Categories of Skills, and Recipe for Skills
- Clear Picture
- On-Track Thinking
- On-Track Action
- Safety Plan
- New-Me Activities
- Problem Solving
- Expressing Myself
- Getting It Right
- Relationship Care

TABLE 4.4. Targeted Instruction

Type of instruction	Instruction objectives	Instruction format	Primary teaching resources	Focus of instruction
Targeted instruction (Chapter 9)	Instructors teach how to apply skills in real-life. Note: Targeted instruction is crucial for individuals with lengthy histories of behavioral dysregulation to address specific skills gaps.	Format options: • Individual therapy • One-on-one instruction • Small groups	Targeted instruction worksheets (Reaching Goals, pp. 227–238): • Skills Plans • My Progress • Back-Track • Re-Track	Facilitate generalization of skills: • Create skills plans. • Review progress to goals. • Back-Track: Get a Clear Picture of a specific situation. • Re-Track: Adjust strategies for a similar future situation.

behaviors he needs to increase or decrease to reach his goals (targets). Clarifying goals and targets offers a concrete context in which to apply skills, thus facilitating learning and enhancing motivation. A detailed explanation of structured and informal targeted instruction strategies is presented in Chapter 9, and the accompanying *Emotion Regulation Skills System Workbook, Second Edition* (sold separately), contains worksheets and worked examples to be used during targeted instruction.

A-la-Carte Instruction

A-la-carte instruction is when the instructor teaches one skill concept or a few skills concepts at a time, rather than in the standard topic progression (Table 4.5). For example, the instructor may begin by teaching the strategy of Move Away by encouraging an individual to go to her bedroom to avoid an argument with staff. When in her room, the instructor may suggest she listen to music using her headphones. Alternatively, a standard approach would focus on the individual getting a Clear Picture, doing On-Track Thinking, taking On-Track Actions that would include doing a Safety Plan and a New-Me Activity. The Skills System Targeting Strategy (presented in Chapter 5) helps coaches and instructors decide what skill and/or subskill is best to address.

Instructors may teach a skill in its explicit form (using Skills System terms) when doing a-la-carte instruction. For example, if there is an adolescent who wants to get something from a parent or teacher and the youth refuses to engage in standard instruction, teaching Getting It Right can be useful. This approach gives the individual relevant information and can be a gateway to learning other skills. For example, if the dyad discusses when the youth should use Getting It Right (Right Time), it can be an opportunity to introduce the concept of the Feelings Rating Scale. It may be also be a chance to talk about the Categories of Skills (explicitly or implicitly), discussing how at Levels 0–3 we are in the Right Mind to Get It Right.

A-la-carte instruction is necessary in multiple situations. For example, if the instructor

TABLE 4.5. A-la-Carte Instruction

Type of instruction	Instruction objectives	Instruction format	Primary teaching resources	Focus of instruction
A-la-carte instruction	Instructors teach a single skill concept or a few skills concepts (e.g., Move Away; New-Me Activities).	Format options: • One-on-one instruction • Individual therapy	• Skills summary sheets • Handouts • Worked examples • Worksheets	Helping an individual who is unable to do standard instruction or an individual who is not ready for standard instruction, a-la-carte instruction offers a sample of skills to get an initial buy-in to learn more. • Teach any of the nine core skills (e.g., Safety Plan) • Teach any of the subskills (e.g., Move Away) • Teach any of the System Tools (e.g., Feelings Rating Scale)

has limited time to teach, an a-la-carte approach can help the individual learn key strategies that will help him manage Level 4 feelings without going to Level 5. A-la-carte is also helpful when the individual has more cognitive challenges. Additionally, an a-la-carte approach may be best when the individual is early in treatment or lacks motivation to do standard one-on-one or group skills training. If the a-la-carte instruction (1) works and (2) is reinforcing to the individual, this approach can be an appetizer, which entices the individual to partake in the standard instruction process.

Instruction during Coaching

Instruction during coaching (Table 4.6) involves instructors using the A + B = C coaching framework to help the individual use their skills (see Chapter 8). A + B = C helps the individual get a Clear Picture, do On-Track Thinking, and make a skills plan to take On-Track Actions. If the individual's plan appears to align with his goal, the coach does not give feedback; the coach just asks the individual to clarify his next steps and offers positive reinforcement for the plan. When the individual's plan does not appear to align with the stated goal, the coach asks permission to share observations about the misalignment. If the individual consents, the coach offers her two cents and listens to the individual's perspective. If the situation dictates, the coach invites the individual to collaborate to develop a new skills plan. If the individual consents, the coach and individual review the situation, brainstorm about alternatives, and create a skills plan that aligns with the individual's goals.

If the individual has the knowledge and ability to execute the skills plan, no skills instruction is needed. If the individual has a skills gap, the coach may determine that instruction

TABLE 4.6. Instruction during Coaching

Type of instruction	Instruction objectives	Instruction format	Primary teaching resources	Focus of instruction
Instruction during coaching (A + B = C +)	Coaches or instructors teach skills concepts during in-life skills coaching conversations.	Format options: • Any setting when all involved are 0- to 3-level feelings.	• A + B = C + Coaching Conversations ("+" = the instructor asks the individual if the individual wants to learn the skill concept during collaboration [C]) to get consent • Skills visual aids	• Explicit/direct instruction: Teach a skill using skills terms. • Implicit instruction: Help the individual do a skill. • Contextual instruction: Teach concepts without skills terms.

during coaching would be helpful. In that case, the coach asks the individual if she would like to learn a new skill concept that might help her in this situation. For example, perhaps the individual is not sure what the parts of Right Words are. The instructor can explain what SEALS is and how to use it (Sugar, Explaining, Asking, Listening, and Sealing the Deal). The instructor can verbally describe the concepts or refer to a visual aid to review how to use the Right Words. Instruction during coaching integrates an a-la-carte approach with the A + B = C framework to create A + B = C + (coaching plus instruction).

Training coaches to do instruction can be a powerful tool to support the generalization of skills in real-life contexts. To do this on-the-fly teaching, support providers need to know Skills System concepts, the Quick Step Assessment (see Chapter 5), and Skills Coaching Strategies (see Chapter 8). When support providers are able to teach skills, it helps the individual build core emotion regulation capacities.

Environmental Instruction

Environmental instruction teaches skills concepts implicitly through environmental interventions (Table 4.7). Skills concepts and language are integrated into the individual's daily experiences. For example, daily schedules can include opportunities to get a Clear Picture or do New-Me Activities. The Feelings Rating Scale may be commonly woven into conversations and procedures. Support plans may include Skills System terms, like Safety Plans and Relationship Care, and there could be designated Safety Plan areas and New-Me Activity resources.

Individuals who experience higher levels of impairment need higher levels of environmental instruction. If an individual has less verbal ability, the environment will need to provide more scaffolding to help her integrate adaptive techniques. For example, if the person is not able to read, documents (i.e., daily schedules, rules, and Safety Plans) may need to include pictures. As the individual interacts with the environment, she learns skills concepts. When the individual moves to different environments, it may be helpful to have similar structures in place

TABLE 4.7. Environmental Instruction

Type of instruction	Instruction objectives	Instruction format	Primary teaching resources	Focus of instruction
Environmental instruction	The environment teaches skills concepts implicitly through environmental interventions, creating skill-based experiences.	Skills integrated into: • Adding skills terms into daily schedules (e.g., New-Me Activity time) • Visual aids (e.g., Clear Picture handout) • Interactions (e.g., staff or parents receive training to be able to use skills [to self-regulate] and coach skills [co-regulate]). • Support plans (e.g., the individual has a goal to use Safety Plans to manage strong emotions). • Physical site (e.g., a closet that stores New-Me Activities; Safety Plan areas where individuals can go to take space).	Skills System hierarchy is used to ensure adequate supports and triage gaps in supports that increase the individual's emotional vulnerabilities • Medical issues • Psychiatric issues • Environmental factors • Skills development	Build skills into all aspects of a support environment.

to facilitate transitions. For example, if the individual attends a day program, having the staff of that program trained in the Skills System will provide integrated supports. Similarly, if the individual is being discharged to another residence, having the new team trained in the Skills System will help the individual transition more successfully. This type of carry-over can help improve self- and co-regulation within variable life contexts.

Individuals with more verbal and academic abilities may need to have environmental instruction faded as they prepare to transition to other environments. Alternatively, instructors may assist them in developing individualized resources to access in new environments. Often it is the individual's goal to live more independently and free of supports; empowering the individual to build her own resources can help her reach this goal.

USE ALL FIVE TYPES OF INSTRUCTION

As an individual learns and practices skills, his skills knowledge-base is stored in long-term memory. Once there, it reduces the reliance on working memory capacities, which helps him apply skills in real-life situations. All five types of instruction used in conjunction provides the more potent learning experience, particularly for individual with learning challenges or a long history of behavioral dysregulation. In these cases, it may be necessary to implement multiple types of instruction to change patterns from off-track to on-track.

When an individual participates in standard instruction he is able to learn key foundational processes that help him navigate emotions. He builds the ability to create powerful skills chains to manage situations effectively—even challenging ones. For example, the individual learns that the only way to be sure a New-Me Activity is actually new is to do Clear Picture, On-Track Thinking, and On-Track Actions, creating a 1235 skills chain. Adding targeted instruction on top of the standard instruction can help the individual apply those skills in his everyday life. By repeatedly assessing situations, creating skills plans, reflecting on progress, and creating new, more effective plans, the individual hones his skills.

A-la-carte instruction can be an important starting point, but may not be enough to fill skills gaps. If the individual has reinforced patterns of emotional dysregulation, doing a 123 skills chain will be necessary. When she is in standard instruction and is able to use Clear Picture, On-Track Thinking, and take On-Track Actions, augmenting learning with a-la-carte instruction deepens skills knowledge. A-la-carte instruction is crucial, but ideally should not be the only type of instruction that an individual receives, particularly an individual with complex behavioral health/learning challenges.

When an individual receives standard, targeted, a-la-carte, *and* knowledge of specific skills (a-la-carte), she is also receiving in-vivo coaching to learn how to use the skills in real-life situations (instruction during coaching). Adding environmental strategies further strengthens learning experiences, especially for more vulnerable learners who may have more barriers to standard and targeted instruction. The key take-away is: Exposing the individual to many types of instruction enhances learning.

STRUCTURING STANDARD SYSTEM INSTRUCTION SESSIONS: THE E-SPIRAL FRAMEWORK

The E-Spiral is a teaching framework that guides teaching strategies within standard Skills System instruction sessions. It serves only as a general framework to help instructors remember the multiple steps within the learning process. Four phases of the E-Spiral are addressed during a group (or individual) training session: exploring existing knowledge base, encoding, elaboration, and efficacy.

In Phase 1, exploring existing knowledge base, the instructor reviews past learning related to the topic that will be the subject of the session's instruction (e.g., Week 3: Clear Picture). For example, the instructor asks the individual to reflect about a time when he had a clear picture of a situation and a time when he had a fuzzy picture of a situation. Active discussions that highlight relevant issues can prime new learning. Creating a relevant context for learning (i.e., how this learning can benefit the individual) can help increase motivation.

In Phase 2, encoding, individuals participate in direct instruction and multimodal activities to learn the skill topic. The aim is to teach new information in fun, interesting, accessible, and engaging ways. The goal of encoding is to help the individual learn the Skills System terms and concepts. For example, in Week 4 of the 12-week curriculum, the instructor introduces On-Track Thinking, including Check It, Turn It, Cheerleading, and Making a Skills Plan, and creates simple exercises to demonstrate one or more parts. The individual learns and practices each of these tactics to understand each component and how do put them together in real time.

In Phase 3, elaboration, the individual learns how the concepts are used in conjunction with skills she has learned before. Since the Skills System is a system, it is important to review how the new learning fits into the past learning. Ultimately, the individual needs to know how to combine strategies to navigate situations. The elaboration phase helps the individual expand and link knowledge to enhance skills application and generalization. For example, the instructor discusses how different skills are used to make a Skills Plan to elaborate the individual's understanding of On-Track Thinking and the Skills System.

Phase 4, efficacy, helps individuals practice skills to build self- and skill-efficacy. Activities such as role playing and practice exercises give the individual opportunities to demonstrate skills. At this point, the individual has experience with the skill, so there are discussions that weigh the benefits and costs of using and not using the skill. Reflecting on the learning helps exercise identity, consolidate commitment, address existing barriers, and facilitate generalization in the real world. When an instructor leads the individual through these four phases, it broadens and deepens the individual's skills knowledge base.

The 12-week Skills System curriculum (presented in Chapter 7) provides lesson plans that are broken down to address each of the E-Spiral steps. As learners move through these phases and activities, their knowledge about the topic is broadened and deepened. This learning process guides people through steps that naturally transition skills information from short-term to long-term memory. Building skills knowledge in long-term memory can reduce cognitive load demands and increase the individual's abilities to recall skills in high-stress situations. The E-Spiral multilayered learning experience helps intellectually impaired individuals gain mastery that promotes generalization of skills.

The E-Spiral functions as a guide for teaching practices. While issues and time constraints commonly force the instructor to make adjustments, the E-Spiral serves as a template for organizing effective teaching strategies. Even when time frames are limited, instructors learn how to quickly review past learning, teach a new concept, practice it, and make a bridge to real-life contexts. Organizing teaching in this looping progression that layers old and new information, deepens learning, enhances retention, and improves recall. Being mindful of these principles helps instructors avoid truncating the teaching process, which may jeopardize the integration of concepts.

TRANSITION TO CHAPTER 5

Chapter 5 presents foundational strategies that are used during skills coaching and instruction. The chapter presents DBT validation strategies, which are acceptance-based interventions. The chapter also introduces the Quick Step Assessment, a simple framework that coaches and instructors use to monitor and adjust for the cognitive load capacity changes in an individual. Chapter 5 describes a Targeting Strategy that assists coaches and instructors in choosing which skill or subskill to coach or teach. The chapter ends with a review of basic behavioral strategies that enhance skills learning.

CHAPTER 5

Foundational Instruction Strategies

This chapter describes four foundational strategies that are used during coaching conversations and in all types of skills instruction. First, we introduce DBT validation strategies. Validation is an acceptance strategy that is combined with other interventions to support the individual's growth and development. Then, this chapter describes the Quick Step Assessment. Based on cognitive load theory, the Quick Step Assessment helps the coach and instructor plan and adjust their strategies during interactions. Targeting strategies build on the Quick Step and help the coach and instructor make decisions about how to address specific skill gaps to enhance competency. Lastly, behavioral techniques that are often used during instruction and treatment planning to strengthen adaptive behaviors are presented. Understanding these foundational strategies helps the instructor be flexible, maximizes learning opportunities, and promotes generalization.

VALIDATION STRATEGIES

Validation is a core strategy in both DBT (Linehan, 1993a) and the Skills System. Validation is an acceptance-based strategy that communicates awareness and acceptance of something or someone. Coaches and instructors use validation strategies to communicate the acceptance of something the individual is doing or who the individual is in the moment.

If the individual experiences patterns of emotional dysregulation, it is likely she has difficulty self-validating. Instead of having the basic belief that she exists and has the capacity for wisdom, she self-invalidates. Self-invalidation functions like quicksand; it envelops the individual, making it difficult to move in the direction of her personal goals. When the coach and instructor use validation strategies, they can serve as a platform from which the individual can step to change. The validation strategies presented in the text box below are designed to expand the individual's self-awareness in the moment, communicate acceptance from the coach and instructor, and promote the individual's self-validation.

DBT Levels of Validation

1. The skills coach pays attention, listening carefully and observing the individual's behaviors to convey acceptance.
    - Example: Consistent eye contact and staying on topic.
2. The skills coach offers accurate reflection of what the individual is saying. Directly repeating and/or paraphrasing the individual's points (checking with her to ensure accuracy of the assumptions) communicates an understanding of the individual's experience.
    - Example: "So you are saying that you feel anxious?"
3. The skills coach labels unverbalized factors that may be impacting the individual. This strategy can help the individual deepen awareness of internal and external experiences.
    - Example: "The way you are pacing makes me think you might be anxious."
4. The skills coach links the individual's responses to their past learning or a precipitating event. Highlighting that a precipitating event caused an understandable reaction can serve to validate the response without necessarily reinforcing the action taken.
    - Example: "I think that your fear of hearing your biopsy results makes complete sense."
5. The skills coach states that a behavior is a normal response to an event. Universalizing the experience can validate the individual's reaction as justified and human.
    - Example: "Anyone who had those symptoms would be nervous."
6. The skills coach treats the person as an equal beyond the other roles of the relationship. The coach has a person-to-person, genuine response to the individual.
    - Example: "That would really suck. I am going to keep my fingers crossed for you. Would you mind if I said a prayer for you?"

Linehan (1993a) explains that acceptance-based interventions (validation strategies) are paired with change strategies (skills coaching and instruction) to promote "the reconciliation of opposites in a continual process of synthesis" (p. 19). Support staff members using the Skills System are encouraged to combine acceptance strategies and change strategies to provide the individual with key ingredients of growth that will help her develop emotion regulation capacities. Intertwining these strategies helps the individual both co-regulate in the moment and experience longer-term intrapersonal development. *Moving too quickly and consistently to change strategies will likely create patterns of co-dysregulation versus co-regulation.* Balancing may mean offering more acceptance than change comments because of the sensitivity vulnerable individuals can have to guidance or feedback. Linehan recommends "surrounding negative feedback with positive feedback" to reduce negative reactions such as "stimulus overload or discouragement" (1993a, p. 337).

QUICK STEP ASSESSMENT

All people, and especially individuals with complex behavioral health and learning challenges, experience cognitive overload. Unfortunately, in the human service environments, support providers are often forced to address complex, emotional issues with individuals in short time frames. These types of situations contribute to individuals experiencing emotional, cognitive, and behavioral dysregulation.

Most coaches and instructors tend to focus primarily on the content of an interaction and secondarily on the process of an interaction. Overvaluing quantity, productivity, and vertical progress can lead to overload and block skill use and learning. The Quick Step Assessment shifts the primary focus to the planning and adjusting of interventions, so that the content can be processed effectively. It is an ongoing, three-step strategy that the coach and instructor use to optimize coaching and teaching opportunities and reduce factors that lead to emotional, cognitive, and behavioral overload. The terms "Quick Step Assessment" and "Quick Step" are used interchangeably throughout this book.

Coaching conversations and teaching interventions involve back-and-forth communication between sender and receiver. The Quick Step helps the coach and instructor be an effective sender and improves how the individual receives the verbal, nonverbal, or visual communication. When the individual can receive helpful information, the likelihood of learning and executing adaptive skills is higher. When cognitive overload occurs, learning decreases and behavioral dyscontrol increases.

The term "intervention" is used to describe each discrete communication the coach and/or instructor sends. Coaching conversation and instruction sessions involve varying types and numbers of interventions. The coach or instructor uses the Quick Step to (1) proactively plan ahead and (2) reactively change interventions as needed. Figure 5.1 shows the Quick Step process, and each step is explained in the following sections (in Chapter 8 there will be examples of how to integrate the Quick Step into Skills Coaching Strategies).

Step 1: Assess the Cognitive Load of the Intervention

Throughout all interactions, the coach and instructor assess whether the cognitive load of their intervention is high or low. This assessment allows the instructor to proactively and reactively consider the individual's ability to engage without cognitive overload and make necessary adjustments to their intervention. Understanding what types of interventions cause cognitive overload helps the coach and instructor identify situations that may derail interactions and learning.

Figure 5.2 lists factors that contribute to high cognitive load. Simultaneous processing is required when integrating movement, visual stimuli, and auditory information at the same time; it is an activity that taxes working memory. For example, simultaneous processing is

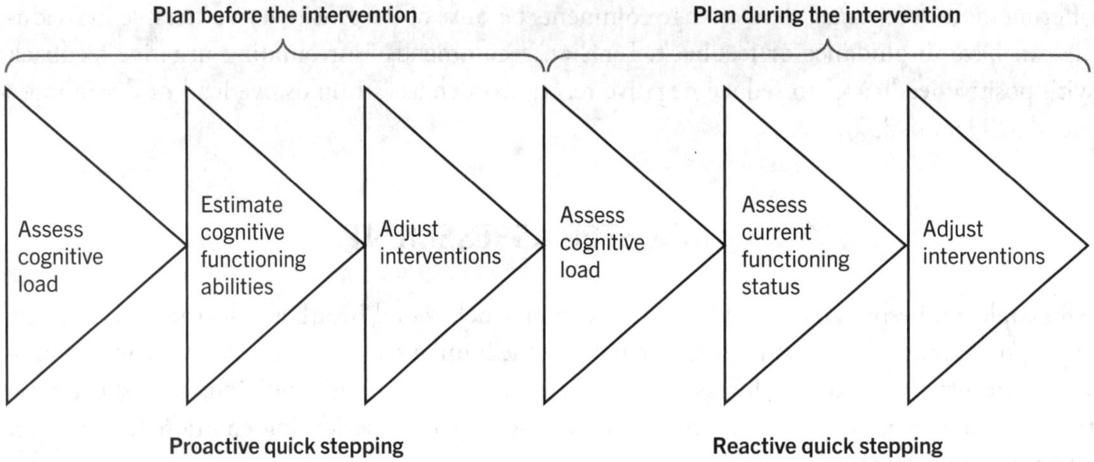

FIGURE 5.1. Proactive and reactive quick stepping.

required when an individual is working at a cash register and interacting with customers. Cognitive load also increases when an individual is asked to understand or recall large amounts of information. This can be compounded when an individual is presented with new information or does not have knowledge of the topic being discussed. For example, an individual may experience overload on the first day of a new job when she is introduced to multiple policies and procedures that must be followed.

The complexity of an interaction also contributes to cognitive load increase. If the individual does not understand the language or words being used in an interaction or it involves abstract concepts, he may become overloaded. Applying for social services that have different requirements, tasks to complete, and platforms to interact with, for instance, can cause cognitive overload. Similarly, if an individual is being asked to process information quickly, it may affect his ability to perform tasks.

The context in which information is given must also be considered when assessing cognitive load. Information is "divergent" when it is learned at a different time or place than the

- Simultaneous processing of information
- High volume of information
- Novelty of information
- Complexity of concepts
- Speed of interactions
- Divergent information
- Rapid shifts without transition from one topic to another
- Information or an intervention that inspires a strong emotional response

FIGURE 5.2. Factors that increase cognitive load.

individual is accustomed to. If an individual learns a piece of information in group and associates that information with specific elements of that experience, it may be challenging to recall the information in a work setting. Quick movement from topic to topic or context to context also increases cognitive load. Individuals with learning challenges and/or executive functioning deficits may have difficulty transitioning from one event, location, activity, and relationship to another.

Finally, it is important to consider the individual's response to the information and the way in which it is provided. If the individual experiences strong emotional responses while processing information, cognitive demands increase. For example, if the skills group discussion addresses "hot" topics, such as living with impairments, victimization, losses, and/or processing past behavioral problems, strong feelings may result. Similarly, if an intervention is not designed properly—such as a case manager informing the individual in passing that his discharge plans have been canceled—it can cause cognitive overload.

Step 2: Evaluate Cognitive Functioning Abilities

In the second step of the Quick Step Assessment, the coach and instructor evaluate the individual's ability to cognitively process an intervention. As in the assessment of cognitive load, this happens both proactively (estimating the ability to process a proposed intervention) and reactively (evaluating cognitive processing during an intervention).

Proactively Assessing Cognitive Challenges

Individuals have unique constellations of strengths and deficits. In an ideal world, psychometric testing clarifies capacities, but practically speaking, coaches and instructors often rely on scant documentation and limited experience with the individual to make estimations of her abilities. Figure 5.3 presents some preexisting conditions that affect cognitive regulation. These are conditions that can make weighing benefits and costs, orienting to goals, recalling strategies, and organizing/executing tactics more difficult. Cognitive processing impairments are also associated with many mental health disorders (Laurinaitiene & Steibliene, 2019; Hamid & Darweesh, 2020; see Figure 5.4).

If an individual has a known preexisting condition, the coach and instructor should anticipate that it will be necessary to adjust interventions to reduce cognitive load. If they are not aware of any preexisting conditions, they still must continually assess the individual's functioning during interactions.

Reactively Assessing Cognitive Functioning

The coach and instructor continue to assess the individual's level of cognitive regulation during interventions. As cognitive demands increase and capacities decrease, emotional and behavioral dysregulation can happen. As the individual begins to become cognitively stressed, there are early warning signs. As the dysregulation progresses, more clear behavioral expressions often follow (see Figure 5.5). For example, the coach or instructor may initially notice the individual

Patterns of emotional dysregulation
- High sensitivity
- Rapid escalation
- Slow return to baseline

Cognitive difficulties
- Executive functioning deficits (planning, problem solving, goal-directed behavior, organizing, time management/sequencing, reasoning, abstract thinking, and flexibility)
- Memory/working memory deficits
- Attention deficits (ability to sustain and shift attention)
- Verbal deficits (receptive and expressive)
- Difficulty processing nonverbal information
- General knowledge deficits
- Difficulty orienting to time, place, and people.

Patterns of behavioral dysregulation
- Inability to do self-care
- Difficulty following rules
- Verbal escalation and abuse
- Property destruction
- Physical assaultiveness
- Sexually problematic behaviors
- Self-injury/suicidality

Additional conditions
- Medical problems
- Mental health diagnoses
- History of trauma
- Power differentials/conflict in the environment
- Low self-efficacy
- Low skill efficacy

FIGURE 5.3. Preexisting conditions that can increase cognitive vulnerabilities.

having difficulty tracking topics within the conversation, and as the cognitive dysregulation increases the instructor may observe flight–fight–freeze responses. If the instructor notices early warning signs, it is important to assess the individual's cognitive status and adjust the intervention. Waiting until the individual is cognitively dysregulated to switch tracks increases the chances of emotional and behavioral escalation.

It is important to remember that cognitive dysregulation is an involuntary experience. The individual is often caught off guard and is not consciously aware of the dysregulation. The nature of cognitive dysregulation impairs the individual's ability to have intra- and interpersonal clarity. Therefore, it is unlikely that the individual will communicate to the coach or instructor

- Mood disorders
- Anxiety disorders
- Psychotic disorders
- Trauma- and stress-related disorders
- Substance abuse disorders
- Acquired brain injury/traumatic brain injury
- Dementia/Alzheimer's disease
- Intellectual disabilities
- Medical problems (e.g., thyroid dysfunction, vitamin deficiencies, sleep disorders, kidney or liver dysfunction, and infection)
- Side effects of medications

FIGURE 5.4. Examples of diagnoses that commonly include cognitive impairment.

that his cognitive capacities have diminished. In fact, he may try to appear competent, so as not to experience shame related to feeling lost and/or confused. The individual may be interested in participating in the interaction but lack the skills to inform the coach or instructor about the cognitive processing decline. The instructor may misperceive cognitive dysregulation in a number of ways, including:

- The individual has a poor attitude.
- The individual lacks motivation.

Early warning signs of cognitive dysregulation

- Nod of incomprehension: agrees without understanding
- Confusion/unfocused: glancing around or being fidgety
- Verbalizing inaccurate information
- Rumination: stays focused on one topic, resists redirection
- Expresses discomfort, verbally or nonverbally
- Verbalizing physical/psychiatric symptoms

⇩

Signs of cognitive dysregulation

- Avoidance: withdrawal, "shut down," staring
- Resistance/willfulness
- Resignation: stops engaging, gives up, returns to default behaviors
- Frustration/anger, including verbal threats or physical aggression
- Self-injury: nonsuicidal self-injury, suicidal ideation, or suicidal behaviors

FIGURE 5.5. Signs of cognitive overload.

- The individual is just seeking attention.
- The individual is intentionally avoiding responsibilities.
- The individual is choosing to have a behavior problem.
- The individual is intentionally manipulating people around her.

Any of these common misperceptions can cause negative transactions to happen within the relationship, which may lead to co-dysregulation between the individual and coach/instructor.

Step 3: Adjust Interventions

When the coach and instructor adjust interventions and decrease cognitive load demands, it may allow the individual to remain focused and present in the moment. Being present is important because it helps him remain aware and able to effectively manage the microtransitions across feelings (as opposed to avoiding and escaping prematurely). When present, the individual is better able to plan and use adaptive skills. Additionally, when the coach and instructor respond to his needs, it fosters co-regulation and improves the relationship between them. Table 5.1 lists strategies that can be used to reduce cognitive load demands.

TARGETING STRATEGY

The System Tools help the individual create Skills Plans during On-Track Thinking. Optimally, the individual can do 123 Wise Mind, meaning that the individual does Clear Picture, On-Track Thinking, and various On-Track Actions that include other skills. While that "standard" approach offers the strongest base for emotion regulation, it is not always possible for the individual to execute that type of plan due to high cognitive load. In high-load situations, coaches and instructors use the Quick Step Assessment to make adjustments. The Targeting Strategy guides coaches and instructors to help the individual create and execute optimal Skills Plans given the situation, level of feeling, and cognitive load status. The targeting strategies help coaches and instructors create a-la-carte interventions.

To effectively co-regulate and teach, the coach and instructor provide scaffolding for the individual so he can use and expand his competencies. The Skills List, System Tools, and the Quick Step Assessment offer support for the coach and instructor to make decisions that optimize opportunities. When targeting, the coach and instructor experience the situation, reflect on skill options, and channel possibilities to an On-Track Action that begins the Skills Plan chain. The Skills System Targeting Strategy helps the coach and instructor guide this funneling or zooming-in process.

The Skills System Targeting Strategy has three basic steps (see Figure 5.6 for examples):

1. *Brainstorm:* The coach or instructor brainstorms skill options that could help the individual manage the situation.
2. *Skills Plan:* The coach or instructor imagines a Skills Plan to manage the situation.
3. *Start:* Do the Quick Step Assessment to target where the Skills Plan should start.

TABLE 5.1 Adjust Strategies to Reduce Cognitive Load Demands

Use simple language	Abstract, complex, and interconnected information creates high cognitive load.
Present information slowly	Moving quickly increases cognitive load.
Present one thing at a time	Going step-by-step, presenting one concept at a time reduces cognitive load.
Engage with "cool" versus "hot" topics or activities	Stress-producing topics increase load.
Ask clarifying questions	The coach/instructor should ask clarifying questions to ensure being on the same page and reduce opportunities for misunderstandings and co-dysregulation.
Repeat concepts	Repeating key concepts reduces cognitive load and helps the individual understand contextual skill application.
Organize/summarize concepts	Divergent information increases cognitive load. Providing a clear framework helps the individual manage multistep processes.
Use chunking	High volume of information causes high load, so breaking concepts down into understandable chunks is helpful.
Use metaphors	Simple metaphors can help the individual understand complex concepts by bridging the topic to existing knowledge.
Use mnemonics	For example, the acronym SEALS helps the individual remember to use Sugar, Explaining the Situation, Asking for What You Want, Listening, and Sealing the Deal in Getting It Right.
Analyze tasks	By reducing multicomponent concepts into a progression of single elements, the individual can complete the entire task one step at a time.
Orienting to transitions	Orienting to changes in topics and activities can facilitate transitions and decrease the fear of the unknown that blocks progress.
Confirm readiness	Rushing and assuming an individual is prepared to progress can create confusion and disengagement.
Use visual aids	Visual aids can help (a) explain concepts during instruction and (b) provide scaffolding/reminders after instruction to support skill recall in real-life contexts.
Model the skill	The coach and instructor model skills during all interactions to provide an example of skills application for the individual.
Use worked examples	Worked examples (completed versions of a worksheet) provide accurate information that can be stored in long-term memory, which decreases working memory demands and cognitive load.

(*cont.*)

TABLE 5.1 *(cont.)*

Provide demonstrations	When the coach or instructor demonstrates a skill, it provides a tangible example to model.
Rehearse tasks	Once an individual has learned a skill, rehearsing it prior to using it in context can improve the real-life performance.
Practice in the context	Practicing a skill in the real-life context can increase the likelihood of generalization following the practice.
Use New-Me Activities to focus or reduce discomfort	In low-risk situation when the individual wants to remain engaged in a situation, it may be helpful to do a Focus or Feel Good New-Me Activity to increase focus and/or to reduce discomfort.
Provide scaffolding (e.g., check-ins in-person or via phone or text)	The individual is likely to experience unexpected challenges in real-life contexts. Having access to a skills coach or instructor for in-the-moment support can reduce cognitive load and increase skill application.
Hold regularly scheduled meetings to address ongoing issues	Having periodic meetings to review skill use and address challenges with a practitioner who is familiar with the Skills System can help address underlying issues that create high cognitive load.

The Targeting Strategy is a tool to help the coach and instructor be strategic when collaborating with the individual during coaching conversations and skills instruction. Since emotional dysregulation can affect the individual as well as the coach and instructor, having a framework in place to clarify courses of action can support co-regulation, learning, and generalization. Additionally, using the Targeting Strategy, the coach and instructor can help the individual manage the current situation effectively, building self-efficacy and skill-efficacy in the process.

BEHAVIORAL STRATEGIES

It is helpful for the coach and instructor to understand behavioral strategies, including positive reinforcement, shaping, contingency management, intermittent reinforcement, informal exposure, and Back-Track and Re-Track (the Skills System's version of functional behavioral assessment). Information gleaned from Back-Tracking and Re-Tracking can be integrated into individual support and behavioral treatment plans.

Behavioral interventions and the Skills System are integrated by practitioners in different ways. For example, they are used in environments that include positive behavior supports and by people who are trained in applied behavior analysis (ABA). My intention in this section is not to educate the trainer about behaviorism, but rather to highlight several ways to integrate elements into Skills System instruction.

Brainstorm: The coach/instructor brainstorms skill options, thinking about skills that would help the individual deal with the situation.

Example: The individual is having a problem with a coworker who is gossiping about him. The coach/instructor believes he will need All-the-Time skills to manage his emotions, as well as Calm-Only skills to address the underlying issue with the coworker.

Skills Plan: The coach/instructor imagines a Skills Plan that would manage the situation.

- *What are the individual's capacities in the moment?* (Use the Feelings Rating Scale.)
- *What skills would help in this moment?* (Use the Categories of Skills and the Recipe for Skills.)

Example: The individual reports he is at a Level 3 frustrated. The coach/instructor evaluates that although between 0 and 3, he may have difficulty doing Calm-Only skills at this time due to high cognitive load. The coach guides the individual toward a Skills Plan that includes his All-the-Time Skills (e.g., Clear Picture, On-Track Thinking, On-Track Action, Safety Plan, and a New-Me Activity—a 12345 skills chain).

Target: Do the Quick Step to target where the Skills Plan should start.

- *Assess the cognitive load demands of the Skills Plan to determine where to start coaching/teaching.*

Example: The 12345 skills chain includes All-the-Time Skills that the individual has used before, so the strategies are in his repertoire, which reduces cognitive load demands. Alternatively, three factors increase cognitive load demands. He is at work where there are time constraints, there is conflict with the coworker, and there is no skills coaching available to provide scaffolding. The coach adjusts the coaching suggestions to accommodate for the situational high-load factors. For example, tactics have to fit the constraints of the work environment, work-around the coworked conflict, and ensure the individual has visual aids that supply scaffolding.

Lower cognitive load demands	***Higher cognitive load demands***
☑ *All-the-Time skills*	☐ *Calm-Only skills*
☑ *The skill is in the individual's repertoire*	☐ *New skills*
☐ *No time constraints*	☑ *Time constraints*
☐ *Lower social demands*	☑ *High task demands or conflict*
☐ *There is available scaffolding (e.g., coaching)*	☑ *No scaffolding or coaching*

(cont.)

FIGURE 5.6. Targeting Strategy.

<table>
<tr><td colspan="2">

- *Assess the individual's abilities to complete the chain.*
- *Consider preexisting conditions that increase likelihood of cognitive overload.*
- *Assess current cognitive functioning (experiencing low or high cognitive load).*

Example: The individual is diagnosed with autism spectrum disorder and has a history of demonstrating aggressive behaviors in the community. The coach/instructor assesses what barriers will he experience completing one or more skills. For example, the coach examines whether the hectic work environment may increase sensory discomfort for the individual.
</td></tr>
<tr><td colspan="2">

- *Adjust the intervention to maximize emotion regulation processes, given the individual's abilities in the moment.*
</td></tr>
<tr><td>

Lower load situation (higher abilities to do cognitive processing)

☐ *Standard approach: Start with Clear Picture.*

Example: The coach suggests the individual begin with Notice the Breath and move through the other Clear Picture Do's, On-Track Thinking, On-Track Action, and the other skills.
</td><td>

Higher load situation (lower abilities to do cognitive processing)

☐ *A-la-carte approach: Focus on one skill that would help the individual reach his goal.*

Example: Perhaps the coach could suggest the individual go to the bathroom (Safety Plan—Move Away) and put cold water on his face (Solo New-Me Activity).
</td></tr>
</table>

FIGURE 5.6 *(cont.)*

Positive Reinforcement

Skills coaches and instructors provide positive reinforcement for on-track behaviors to increase the individual's skill use and adaptive functioning. Examples of positive reinforcement include verbal praise (e.g., "Great job getting a Clear Picture!"), nonverbal gestures (e.g., smile, head nod, clapping hands, thumbs up, high five, and fist bumps), and written/tangible feedback (e.g., stickers, sticky notes, and cards).

Offering specific positive reinforcement (e.g., "Great job noticing your breath!") helps differentiate and target the reinforcement, which increases the effect of the intervention. The coach and instructor must continually scan interactions with the individual to notice when he is making effort and demonstrating new skills. Clearly labeling a skillful behavior, highlighting the context, and adding positive reinforcement is important (e.g., "I saw that you put your book away and turned your attention to our activity. Great On-Track Action—Switch Tracks!"). Emotion regulation is a series of small steps, so it is important that the coach and instructor take available opportunities to reinforce as many as possible.

Shaping

An individual with behavioral health/learning challenges may need to be taught complex tasks through a gradual process. "Shaping" is a behavioral technique that reinforces steps of successive approximations. The individual is reinforced for reaching objectives that are steps toward a larger goal. For example, a learning progression may take steps: A, B, AB, C, and ABC. This type of practice helps the cognitively impaired individual learn to integrate information; schema acquisition is facilitated through this repeated pattern of shaping. Teaching ABCDEFG may introduce more information, yet the person may not have reinforced connections between steps.

There are times in coaching and instruction when it is not possible—due to time constraints, circumstances, or ability levels—to discuss or teach all the necessary elements of multicomponent concepts. The coach and instructor individualize and prioritize elements that help most in the immediate situation, trusting that other opportunities will arise to teach the remainder of the concept at another time. The coach and instructor use the Quick Step to decide what to address in the current moment and what to address later.

Contingency Management

The coach or instructor frequently faces challenges in interactions with the individual that slow or stop the coaching and instruction processes. When this occurs, the instructor adjusts interventions using the Quick Step Assessment to keep the process moving ahead; she may simplify or slow down the intervention and/or offer access to a Focus or Feel Good New-Me Activity.

With certain behaviors, the coach or instructor may choose to use extinction by refusing to reinforce a specific behavior. In a case like this, the coach or instructor would continue focusing on productive aspects of the interaction and not attend to behaviors that are less adaptive. The individual may respond by exhibiting an extinction burst. An extinction burst is when the individual increases the intensity, frequency, or duration of a behavior to receive reinforcement. When using extinction, it is important that the coach or instructor not reinforce the escalated behavior and remain consistent with the intervention.

Intermittent Reinforcement

Intermittent reinforcement is when a behavior is reinforced on a random versus consistent schedule. Intermittent reinforcement strengthens both the frequency and intensity of a behavior (e.g., slot machines). If the coach or instructor intermittently reinforces an individual when he is demonstrating maladaptive behaviors, it increases the likelihood that the behaviors will happen more and in a more intense way. Similarly, if the coach or instructor intermittently reinforces On-Track Actions, those behaviors are strengthened.

It is important to observe and address situations when escalating feelings levels are being intermittently reinforced. For example, if some support staff are engaging in Calm-Only skills (e.g., Expressing Myself, Problem Solving) with the individual when she is over a Level 3 feeling, it will intermittently reinforce using Calm-Only skills at a time that will increase the likelihood of escalation and conflict. In this situation, the coach might be encouraging a conversation with the individual who is yelling about a housemate being impossible to live with (i.e., Expressing Myself) and she is threatening to run away (i.e., Problem Solving), reinforcing misusing Calm-Only skills at a Level 4 feeling, rather than shifting to All-the-Time skills.

It is important for all support staff and family members to follow the Skills System and the plan the individual has created with her coach or instructor. If some support people are following written de-escalation procedures carefully and others are not, it sends mixed messages to the individual. If she believes she can persist in less adaptive behaviors and be reinforced (i.e., get what she wants), the individual's off-track behavior will not only persist, but will likely increase in frequency and intensity.

Intermittent reinforcement can be difficult to find and root out. It will be necessary to look carefully at interactions. We can all be culprits—I know I have been! Creating support environment that reinforce self-reflection, group reflection, and open discussions to explore how interactions are functioning will support a focus on "doing what works."

Informal Exposure

It can be challenging to determine the best course of action in some situations. There are times when facing challenges has benefits that outweigh the costs; similarly, there are times when avoiding a situation has benefits. If an individual demonstrates reinforced behavior that has high costs and low benefits, it may be advantageous to use the behavioral strategy of informal exposure to change that pattern. Informal exposure involves the individual experiencing a cue and executing adaptive skills, rather than engaging in the default behavior. Over time, as the individual experiences the cue and engages adaptive responses, the cue no longer automatically elicits the default behavior.

The skill On-Track Actions—Switch Tracks can help the individual create different responses, particularly when doing the opposite of the off-track urges (like Opposite Action in DBT). For example, if the individual wants to have a romantic relationship, but avoids contact with potential partners, it may be helpful to explore acting opposite to the urge. The individual may want to introduce himself to people he finds attractive, rather than admiring them silently and skulking away. Instead of staying home playing with his cats, he might shower, shave, put on cologne, and join a community social event, fully embracing his potential and freeing himself from his self-imposed limitations. As the individual expands capacities without experiencing his worst nightmares, the avoidance cues decrease.

The coach and instructor continually use the Quick Step to assess the individual's abilities to manage situations. The instructor must be aware of the delicate balance between reinforcing avoidant behaviors and flooding the individual by continuing with a high-demand activity that is overwhelming. Helping individuals consider the long-term benefits of adaptive behaviors, rather than valuing the short-term benefits of avoiding discomfort, may help the individual reach his long-term goals more effectively.

Back-Track and Re-Track

In DBT, a functional behavioral assessment is referred to as a behavioral chain analysis (understanding the antecedents and behaviors during an event) and solution analysis (highlighting adaptive alternatives for future events). The same concepts in the Skills System are referred to as doing a Back-Track and Re-Track. Understanding patterns of behavior helps support providers create plans that reinforce behaviors that are in service of the individual's goals.

Doing a Back-Track involves getting a Clear Picture of each level of feeling during a past event. For example, if the individual had a Level 5 behavior (e.g., assaulted staff), the Back-

Track would examine what was happening from when he was at baseline or low feelings up to the Level 5. A Re-Track is the process of exploring additional skills that could enhance the individual's experience navigating a similar event in the future. Re-Tracking involves enhancing existing on-track behaviors and introducing additional strategies that would be off-ramps, while assessing the individual's ability to manage the situation without harming self, others, or property (Level 5).

Back-Track and Re-Track are used in multiple ways, some impromptu and brief. For example, an instructor, coach, or family member might ask an individual to describe her experience of an event (e.g., a holiday family visit), guiding her to examine what went well and what didn't. The coach may informally ask the individual to explore how the Skills Plan could be enhanced to more effectively reach her goals in a similar situation in the future.

Other Back-Tracks and Re-Tracks are done consistently during targeted instruction sessions (described in detail in Chapter 9). Below are the steps of targeted instruction, showing where Back-Track and Re-Track fit in the process:

- Pre-Learning activities: Set goals and specific behaviors (targets) to increase or decrease in order to reach her goals.
- Reaching Goals:
  - Skills Plan: Create a Skills Plan for an upcoming period of time (e.g., 1 week) that outlines skills the individual will use to reach her goals.
  - My Progress: The instructor and individual review the previous time period, exploring On-Track Actions, off-track urges, and off-track actions.
  - Back-Track and Re-Track: The dyad choose one situation to Back-Track and Re-Track. This allows them to zoom in to assess antecedents of unwanted escalation and discuss and practice adaptive replacement behaviors.
  - Create a new Skills Plan: The instructor and individual create a revised Skills Plan that integrates additional, more targets skill options that increase On-Track Actions.

Individual Support Plans

As patterns are clarified during formal and informal Back-Track and Re-Tracks, the information can be integrated into general individual support plans and/or behavioral support plans that address specific challenging behaviors. Generally speaking, support plans often describe the individual's goals, current functioning, strengths and resources, challenging behaviors or barriers to goals, changes the individual needs to make to reach his goals, and how the support team will help him demonstrate the new behaviors.

When assessing various types of past and current functioning, it is useful to segment information in the different sections by functioning (e.g., communication, relationships, behaviors) at different levels of feelings. It helps to create three subsections of the feelings levels:

- Levels 0–3: Baseline; regulated functioning
- Level 4: What adaptive strategies are used to manage strong feelings? What behaviors are demonstrated during emotional escalation?
- Level 5: Behaviors that harm self, others, or property

For example, at Levels 0–3 the individual may have the ability to communicate needs in a respectful way. At a Level 4, she takes space in her bedroom when she is well-rested and taking her medications. Alternatively, when she is experiencing emotional vulnerability at a Level 4, she raises her voice and threatens people. At a Level 5, the individual tends to bang her head, break her devices, and/or assault staff.

By differentiating levels of functioning, the evaluator can systematically assess antecedents, setting events, precursors, and influencing factors that (1) affect the individual at the different feelings levels and (2) lead to changes in feelings levels. Examining what internal and external factors are associated helps the team enhance the individual's strategies at Levels 0–3 to reduce escalations to Level 5 feelings.

When an individual exhibits high levels of dysregulated behaviors, people (e.g., family members, support staff) in the environment can often over- or underestimate the frequency and intensity of behaviors. Integrating levels of feelings and factors that contribute to increases, allows them to target specific replacement behaviors earlier in the chain to improve emotion regulation capacities and address environmental factors that contribute to escalation. Figure 5.7 presents an example that integrates these strategies. It is valuable to gather the information presented in the figure from the individual, evaluator, and collateral support providers (e.g., family members, staff, instructors).

Behavioral Support Plan

Individuals who demonstrate patterns of dysregulated behaviors may have behavioral treatment plans that outline strategies for the individual and support providers to use. Information from doing informal and systematic Back-Tracks and Re-Tracks can aid in the process of developing and adjusting behavioral treatment plans. For example, once the instructor has collected the necessary data, she defines target behaviors that the behavioral treatment plan will be designed to increase or decrease. It can be helpful for her to address precursors (i.e., observable behaviors the individual may demonstrate) using the Levels 0–3, Level 4, and Level 5 breakdowns to help staff and parents better understand where the individual is in the escalation process. The Targeting Strategy, discussed earlier in this chapter, can help explore, prioritize, and create interventions designed to fill skill gaps.

ABA Plans

ABA evaluators make a series of hypotheses about the function of the target behaviors. While the Skills System does not use this exact framework of functions of behaviors, the skills can be integrated into ABA behavioral treatment plans as replacement behaviors. Table 5.2 highlights the functions of behaviors and several Skills System options for replacement behaviors.

Much like functional behavioral assessments, even ABA behavioral treatment plans can take many different forms. Figure 5.8 lists common elements of an ABA behavioral treatment plan. The ABA Skills System integration described in this chapter offers general principles to help ABA and Skills System practitioners integrate the two models. Each of these models can help the other, if thoughtfully combined. The Skills System can help ABA evaluators elaborate patterns of behavior and target interventions to build areas of need. ABA strategies can help

<table>
<tr><th colspan="2">Background information and interviews</th></tr>
<tr><td colspan="2">Describe how you/the individual communicates at:
Levels 0–3:
Level 4:
Level 5:</td></tr>
<tr><td>Describe your/the individual's Relationship Care with themselves at:
Levels 0–3:
Level 4:
Level 5:</td><td>Describe your/the individual's Relationship Care with others at:
Levels 0–3:
Level 4:
Level 5:</td></tr>
<tr><td colspan="2">Describe your/the individual's behaviors at:
Levels 0–3:
Level 4:
Level 5:</td></tr>
<tr><td colspan="2">What are common antecedents (i.e., stimuli that precedes events) that tend to increase responses from Levels 0–3 to a Level 4?</td></tr>
<tr><td colspan="2">What are common antecedents that tend to increase responses from Level 4 to Level 5?</td></tr>
<tr><td colspan="2">What strategies do you/the individual prefer to use to manage emotions at:
Levels 0–3:
Level 4:
Level 5:</td></tr>
<tr><td colspan="2">What strategies help/the individual de-escalate from a Level 4 to Levels 0–3 feelings?</td></tr>
<tr><td colspan="2">What strategies help/the individual de-escalate from a Level 5 to Level 4 feeling?</td></tr>
</table>

(cont.)

FIGURE 5.7. Example of an individual support plan.

Direct observation (3+ months)
• Use the Feelings Rating Scale to describe behaviors that happen from baseline through the highest level of emotion (e.g., 0–3 = Engaged in activities, 4 = Paces, raises voice, and swears at staff, 5 = Hits staff). • Track the *days of the week* when behaviors happen to understand patterns that contribute to the escalation. • Track *times of the day* when behaviors happen to understand patterns that contribute to the escalation. • Track *people involved* when behaviors happen to understand interpersonal factors that contribute to the escalation. • Track the *activities or events* that are happening to understand environmental factors that contribute to the escalation. • Describe factors that increase vulnerability (e.g., lack of sleep, medication side effects) that contribute to escalation. • Describe setting events and bidirectional influencing factors (e.g., home visit was canceled, conflict with staff/peer) that contribute to the escalation.

FIGURE 5.7 *(cont.)*

certain individuals who need this level of support to learn and generalize Skills System concepts within treatment environments.

TRANSITION TO CHAPTER 6

Chapter 6 presents information about planning skills instruction, conducting pre-instruction activities, and structuring group or one-on-one skills instruction.

TABLE 5.2. Functions of Behavior

Hypotheses about the functions of behavior	Replacement behaviors
1. The behaviors help the individual communicate with others.	• Learn to use standard 123 skills chains (i.e., doing Clear Picture, On-Track Thinking, and On-Track Actions). • Learn to do Safety Plans (Skill 4) to manage risk effectively. • Learn to do New-Me Activities (Skill 5) to manage feelings. • Learn Expressing Myself (Skill 7) to improve abilities to communicate.
2. The behaviors help the individual obtain a preferred item.	• Learn to use standard 123 skills chains. • Learn to do Safety Plans to manage risk effectively. • Learn to do New-Me Activities to manage feelings. • Learn Getting It Right (Skill 8) to get things from other people.
3. The behaviors help the individual to escape or avoid a setting or activity.	• Learn to use standard 123 skills chains. • Learn to do Safety Plans. • Learn to do New-Me Activities to manage feelings. • Use Calm-Only skills to increase abilities and opportunities to self-advocate and self-direct in life contexts.
4. The behaviors help the individual gain power and control when feeling powerless.	• Learn to use standard 123 skills chains. • Learn to do Safety Plans. • Learn to do New-Me Activities to manage feelings. • Learn Problem Solving (Skill 6) to address underlying issues that disempower the individual. • Learn Relationship Care (Skill 9) to address relationship conflicts that lead to disempowerment.
5. The behaviors help the individual get attention from someone.	• Learn to use standard 123 skills chains. • Learn to do Safety Plans • Learn to do New-Me Activities to manage feelings. • Learn Problem Solving to address underlying issues that disempower the individual. • Learn Expressing Myself to improve abilities to communicate perspectives and needs. • Learn Getting It Right to ask for attention and other things that are needed in effective ways. • Learn Relationship Care to address relationship conflicts.
6. The behaviors help the individual to manage internal stimuli.	• Learn to use standard 123 skills chains. • Learn to do Safety Plans. • Learn to do New-Me Activities to manage stimuli.

Objectives: To increase adaptive behaviors (e.g., replacement behavior or skill) and/or decrease maladaptive behaviors (e.g., physical assault, self-injury) during a specified period.

Example: The individual will use Safety Plans effectively to manage risk, as evidenced by having no incidents of physical assault for 3 months.

Baseline frequency: The number of incidents of the target behavior the individual was demonstrating prior to the behavioral treatment plan.

Example: During the past 3 months the individual averages 1.5 incidents that included physical assault.

Data collection: The treatment planner offers staff and/or parents criteria for responding to behaviors and requires documentation of interventions. Using the 0–3, 4, and 5 levels help clarify how and when people in the environment intervene.

Example: When the individual is between Level 0 and Level 3 feelings, the support staff will use skills and the A + B = C Skills Coaching Strategies (Chapter 8) to proactively support him to manage situations. If the individual escalates to a Level 4 or 5, the support staff will use the agency's nonviolent crisis intervention model to manage de-escalation and emergency procedures (e.g., Crisis Prevention Institute, Safety Care). The support team will use All-the-Time skills (versus Calm-Only skills when interacting with the individuals when he is over a Level 3 feeling.

Antecedent interventions: Antecedent interventions are proactive strategies (replacement behaviors) that the environment uses to increase the likelihood that the individual can self- and co-regulate with people around them. The behavioral treatment plan should integrate ample proactive skills early in situations (Levels 0–3) so that high levels of escalation (Levels 4 and 5) are not reached. The goal of integrating emotion regulation skills is to change the trajectory and duration of emotions, so that emotional and behavioral dysregulation does not happen. Additionally, the goal is to reinforce skillful behavior, rather than reinforcing escalated behavior or intermittently reinforcing maladaptive patterns of behavior.

Examples:

- The individual has access to Skills System visual aids whenever possible.
- The individual has places he can go to remove himself from risks (e.g., access to his bedroom and/or sensory space).
- The individual has opportunities to do Solo and Partnership Focus, Feel Good, Distraction, and Fun New-Me Activities when at Levels 0–3 feelings.
- When over Levels 0–3, the individual has access to Solo New-Me Activities. It is important that he not have access to preferred New-Me Activities at a Level 4 or 5 (engaging in preferred activities at a Level 4 or 5 will positively reinforce escalation).

(cont.)

FIGURE 5.8. Elements of behavioral treatment plans.

Intervention technique: It is important that coaches (including staff and parents) have clearly outlined procedures to teach, practice, coach, and reinforce replacement behaviors. Teachable moments are between Level 0 and Level 3 feelings. Teaching skills when the individual is over a Level 3 will cause high cognitive load, and may increase escalation.

Examples:

- In the morning, before getting on the van to go to his day program, the individual will meet with staff for 15 minutes to get a Clear Picture, discuss goals for the day, review any Safety Plans, and list New-Me Activities he will do.
- The individual will carry his New-Me Activity backpack to and from day program, so he has activities to do on the van and at work.

Back-Track and Re-Track procedure: People in the individual's environment need to know how to respond if the individual demonstrates maladaptive behaviors. Doing a Back-Track (to review the escalation process) and Re-Track (to map potential ways to improve supports for the individual) helps people in the environment understand how to respond effectively in future situations. (In the Reaching Goals section of the *Skills System Workbook,* Worksheets 4 and 5 and Worked Examples 4 and 5 on pp. 235–238 show how to conduct Back-Tracks and Re-Tracks.)

FIGURE 5.8 *(cont.)*

CHAPTER 6

Providing Standard Instruction

This chapter helps the instructor provide standard instruction (i.e., teaching all nine skills in a group/one-on-one setting). We first review logistical considerations to aid in the instruction planning process, then introduce pre-instruction strategies. The chapter also describes how standard instruction can be structured using the E-Spiral framework for group or one-on-one sessions. The final portion of this chapter presents teaching strategies that fulfill the functions of the E-Spiral framework to deepen and broaden learning.

PLANNING STANDARD INSTRUCTION

Skills can be taught to an individual in a skills group or a one-on-one setting. Although skills group offers many advantages, including sharing experiences, offering support, opportunities to practice, and socialization, it may not always be possible to run a group. The individual may not be able to manage in a group setting without experiencing high levels of emotional, cognitive, and/or behavioral dysregulation. Having a consistently dysregulated individual in group will hinder his learning and impede the learning of the other people in group. In this case, one-on-one instruction may be a better option. It is also possible for the individual to begin in one-on-one skills instruction and shift to a skills group once he is able to do basic Safety Plans. Once the instructor has decided that a skills group is the appropriate setting for standard instruction, there are a number of factors to consider.

Size of a Skills Group

Skills System groups do not need to have a specific number of participants. It may be ideal to have multiple options for group sizes to suit the needs of the individuals. Small groups of two to four participants offer more individualized training and coaching. Groups of four to seven people allow for individual participation and opportunities for social interaction. Larger groups (seven to 10 participants) allow the individual to practice skills in a more complex social setting but may provide fewer opportunities for individual sharing and practice. Logistics and resources can dictate group size, but by understanding factors that impact learning, the skills instructor can advocate for group sizes that optimize learning. The cognitive load of the instructor is also a consideration. If the instructor has not conducted a Skills System group before, it may make sense to start with a smaller number of participants. In DBT, skills groups have co-leaders: The primary leader focuses on teaching content and the other is available to assess and support individuals who are experiencing difficulty. Whenever possible, particularly in larger groups, the Skills System follows this same co-leader model to offer augmented scaffolding for participants.

Time Frames of Group Sessions

Group sessions generally meet for 1 hour per week. Group skills training places high cognitive and emotional demands on participants and skills instructors, so fatigue is a legitimate concern as time frames lengthen. In residential settings, it may be useful to run multiple 1-hour skills groups per week. Meeting more than once per week may create opportunities for heightened integration of the Skills System concepts. This exposure may foster improved generalization of skills. Shortening groups to less than one hour and increasing the frequency may also be workable. Having a standard skills group that meets once per week plus shorter ones on topics such as a Safety Plan, New-Me Activities, Problem Solving, or Getting It Right can offer opportunities for practice. It is important to design groups so that there is sufficient time for all aspects of the E-Spiral learning process to occur.

Location for Group

The instruction space should be big enough to allow people to maintain their personal space. Having a table that people sit around can allow them to write, do activities, and sort skills cards. A large whiteboard can also be useful. As participants discuss skills applications, the instructor can diagram levels of feelings, events, time frames, and skills use on the board. Creating a scenario map can help group members better understand the situation and options.

It is often beneficial for there to be a waiting area that allows an individual to leave the group and do a Safety Plan. This area might also include various New-Me Activities so the individual can focus and prepare to reenter group. If the group includes individuals with histories of Level 5 behaviors, it is prudent to use a location that has two exits. If an individual becomes behaviorally dysregulated, it may be necessary to evacuate the other group members safely. It is helpful to be sure all involved with the individual's support are familiar with his safety plan and de-escalation procedures. Because the individual may experience heightened cognitive load during group, it is important that he practice executing Safety Plans when cognitively regulated. This increases the likelihood that he will be able to do a Safety Plan within the group context.

Staff or Family Members Attending Group

Staff and/or family members may ask to attend group. The instructor needs to weigh the benefits and costs of this option. She uses the Quick Step to proactively plan how to structure the comingling of individuals and collateral supports. It is important for individuals to be able to talk openly about challenging situations to assemble effective skills chains; having family or staff in group can inhibit the exploration of factors that are essential to manage these relationships. Rather than inconsistently inviting outsiders in, the format should be clear, as in DBT for adolescents' multifamily groups (Miller, Rathus, & Linehan, 2007). Parallel (a group for individuals and a group for family/staff) versus integrated skills training for collateral support providers may be a useful option.

Homogeneous and Heterogeneous Aspects of Group

The instructor may need to decide what aspects of the group will be heterogeneous and homogeneous. Frequently, participants have commonalities in one area while being diverse in others. For example, the group may include participants who all live in the same residence or attend a specific day program. The people in these settings, however, may be various ages and have different abilities to communicate and levels of impulsivity. The instructor may decide that the group benefits from having a more heterogeneous make-up—inviting everyone to join—or he may choose to have more homogenous groups with narrow attendance (e.g., creating a women's or men's group; a group exclusively for people in substance abuse treatment). Mixing perpetrators of abuse and victims of abuse in the same group is not recommended.

There may be benefits to grouping participants by academic functioning level. This distribution may allow individuals with more cognitive capacities to move through material at a faster rate and in greater depth. While reading and writing are not prerequisite skills for participating in the curriculum, clustering individuals who can read and write may increase options for instructors to utilize activities that integrate these media.

Open versus Closed Groups

Skills System groups can be either open (accepting new members) or closed. There is often variability in attendance due to logistical factors; participants may frequently miss sessions or drop out of skills instruction. These factors dictate that group be constructed in a way that allows an individual to miss a meeting or join in the middle of a cycle without experiencing a significant gap in learning. Instruction needs to be adjusted to accommodate this flow.

The instructor must address the learning needs of both the new person and the participants who have already been studying skills. Individuals who have been in group will be familiar with skills concepts and will be able to delve into elaborated discussions about more nuanced skills concepts. For example, a discussion of a scenario with a more experienced learner might examine Safety Plan application. Is the risk low, medium, or high? Should the person do a Thinking, Talking, and/or Written Safety Plan? The individual just joining group will not be familiar with levels of risk and types of Safety Plans, so it will be necessary for the group to explain the basic concepts and application.

Often, more seasoned participants enjoy teaching and coaching newer members. This is a great opportunity for participants to consolidate learning and demonstrate to newer participants that skills are learnable, fun, and cool (particularly important when teaching clients who are communicating less readiness to learn skills). Peer teaching creates an on-track culture that builds self-efficacy and is a chance to practice Relationship Care. It is a win–win–win!

Participants Revolve Multiple Times through the 12-Week-Cycle Curriculum

The pace at which the group and individuals progress through the Skills System materials is variable. Generally, the basic Skills System material cannot be integrated by individuals with cognitive challenges within a single 12-week cycle. Such individuals require repetition of the Skills System curriculum to learn and generalize the information. It is recommended that an individual with an intellectual disability participate in the Skills System for a minimum of 1 year, so he would cycle through the material four times. This format allows ample time to introduce the basic Skills System concepts and offers opportunity for repetition.

It may be beneficial for the individual to remain in a skills group on an ongoing basis or have the ability to return to group to deepen and broaden skills competency needed. As people increase capacities, often they accept more personal responsibilities. For example, the individual may move from working in a vocational site to being employed in the community. Skills group helps her develop improved coping skills as she is participating in more demanding tasks. Each accomplishment brings new challenges, and the group helps her face transitions and continually progress toward her personal goals. Perhaps attending a skills group on a monthly or biweekly basis could address these needs.

Training Skills Coaches in the Individual's Environment

When people in the individual's environment (e.g., staff, family members) know the skills and skills coaching strategies, it offers important scaffolding to the individual. Although the individual will likely be able to apply some skills on their own, having effective coaching supports will allow him to plan and execute more complex skills chains within his life context. If multiple people within the environment know skills and coaching strategies, coaches can be interchangeable, increasing the availability of coaching. Skills and coaching strategies (presented in Chapter 8) create a common language that helps the individual and the people supporting him to co-regulate.

Handouts and Visual Aids

The Emotion Regulation Skills System Workbook, Second Edition, is designed for instructors to utilize with individuals. The *Skills System Workbook* includes handouts, worked examples, and worksheets. Information in this book helps demonstrate how to integrate the materials into instruction. Even if the individual does not read or write (independently completing worksheets), instructors can fill out worksheets collaboratively with her. Having visual aids and cue pictures can help all participants to follow along, be engaged, and better understand concepts.

Copyright restrictions affect the duplication of these materials. The copyright rules allow the instructor to copy the *Skills System Workbook* for people on their own caseload. If resources allow, it is recommended that each individual have their own complete workbook.

PRE-INSTRUCTION SESSIONS

Before skills instruction can begin, the instructor or individual therapist meets with the individual for one or more pre-instruction sessions. The transtheoretical model of change outlines five phases the individual must progress through in order to change their behavior: precontemplation, contemplation, preparation, action, and maintenance (Prochaska, DiClemente, & Norcross, 1992). This section explores ways to help the individual move through each of these phases, from not being aware of skills to engaging in skills instruction.

Precontemplation to Contemplation

To encourage contemplation, the instructor engages in dialogues that help the individual self-reflect about his goals and barriers to the goals. The instructor highlights resources that are available to help him reach his personal goals and explore the possibilities of living aligned with his values. Figure 6.1 provides some talking points for these dialogues that can help instructors encourage the individual to contemplate learning and using skills.

Ask about Goals, Abilities, and Barriers

In a preliminary conversation about goals, as a warm-up for goal setting, the instructor asks the individual about what she wants, what she values, and what aspects of her life are moving her in the direction of her goals. This is a strength-based approach that focuses on increasing efficacy. The instructor also asks about barriers to the individual's goals. By asking about the gap between her current situation and her desired situation, the instructor assists the individual in reflecting on these barriers. This awareness lays the groundwork for setting targets to work on and mobilizing motivation to change behavior.

The individual may not have clarity about how his feelings are linked to his difficulties. In this case, the instructor may want to explain the effects of emotional dysregulation. The Relationship Care—Getting to Know My Feelings worksheet, available in the *Skills System Workbook* (p. 6), can be used to facilitate a discussion about the individual's experiences with their feelings. Figure 6.2 lists common difficulties that are the results of skill gaps that the individual may experience.

- Ask the individual to talk about his goals and values.
- Ask the individual to reflect about his abilities to reach his goals.
- Ask the individual to reflect about barriers he experiences related to reaching his goals.
- Explain the skills gaps that commonly create barriers.
- Share information about Skills System resources.
- Explore the potential benefits and costs of addressing or not addressing abilities and barriers.

FIGURE 6.1. Ways to foster contemplation.

- Difficulties balancing self-care (e.g., sleep, taking medications as prescribed, healthy eating, exercise, hygiene)
- Difficulty facing demands (e.g., chores, homework, work tasks)
- Difficulty managing time and being organized
- Not able to access resources/supports/ treatments
- Difficulty taking responsibility and being accountable
- Unstable relationships
- Difficulty managing money
- Difficulty balancing social media and technology use
- Difficulty managing stress and anger
- Excessive risk taking
- Patterns of over/underregulating (e.g., verbal abuse, isolation)
- Physical aggression
- Self-injury/suicidality
- Property destruction
- Stealing
- Substance abuse

FIGURE 6.2. Common challenges associated with emotion regulation skill deficits.

Skill Gaps and Skills System Resources

James Gross (2024) highlighted that when people have skills gaps they are less likely to engage adaptive strategies. During the pre-instruction process, the instructor explains that as the individual develops skills, he can increase his abilities to manage his feelings and his life. As the individual may hesitate to learn skills, the instructor introduces the Skills System and the available opportunities for instruction. The instructor helps him see that learning skills is manageable and beneficial.

To cultivate the urge to participate, the instructor explains the Skills System as a simple, user-friendly way to fill skills gaps and reach the individual's personal goals. The instructor can use handouts and/or online resources to introduce the model. Keeping the messaging aligned with relevance and fun may help the individual see there are accessible ways to address these long-standing, seemingly unsurmountable, pervasive problems. The instructor creates two-way-street communication and uses validation strategies as the individual contemplates.

Weigh Benefits and Costs

During the contemplation-provoking conversation, the instructor offers information about the benefits and costs of engaging in skills instruction. Additionally, she highlights the benefits and costs associated with not learning new adaptive emotion regulation skills. Table 6.1 outlines some of the benefits and costs of learning and not learning skills that the instructor can highlight.

TABLE 6.1. Benefits and Costs of Learning and Not Learning Skills

Benefits of learning skills	Costs of learning skills
• I may feel better, sooner. • I may be able to manage all sizes of emotions and be present. • I may expand my comfort zone and do more things. • I may be able to stay on-track or get back on-track to goals.	• I will need to invest time and energy into learning and practicing skills. • I will need to try new things; get out of my comfort zone.
Benefits of not learning skills	**Costs of not learning skills**
• I will not have to go to group or do one-on-one skills instruction. • I will not have to learn new skills. • I will not have to share about my issues.	• My emotions will continue to overwhelm me. • I will continue to experience difficulties reaching goals. • I will continue to have a hard time in balancing relationships with myself and/or others.

Preparation to Action

When an individual is oriented to the process of learning, it reduces her cognitive load demands and facilitates her participation. It is important to explain aspects of the learning experience and create a dialogue about the individual's concerns. Partnering to troubleshoot barriers creates a foundation for the learning process.

Often, individuals who experience complex learning challenges live in systems of support that involve multiple support providers and limited access to resources. For example, the individual may not have transportation to instruction sessions. There may be barriers that make it difficult for her to access a computer or the internet for remote learning. It is essential that the support system facilitate the individual and her team in learning skills. Support providers may need to reduce barriers on their end related to logistics and motivation in order to consistently support learning the Skills System.

Creating an Instruction Plan

Once the individual agrees to participate in instruction, she works with the instructor to create an instruction plan. The individual will be more likely to follow a plan she helps create. The dyad discusses logistics and expectations. For example, the planning process may involve communicating certain logistics to other programs and/or family members; the pair agrees how this communication will happen (preferably the individual should be involved in these communications).

The individual may have various instruction options (e.g., joining a group or meeting one-on-one with an instructor), or she may only have one option. Various factors affect the available opportunities, such as transportation, other participants, or administrative requirements. It is helpful if the instructor orients the individual to logistical concerns that may affect her and her experience. Reviewing the benefits and costs related to the different learning experiences, potential positive outcomes, and challenges will help the individual be in the driver's seat of her supports and prepared to begin instruction.

The individual's initial plan may evolve over time. The more skills she develops, the more challenging social settings she may be able to tolerate. Additionally, when a Two-Way-Street relationship with the instructor develops, the individual may increase her willingness to participate in other recommended learning opportunities.

Setting Specific Goals to Build Skills Competency

The self-regulation process relies on goal activation, so it is important to help the individual clarify her goals and values. Once the individual has agreed to participate in skills instruction, the instructor helps her explore and set goals. The goal setting is an individual process; there are different ways to state goals. For example, the individual may list out things, people, or situations she wants in her life, like getting an apartment or a full-time job. She may want to have certain experiences, like going to school or entering a romantic relationship. The individual may have goals to avoid specific circumstances, such as not getting hospitalized or incarcerated.

An emotion regulation goal is a specific goal that the individual sets related to the intensity and duration of feelings and moods. For example, the individual may want to be less anxious and/or depressed. She may set a goal to have more peace, more often, or a goal to not remain as angry for as long when she gets mad.

There are four Pre-Learning worksheets and worked examples in the *Skills System Workbook* that can be used to help the individual clarify her goals (Getting to Know Me, My New-Me and My Old-Me, Exploring My Goals, and My Goals). The instructor uses the Quick Step and Targeting Strategy to determine whether to do the worksheets in order or to choose a specific one that fits the individual.

Action to Maintenance

As the individual learns skills, it is important that she practices and integrates those skills into her daily life. The Pre-Learning, Learning Skills, and Reaching Goals materials in the *Skills System Workbook* are designed to help the individual fill skills gaps. As she increases competency the individual can increase demands, take on more responsibilities, and improve quality of life. Support providers reinforce skillful actions to increase the frequency and effectiveness of skills use. Additionally, coaches provide scaffolding to help the individual increase skill application to maintain adaptive functioning.

STRUCTURING STANDARD INSTRUCTION

The instructor engages in many different types of preparation for providing well-designed Skills System instruction. For example, the instructor uses the 12-week curriculum to guide her through a week-to-week progression of the nine core skills and the System Tools (see Chapter

7). Each weekly skills instruction session integrates the E-Spiral framework. This framework (explored in Chapter 4 and in further detail later in this chapter) guides the instructor through phases of teaching that broaden and deepen learning. The instructor creates lesson plans and uses specific teaching strategies to address the functions within the E-Spiral framework for each week of the curriculum.

Skills System 12-Week-Cycle Curriculum

The Skills System curriculum revolves in a 12-week cycle. Each time a participant revisits familiar concepts from a previous cycle, understanding and awareness deepen and more information is stored in long-term memory. Through this spiral process, the individual continually integrates new facets of the skills, gaining the ability to utilize skills in increasingly complex situations. Figure 6.3 presents Skills System topics that are covered during each of the 12 weeks, and Chapter 7 presents detailed explanations of how topics may be reviewed, introduced, practiced, and integrated.

It is unrealistic to expect group members to learn a skill completely in a 1-hour group session. The 12-week-cycle curriculum forces the group to keep moving through content related to each of the skills. The instructor may have the urge to spend weeks on one skill to ensure comprehension. Rather than focusing in-depth on one skill for several weeks, the 12-week-cycle curriculum is designed to continually broaden skills knowledge.

In its entirety, the Skills System is vast. An instructor knows the complete Skills System, but an individual in the group can progress at different rates through the material, building mastery over time. To reduce cognitive load and facilitate recall, the system itself and the teaching process are broken into more manageable chunks of information.

During a group's first cycle through the Skills System material, it is important to introduce basic skills information. For example, the instructor may plan on reviewing the several handouts

- Week 1: Skills List
- Week 2: System Tools
- Week 3: Clear Picture
- Week 4: On-Track Thinking
- Week 5: On-Track Action
- Week 6: Safety Plan
- Week 7: New-Me Activities
- Week 8: Problem Solving
- Week 9: Expressing Myself
- Week 10: Getting It Right
- Week 11: Relationship Care
- Week 12: Skills Review

FIGURE 6.3. Skills System topics in the 12-week curriculum.

in minimal detail to offer a general overview of concepts. Exercises and discussions may be more brief; in-depth exploration of the material will occur in later cycles. As the individual progresses through multiple cycles of the Skills System curriculum, more time is spent on lateral exploration of topics. At that point, the quantity of material introduced is far less important than the quality of the discussions and practice exercises that help an individual integrate concepts.

Evaluating comprehension can be challenging. In the Learning Skills section of the *Skills System Workbook,* there are two resources that can be used to evaluate basic Skills System knowledge: System Tools Review Questions (p. 47) and Using Skills in My Life, Skills Quiz (p. 217, with corresponding answers on p. 218). People with learning challenges may understand and use concepts yet have difficulty recalling and communicating information. A more qualitative approach may be helpful. Discussing scenarios and real-life situations with the individual, with particular attention on whether he is integrating concepts, is also a viable way to assess. Although there are many contributing environmental factors, monitoring for improved quality of life (e.g., social engagement, lower levels of supervision) and reductions in behavioral dyscontrol (e.g., aggression, self-injury and hospitalization) may be the best way to gauge comprehension and generalization.

Structure of Instruction Sessions: The E-Spiral Framework

Once the individual has completed any necessary pre-instruction activities, she may join a skills group or begin one-on-one skills instruction. As introduced in Chapter 4, the E-Spiral is a teaching framework that is used to structure both group and one-on-one instruction sessions. The four phases of the E-Spiral are Exploring Existing Knowledge Base, Encoding, Elaboration, and Efficacy. It is helpful for the instructor to understand the E-Spiral when planning for and engaging in skills instruction.

In Phase 1, Exploring Existing Knowledge Base, the group reviews past learning related to the topic that is introduced in order to create a relevant context for learning. In Phase 2, Encoding, individuals participate in direct instruction and multimodal activities to learn the skill topic. The aim is to teach new information. In Phase 3, Elaboration, individuals engage in practice exercises and discussions that expand and link new information to their existing knowledge base. The elaboration process is a vital yet fun step toward deepening understandings about skills. Finally, in Phase 4, Efficacy, participants continue to build mastery and confidence through contextual learning activities that promote skills integration in real-life contexts. Activities such as role play, *in vivo* practice, addressing commitment, and troubleshooting challenges facilitate generalization. It is critical that individuals with intellectual impairment experience a sense of self-efficacy as part of the learning process. The E-Spiral is designed to provide contextual learning opportunities that maximize retention and generalization of skills.

Benefits of the Skills System Teaching Model

The 12-week-cycle curriculum creates breadth of skills knowledge, while the E-Spiral creates depth of learning. Skills instructors utilize both constructs simultaneously. The broadening and deepening of learning creates a foundation in long-term memory that enhances the generalization of skills. Figure 6.4 exemplifies how an individual's knowledge grows in a web shape using these teaching techniques.

As the individual learns, practices, and generalizes information, linkages between skills fortify over time. The increased connectivity of the knowledge base enhances recall and recognition of information. Adaptive responses become more automated, requiring fewer cognitive resources. As the individual builds a foundation of knowledge, cognitive load demands related to skills use decrease. The person becomes able to master complex skill behaviors because of the integrated skills knowledge base.

The Skills System session format presents the various tasks within each phase of the E-Spiral. The instructor follows these guidelines and designs activities to complete the function of the E-Spiral phase. As the group flows from one discussion point and activity to another, learning happens. Figure 6.5 presents the curriculum tasks that occur during E-Spiral phases in a skills group.

Creating Lesson Plans

The instructor creates a lesson plan that covers each week's topic within the time frames that are available. The Appendix includes an easy-to-use Lesson Planning worksheet and worked example. Instructors use the Quick Step to prepare the lesson plan in advance of the group or one-on-one session and then make adjustments to the plan as the learning experience unfolds.

The instructor may want to create a written plan for the group. It can also be helpful to photocopy the pages from this book that explain the week's curriculum, along with the corresponding worksheets from the *Skills System Workbook.* The instructor can use these pages to highlight specific instructions, discussion questions, activities, and visual aids that are part of their lesson plan. Although some instructors teach directly from this book, it is sometimes easier to have a small packet that addresses only the topic at hand.

Within each week's lesson plan, unplanned teaching opportunities and challenging events may emerge. It is important to be able to utilize contextual circumstances (e.g., holidays, events in the news) when possible, although contextual learning can increase cognitive load demands. It is necessary for the instructor to be prepared for the unexpected. It is critical that the instructor know the Skills System inside and out and have an ample bag of tricks to create teachable moments during all eventualities.

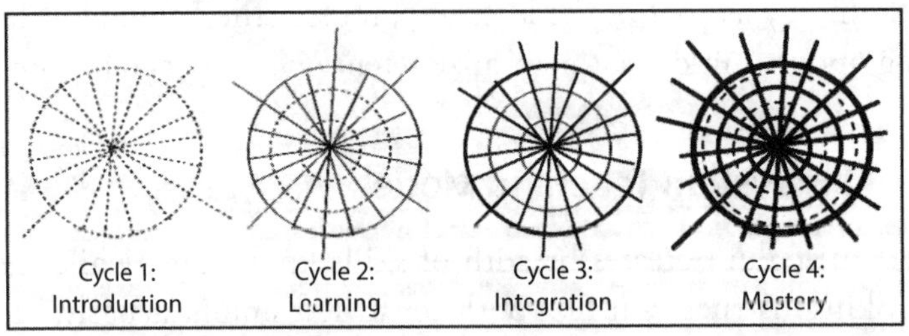

FIGURE 6.4. Learning the Skills System.

1. Exploring Existing Knowledge Base: *Recalling past learning.*
   - Mindfulness activity to focus attention; describe the experience.
   - Review Skills System terms and Skills Practice Review.
   - Introduce new skills topic.
   - Discussion: Assess existing knowledge; highlight the need for skills.
   - Orient to the relevant context of the new learning.
2. Encoding: *Teaching the new topic.*
   - Direct instruction: Lecture, write on the board, handouts and worked examples.
   - Discussion: Test comprehension of content; prompt clarification.
   - Multimodal tools: Use diagrams, cue pictures, gestures, objects, and video.
3. Elaboration: *Practicing new learning and linking it to previous learning.*
   - Practice: Practice exercises, worksheets.
   - Discussion: Describing the experience; some self-disclosure; expand awareness.
   - Skills Chains: Link the new skill with other skills in skills chains.
4. Efficacy: *Bridging to real life.*
   - Contextual learning activities: Role play, psychodrama, and *in vivo.*
   - Discussion: Highlighting barriers; personal commitment; troubleshooting for future use of the skill.
   - Plan for home-study activities.
   - Group ending: Mindfulness breathing.

FIGURE 6.5. Tasks within E-Spiral phases in a skills group.

E-SPIRAL TEACHING STRATEGIES

This section highlights the general structure of each Skills System group. There are four phases that provide different instruction activities to deepen and broaden learning during the session. The instructor progresses through the E-Spiral, shifting from welcoming, highlighting logistics, review, to teaching new material, linking the new material to previous teaching, practicing, and troubleshooting.

E-Spiral Phase 1: Exploring Existing Knowledge Base

Figure 6.6 outlines E-Spiral Phase 1: Exploring Existing Knowledge Base and the teaching strategies in each section.

Welcoming the Group

Greeting people is an important initial element of a skills training session. The instructor engages in lighthearted conversation to initiate a pleasant, egalitarian rapport with participants.

Exploring Existing Knowledge Base: Recalling past learning (review)

- Welcome
- Orient to logistics
- Mindfulness activity to focus attention
  Describe questions
- Skills System review
- Homework review
  Disclosure questions
  Clarifying questions
- Orient to new skills topic
- Discussion: Exploring existing knowledge on new topic
  Assessment questions
- Discussion: Orient to the relevant context of the new topic
  Relevant context questions

FIGURE 6.6. E-Spiral Phase 1: Exploring Existing Knowledge Base.

During this unstructured time of interaction, the instructor uses the Quick Step to evaluate the status of each individual prior to initiating any skills training activities. For example, as the skills instructor engages in chitchat, he can evaluate the individual's feelings rating. The instructor monitors for cognitive overload and immediately begins the process of shaping interventions that reflect the current status of the individual.

It is important to be aware that attending a group can elicit strong feelings. If the individual is demonstrating escalated negative behaviors prior to group, it is best to address them before they develop into safety concerns. The individual can be prompted to sit in a quiet area, do a focus New-Me Activity, or take a walk to reduce arousal.

Orienting to Logistics

Once the group members are seated, the instructor may choose to review the rules for the group and explain any logistics (e.g., time frame of group, schedules, restroom use, cellphone use, breaks, snacks, and transportation). The group discusses any issues that are relevant to be sure all members understand clearly. The instructor may want to orient the group to the format of each session to help reduce the cognitive load of transitions.

Mindfulness Activity

The skills instruction session formally begins with a mindfulness activity to help participants focus attention in the present moment. Specific activities are described in the sample curriculum provided in Chapter 7. The goal of these exercises is to orient the person to the current context, as well as to teach the skill of controlling attention.

The mindfulness exercises in the curriculum utilize tapping a Tibetan singing bowl (or some kind of chime) to begin and end the practice or throughout the exercise to cue attention. It is possible to do the mindfulness exercises without a singing bowl or chime (but most members like it). If an instructor wants to purchase a Tibetan bowl, they are available online for around $50.

Following the mindfulness activity, the participants have a discussion, sharing observations made during the exercise. By allowing an opportunity for everyone to describe the experience, individuals practice self-awareness (observing) and self-expression (describing). Mastery of self-awareness behaviors is a crucial primary step that allows for the development of self-acceptance, self-value, and self-trust.

It is crucial that the instructor fully explain all activities. Clear, step-by-step directions are necessary to be sure that participants fully understand what the activity is and what they are invited to do. It is also helpful to highlight any challenges they may experience and possible solutions for difficulties. For example, when explaining how to do a breathing activity, the instructor may want to discuss how the participants' attentions will drift from the breath; the solution is for them to notice their attention wandering and bring it back to their breathing.

"Describe" Questions

"Describe" questions are asked to elicit participants' observations related to group activities or experiences. For example, after the mindfulness breathing exercise, the instructor may ask describe questions to draw out each group member's experiences of the activity. Instructors query, "What did you notice during that activity?"

Skills System Review

Following sharing about the mindfulness activity, the group reviews the Skills List and the System Tools. The instructor can review the Skills System Review Questions (p. 47 of the *Skills System Workbook*) or create fun games that prompt the participants to recall the names and numbers of the skills, as well as the Feelings Rating Scale, Categories of Skills, and Recipe for Skills. Giving newer members the option of looking at their skills notebooks or the Skills Plan Map (p. 219 of the *Skills System Workbook*) during the review offers worked examples that increase participation.

The individual may need hints. Having the cue pictures, inventing gestures, using the initial of the skills, and making sounds can prompt recall and be fun during the review. The goal of the skills review is to store skills knowledge in long-term memory. It is also useful for newer members, who may have joined the group mid-cycle, to review terms of previously covered skills.

The instructor uses the skills review activities as an opportunity to evaluate each participant's skills knowledge. Therefore, it is useful to have every group member participate in this process. Optimally, the individual will move from relying on visual aids to contributing without the materials. The instructor hopes the individual will move from knowing a few skills to knowing all of them. The capacity for expanding knowledge of the terms and independent recall increases the likelihood that skills will be utilized in the natural environment.

Homework Review

Following the Skills System review, the individuals share experiences related to using the skills during the previous week. The instructor can ask a general question, like "Who can tell us about a skill they used this week?" Alternatively, the instructor may want to ask about the specific skill that was taught the previous week: "Who used their Safety Plan this week?" The goal is to cultivate a dialogue about skills application.

During the homework review in group, it may be helpful to use a whiteboard to write down each person's name and the skills chains they used. It is important to reinforce adaptive skills use and individual progress positively. Writing down information allows the instructor to link commonalities between individuals' scenarios.

The homework review process serves to prime the individual's memory to retrieve skills information in preparation for new learning. Building on existing knowledge schemes places lower cognitive load demands, as compared to learning novel information. Review helps promote connections and linkage between concepts in long-term memory; continual usage facilitates recognition and recall.

It is important to use the Quick Step Assessment to evaluate whether scenarios generated in group are useful as teaching examples. If the topic is interesting and applies, it may strike the balance between holding the group's attention and being a good example for skills application. Conversely, if the topic is too provocative and elicits high feelings, cognitive load demands may increase, impeding learning.

Disclosure Questions

The instructor may want to ask participants to share more detail about internal and external factors related to their experiences. Personal examples help the group broaden and contextualize learning. For example, it can help to ask questions such as "Has anyone ever had difficulty doing a Safety Plan? What was difficult about it?" Delving into a personal disclosure can educate the group about challenges and factors that need to be managed in the natural environment.

It is important to help the individual be efficient with disclosures; instructors guide content and time management with the group to ensure that the discussion is focused and allows everyone to participate. While it is often necessary to address human issues that are relevant, detailing highly personal or arousing events may lead to dysregulation of group members.

Clarifying Questions

Clarifying questions may be helpful during homework reviews to promote a deeper and more detailed understanding of a topic. For example, the participant may attempt to describe a situation that happened during the week. The details and time frames may be challenging to follow or vague. The instructor can ask clarifying questions, such as "Can you tell us a little more about that so we can clearly understand?" or "Help me understand. On Tuesday you first had an argument with your coworker, and on Wednesday you called your boss?" The participant may need assistance recalling the chain of events due to sequencing deficits.

Additionally, clarifying questions can help the individual improve self-awareness—for example, "What body sensations did you notice just before you walked in to meet with your boss?" The instructor helps the individual and the group gain clarity and improved understanding; experiencing the process of becoming clearer is an important aspect of learning.

The instructor asks describe, disclosure, and clarifying questions and makes linking statements that highlight commonalities between participants' experiences: "It is interesting that Kevin, James, and Mary were all dealing with challenging coworkers this week." The instructor consolidates points and moves discussions toward the skills topics that are on the agenda for the group. For example, the instructor may choose to focus on work relationships as a relevant context for learning about the skill for the week. Finding common threads helps create a synthesized body of material that is generated from diverse sources. Additionally, linking provides validation that others are having similar experiences.

Orienting to a New Skills Topic

Once the participants have reviewed skills, it is time to introduce the topic for new learning (e.g., Week 4—On-Track Thinking). The instructor gives only a brief overview of the subject. The goal of this introduction is not to teach the material but merely to begin the process of exploring existing knowledge related to the topic.

Discussion: Exploring Existing Knowledge

The instructor cultivates a discussion about the new topic, expanding information that emerged from the homework review. For example, the homework review may have covered the group's experiences using Clear Picture. The discussion that transitions to the new topic (On-Track Thinking) might highlight one or more of those scenarios to prompt more in-depth exploration of what the group members noticed about their thinking and urges in those situations. Focusing on the thoughts and urges in more detail provides the base information for On-Track Thinking—Check It. When the instructor builds from the existing knowledge base and expands the topic to include a small amount of associated new information, cognitive load demands are lower than they are when transitioning to another unrelated topic.

Discussions between group members and the instructors can be useful interventions in Skills System instruction. When participants have an opportunity to self-reflect and express themselves, multiple aspects of growth are served. First, each person is taking skillful action. Additionally, participation in discussions provides an opportunity for the individual to mobilize her core self (self-awareness, acceptance, value, and trust) as she joins in the skills exploration, building self- and skill-efficacy.

Discussions allow participants to witness others grappling with challenges in their lives and applying skills. This process can be validating; discussions can show the individual that she is not the only one who struggles with complex challenges. Hearing other people share their vulnerabilities and use skills to manage situations can model the learning process. The instructor may encourage participation from group members who are actively communicating and engaged with applying skills to reinforce engagement and create examples of others in the group.

Assessment Questions

Assessment questions are designed to assess the individual's existing knowledge of a given topic. For example, if the topic for the session is On-Track Thinking, the skills instructor may ask, "What is the difference between a thought and an urge?" Skills instructors elicit a baseline of information to evaluate each individual's knowledge and abilities.

Participants may offer inaccurate information during discussions. The instructors may choose to positively reinforce the participation and communicate that a more accurate answer is still needed—for example: "Good try . . . almost"; "We are getting closer, but we are not quite there . . . let's keep trying." Using the Quick Step Assessment process, the instructor may adjust his question or give more hints so that group members understand what he is looking for. To ensure that the group knows which information is accurate, the instructor restates key points, offers positive reinforcement, and writes accurate statements on the whiteboard.

The instructor uses verbal praise to reinforce effective behaviors. If the group members worked together to help each other get the right answer, the group can be praised. If one individual offered the correct answer, perhaps targeting him with praise is best. The instructor reinforces both types of on-track behaviors as soon as they happen in group to encourage more adaptive actions.

The instructor can teach a dialectical perspective by carefully constructing her feedback. For example, saying, "Yes, I have noticed that before, too" sends a different message than "You are right." The first option conveys a more dialectical perspective and communicates that there is value or truth in different perspectives. This tactic teaches that there are many sides in a situation versus merely right or wrong alternatives. This dialectical attitude helps teach foundational perspectives that enhance the individual's capacities to engage in reciprocal relationships (being connected with others while maintaining identity). It is more effective to teach dialectics implicitly to individuals diagnosed with intellectual disabilities rather than explicitly. Instructors guide discussions into the gray areas of situations rather than focusing on a black versus white, polarized perspective.

Orienting to Relevant Context

Motivation and interest are key ingredients for learning; relevant contextual questions are intended to highlight how learning new skills will help participants reach personal goals—for example: "How can off-track urges be a problem at work?" and "If you wanted to get a raise from your boss, how would acting on off-track urges impact that?" If the individual sees that managing feelings, thoughts, and action strategically can improve tangible real-life factors, motivation may be increased.

In addition to stimulating interest, using contextual scenarios in group discussions can help store in long-term memory important information about the individuals, the specific context, and more general social contexts. As the group discusses the myriad internal and external facets that comprise the scenario, this behavior and solution analysis process cobbles together a more complete awareness. These bits of information about the situation and skills become integrated into schemata.

During a discussion of relevant context, the instructor leads the group to highlight an important setting (e.g., work). The group members explore their perceptions about effective and ineffective actions in that context (e.g., being focused is on-track; yelling at coworkers is off-track). The individual may understand that learning skills that help him improve focus at work and decrease coworker conflict may increase the likelihood he will get a raise from the employer. The E-Spiral—Exploring Existing Knowledge Base phase provides a foundation for building schemata that new learning and elaboration can expand and strengthen.

Some groups, particularly adolescents, have individuals with high levels of emotional dysregulation (e.g., hypervigilance associated with trauma). Exploring real-life contexts may elicit high feelings and cause immediate cognitive overload. It may be necessary to adjust interventions and create relevant, hypothetical scenarios. Unfortunately, generic situations may not mobilize motivation the way real-life ones do. Perhaps finding stories in the media or about celebrities can be impersonal enough to manage cognitive load demands yet stimulate interest that will sustain learning.

E-Spiral Phase 2: Encoding Activities That Teach the New Topic

Figure 6.7 outlines E-Spiral Phase 2: Encoding Activities That Teach the New Topic. Once the group members have engaged in Exploring Existing Knowledge Base, they are prepared to learn new information. The goal of the E-Spiral—Encoding Phase is to have the participants learn accurate new skills information. A wide variety of encoding activities are used within the Skills System teaching model.

While direct instruction and teaching points are necessary, multimodal techniques are essential as well. Multimodal teaching strategies provide "dual coding" (Najjar, 1996, p. 14) of verbal and nonverbal stimuli, which may improve recall. Handouts, diagrams, cue pictures, gestures, and objects are some of the common strategies used to facilitate encoding of information. Skills instructors must be aware of cognitive load demands when integrating materials; the supplemental information must support familiar points versus presenting divergent infor-

Encoding: Teaching the new topic (new learning)

- Direct instruction that promotes encoding
  - Teaching points
  - Handouts—summary sheets, introductory handouts, and worked examples
  - Diagrams
  - Gestures
  - Objects
- Discussions that promote encoding
  - Content questions

FIGURE 6.7. E-Spiral Phase 2: Encoding.

mation. The Skills System instruction blends encoding visual, spatial, acoustic, and semantic information related to the topic. This multimodal approach helps an impaired learner encode, retain, and retrieve information.

Direct Instruction Activities That Promote Encoding

Teaching Points

Teaching points are excerpts provided within the 12-week-cycle curriculum in Chapter 7. These points are often presented as quotations. The quotes are not intended to prescribe teaching points; rather, they provide a worked example for skills instructors. The teaching points are examples of how to explain the skills concepts. These excerpts are not necessarily meant to be read; rather, they provide the instructor with principles to be translated into her own words. Merely reading the teaching points may be boring and reduce motivation.

Teaching within the Skills System is less oriented around lecture format and more focused on question-and-answer discussions. It is important that correct information be generated during the encoding process. Therefore, the instructor asks clear, directed questions to elicit correct answers—for example: "If you are feeling very upset, is your mind usually clear or fuzzy?" Most participants will state that "fuzzy" is the more accurate answer. Guided discovery questions are not a quiz; they are a way to increase participation and motivation by expanding the individual's existing knowledge. In between questions and answers, the instructor presents teaching points about the concept. Beyond encoding and personal growth benefits, this question–answer format allows the instructor to effectively monitor a participant's integration of concepts.

Handouts

Handouts are useful during Skills System instruction and are referenced throughout the 12-week curriculum provided in Chapter 7. It can be beneficial to print and give each participant a three-ring binder with a set of handouts. Some settings have restrictions on the material that individuals can have; in these cases, the instructor makes the necessary accommodations. Instructors use the Quick Step to determine which handouts to use and how to use them in the teaching.

Basic handouts are available in the *Skills System Workbook,* but instructors can create new ones for groups and individual skills training as needed. For example, it may be helpful for skills instructors to individualize handouts. Integrating digital pictures, using fun clip art, or scanning photographs may increase engagement. The instructor must be careful to keep visual aids simple and clear to help minimize cognitive load demands of the materials.

Most of the worksheets in the *Skills System Workbook* include worked examples. These serve as a guide for how the worksheet could be completed. These are important because they offer instructors scaffolding to understand the concepts being taught. Additionally, worked examples offer a model to the individual that is less personal, allowing her to focus on the skill concept in a way that reduces cognitive load. Reviewing a worked example can facilitate encoding and begin the elaboration process.

Diagrams

Drawing diagrams on a blackboard, large presentation pad, or whiteboard during discussions can be useful. Diagrams provide visual encoding of information. For example, as the group is discussing how a person can use a Safety Plan, the instructor may draw a diagram of an ascending arc marked with a 0, 1, 2, 3, 4, and 5, and show how a person escalated from a Level 1 feeling up to a Level 5 feeling (harming self, others, or property). Figure 6.8 is an example of a simple drawing that can explain intangible concepts more clearly.

The diagram can show the progression from one level to the next and associated behaviors. Then the group may discuss what skills might have been used to change the outcome. A new arc may be drawn to show what the progression could have looked like if the individual had utilized effective skills earlier in the situation. Visually mapping situations can aid comprehension because the diagram implicitly teaches relationships between various factors.

Utilizing different colors makes activities more fun. Use of different-colored markers can help the participants understand associations between concepts. For example, using orange in every Clear Picture handout creates an association between Clear Picture and orange. Using red to represent On-Track Thinking helps the person see the difference between information in orange and in red. Color-coding diagrams can improve organization of information and enhance explicit and implicit learning (Gold, 1972).

Gestures

Gestures are useful techniques during teaching because they can create tangible representations for abstract concepts. Referencing helpful (on-track to the goal) with a thumbs up and not helpful (off-track to the goal) with a thumbs down is an example of using gestures. Gestures can draw on common knowledge that requires minimal cognitive load.

Objects

Objects are fun and useful. For example, a Tibetan singing bowl or bell is a basic tool in a Skills System group. Ringing of the bell is a cue to focus during the mindfulness activity; listening to multiple rings may also engage second-phase processing. Other objects, such as

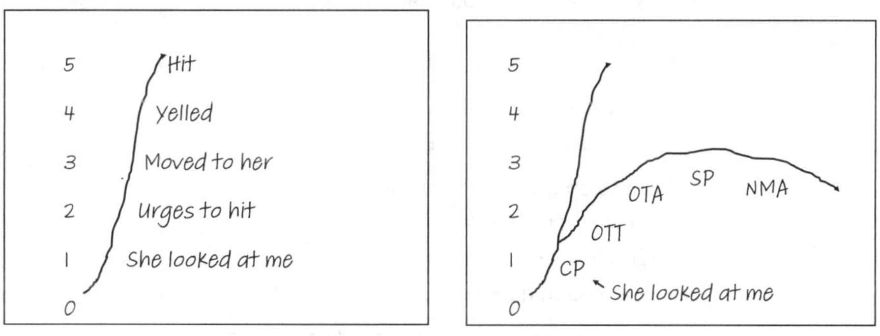

FIGURE 6.8. Examples of diagrams on a whiteboard.

pom-poms, can be used for Cheerleading thoughts, and red flags can be used to signify risks. Skills instructors can find various objects that represent facets of the Skills System and serve to prompt recall.

Discussions That Promote Encoding

Content Questions

Content questions ask the individual to recall information that has been previously introduced: "What is the first step in the Clear Picture skill?" It is important to expose the group to multiple rehearsals of information, so that material is stored in long-term memory. Asking questions about the separate chunks of information can increase the chances the individual learns a concept and is able to assemble it in skills chains. When the individual gets an answer wrong, the instructor remains positive. Statements such as "Almost!" or "You're close—try again!" instead of "No, that's wrong," are helpful.

E-Spiral Phase 3: Activities That Promote Elaboration

Figure 6.9 outlines the E-Spiral Phase 3: Activities that Promote Elaboration. Elaboration is an expanded encoding process that creates "additional memory records that improve the ability of the individual to retrieve the original memory" (Najjar, 1996, p. 14). There are two important aspects of elaboration: (1) expanding knowledge and (2) linking knowledge. In the Elaboration Phase, the participants practice the skills concepts, integrating previous skills knowledge and the new learning.

Activities That Promote Elaboration

Worksheets

There are many worksheets included in the *Skills System Workbook.* While it may be logistically challenging and time-consuming to complete worksheets during group, it can be helpful

Elaboration: Practicing new learning and linking it to previous learning (practice)

- Activities that promote elaboration
  - Worksheets
  - Practice exercises
  - Collaborative feedback
  - Individual instruction
- Discussion that promote elaboration
  - Linking questions
  - Disclosure questions
  - Expansion questions

FIGURE 6.9. E-Spiral Phase 3: Elaboration.

to have individuals list out responses to the prompts on the whiteboard. This group activity can maximize the benefits of collaborative learning and minimize barriers related to participants writing during group. If an instructor is using the curriculum with non-English speakers, this activity can be a way to reduce reliance on handouts and teach the material in the native language.

Individuals in Skills System group often have highly variable levels of academic abilities. Instructors need to personalize the means through which worksheets are completed. One person may be able to complete worksheets independently, while another may require support. The participant may have specific support staff, group members, friends, or family members who help complete paperwork with them. There may be benefits to the person's individual therapist helping to fill out the worksheets. Instructors ask participants about their plan to complete the homework assignment prior to leaving group.

Practice Exercises

Practice exercises are a vital aspect of the learning process. For example, when the group is learning about breathing, it is essential to practice breathing. Talking about breathing teaches about the topic, yet the experience of practicing breathing teaches at a broader and deeper level. Contextual learning that does not lead to cognitive overload facilitates retrieval and generalization. Skills instructors should be creative during group and design practice exercises in the moment that integrate the relevant context and content being covered. Instructors should not be reliant solely on the practice exercises provided in this curriculum. For example, if a discussion comes up about voice tone, the instructor can create an impromptu exercise in which each group member says something using a wimpy, then an aggressive, then an assertive tone.

Collaborative Feedback

It is helpful to offer feedback to the individual during and after a practice exercise. Asking the individual if he would like feedback, before offering it, gives him control in the situation and creates a reciprocal interaction between individual and instructor—for example: "Brian, would you like to get feedback about your voice tone?" The instructor can also ask the individual if he would like feedback from the group. Collaborative feedback is intended to explore whether the individual's actions in the exercise would work to reach his desired outcome. An example of a collaborative approach might be "Brian, I noticed that when you were trying to be assertive, you were looking down. Did you notice that?" The instructor may ask Brian more specific questions or ask the group to delve into a topic to cover the point less directly.

Individual Instruction

During discussions or practice activities, it may be necessary to provide individual instruction for certain participants. If the teaching point is relatively brief, doing the individualized teaching in group is beneficial for the individual and the group. Another participant may have the same issue and would gain from the clarification. If the individual has significant difficulties or if review of the material would disrupt group, meeting with the skills instructor following group to create a plan may be a better option.

Discussions That Support Elaboration

Discussions are another important tool in cultivating elaboration. Once the group has worked on practicing the skill, it is helpful to engage in a discussion that links previous and present learning. During this phase, the skills instructor asks questions that link information, promote personal disclosure, and expand awareness of topics.

Linking Questions

Linking questions are designed to foster elaboration of learning through connecting new with past learning. One example might be, "You mentioned earlier in group that you hit a housemate when she stared at you. How do you think what we learned about the Safety Plan today might have been helpful in that situation?" It is important to be nonjudgmental during discussions; highlighting what behaviors tend to elicit desired results is different than saying a person's choice was good or bad. Skills instructors may comment about experiences but preaching and being overcontrolling are not effective strategies.

Linking questions can also be used to prompt the group to assemble skills chains—for example: "Once Mary does a Safety Plan in that situation, what other skill might be helpful?" Similarly, asking the numbers of the skill chain creates linkages, for example if the instructor wants the group to understand that Safety Plan is a 1234 and adding a New-Me Activity would be a 12345. These types of quantitative activities may be initially challenging, but with practice, quantitative reasoning related to skills can improve.

Expansion Questions

Expansion questions are designed to broaden the scope of the individual's understanding of a concept. For example, the skills instructor may ask, "What other skills would you use in that situation?" Asking the "what–if" questions help the individual learn about various options and the impact on situations. Participants need to know that different actions work well in diverse circumstances. Expansion questions can help a participant understand unusual situations when traditional approaches may be ineffective. For example, the individual needs to know that yelling at people is an important skill in certain situations; the lessons are about using the right skills at the right time. This is an important aspect of learning how to generalize skills in diverse contexts.

E-Spiral Phase 4: Activities That Advance Efficacy

Figure 6.10 outlines Activities that Advance Efficacy. Efficacy-oriented exercises are designed to increase the likelihood that the individual will be able to (and want to) perform a skill in her natural environment. There are two important elements of this phase: (1) being able to use the skill in context, and (2) commitment to using the skill. Retrieval of information is improved if the learning and retrieval contexts are similar. Preparing the individual for real life through situational learning promotes generalization and self-efficacy. Unfortunately, contextual learning and real-life execution of skills creates high cognitive load. It may be necessary to do role

Efficacy: Bridging to real life (real life)

- Activities that promote efficacy
  - Role play
  - Psychodrama
  - *In vivo*
- Discussion promoting efficacy
  - Barrier questions
  - Wisdom questions
  - Commitment questions
  - Coaching questions
- Group-ending activities
  - Homework
  - Mindfulness breathing

FIGURE 6.10. E-Spiral Phase 4: Efficacy.

play, psychodrama, and *in vivo* practice. Although contextual learning may promote improved integration of skills, these activities may elicit higher levels of feelings. It is important to monitor contextual learning activities carefully to manage cognitive load factors.

Activities That Promote Efficacy

Role Play

Role-play activities are important aspects of Skills System teaching. Ideally, each participant will have an opportunity to participate in role play. Time constraints may impact these activities. Dividing into pairs or small groups may increase opportunities for participation.

The skills instructor and the participants work collaboratively to discuss options and solutions in role-play scenarios. The instructors may request that participants act out various action options to help visualize diverse factors and outcomes. The group can explore how things work and what are natural reactions through role plays. This process provides validation and an experience that advances self-efficacy.

Psychodrama Techniques

Psychodrama enactments often expand on traditional role plays by having additional group members play roles that represent various internal and external components within a situation. For example, if an individual role-plays talking to his house manager, one group member can role-play the participant's On-Track Thinking, and another can articulate off-track thinking. This expanded role-play technique is helpful, because the participant can listen to both types of thinking and make an on-track decision. This technique makes intangible forces (e.g., thoughts) more tangible for participants. Additionally, this exercise helps the individual experience real-life pressures and sensations related to the context within which skills will need to be demonstrated. If the person is struggling, he can ask groupmates to assist as skills coaching voices. Behavioral rehearsal under these contextual conditions helps improve the individual's capacity to perform skills outside of group.

It is important to build the complexity of a psychodrama slowly to manage cognitive load demands. Instructors may want to assemble the players gradually so that the activity does not overstimulate the group. It may be useful to pose the rule that one person speaks at a time. Psychodrama techniques "use active/interactive techniques that stimulate more sensory and affective modes of learning than the verbal modality alone" (Tomasulo, 2005, p. 1). While engaging sensory and emotional aspects might have benefits in this process, when working with individuals who experience significant dysregulation, the skills instructor must proceed cautiously.

In Vivo Exercises

In vivo exercises utilize elements of a participant's actual life rather than creating a contrived environment. Support providers and/or family members may be invited to individual skills instruction sessions for *in vivo* activities. For example, the instructor may ask whether the participant wants to practice a skill with her staff, who is in the waiting room. The instructor may function as a skills coach.

Following the exercise, participant and instructor have a rich opportunity to process the experience. The instructor gains a firsthand view of both parties and therefore becomes a more effective skills coach for the participant. *In vivo* exercises may be an important vehicle for generalization of skills into daily life and relationships.

Discussions That Promote Efficacy

Discussions can be designed to improve efficacy. For example, participants can discuss common challenges related to using skills and/or communicating each individual's personal commitment to using skills. Through these discussions, participants communicate personal opinions, make a public commitment, and plan for integrating skills into their lives that strengthen the individual's core self.

Barrier Questions

Generalization of skills may be difficult due to barriers that are encountered in each unique situation. Feelings, thoughts, action urges, and external forces may interplay to create challenges for the individual. The individual must learn to become aware of barriers so that contingency planning is possible. Barrier questions are designed to help him develop a realistic awareness of challenges he may encounter. For example, the instructor might ask, "How closely will you have to work with that person tomorrow at your job?" or "Will seeing her make it harder to stay on-track?" It is useful to explore specific factors that may happen before, during, and after events that affect the individual's ability to focus on or perform skills.

It is important for the individual to understand that all people are impacted by seemingly small issues; everyone faces challenges and skill barriers throughout each day. Self-invalidation can lower self-efficacy in that the individual perceives herself to be more dysfunctional than other people. Barrier questions are a great way to expand knowledge base about the natural environment, provide validation, and help create realistic expectations.

Wisdom Questions

Wisdom questions ask the participant to share personal perspectives about a topic: "Which option do you feel would best fit?" or "As you look at these choices, which is a fit for you?" Helping the individual cultivate self-reflection, consider personal perspectives, and find a sense of wisdom are important self-validating behaviors.

Commitment Questions

Commitment questions are a series of queries that guide the individual in deciding whether he is going to engage in a certain behavior. The question first poses whether the person values taking the action. For example, an instructor might ask, "James, when are you going to practice Getting It Right?" Once the person commits to using the skill, the instructor then tries to get the individual to commit to a plan of action: "James, you mentioned that you wanted to learn to use Getting It Right with your boss. What is your plan to do that?"; "You sound as if you are committed to using skills with your boss. What exactly is your plan?" The instructor can highlight the barriers and double-check whether the individual is willing, ready, and able to start the plan—for example: "We have already talked about all of the things that are going to be difficult about this; are you sure you are ready to give this a try?" It is vital that the individual knows how to seek skills coaching support when challenges are encountered.

Coaching Questions

Coaching questions prompt the participant to consider what skills would be helpful in a situation. Coaching questions are useful during the Efficacy Phase, after the individual makes a public commitment to use skills: "James, what skills are you going to use if your feelings go over a Level 3 when you are talking to your boss?" Coaching questions help create a plan for times when it is challenging to use skills.

Coaching questions may also be helpful when a participant is experiencing stress in skills training. For example, the leader can ask, "What skills could help you handle this exercise?" Depending on the individual's level of skills knowledge, the instructor may offer suggestions to the participant: "Do you think doing a Safety Plan right now would help?" When the individual is over a Level 3 feeling, the instructor may want to ask the individual to go to the waiting area or meet with his support staff individually. If the individual rises above a Level 4 feeling, it may be necessary to move the other participants to another area if there are safety risks.

Group-Ending Activities

At the end of group, the leader assigns homework to be completed between sessions. Home study activities can increase skills knowledge, generalization, and efficacy. As the individual increases knowledge about skills, she is encouraged to participate in ongoing, self-directed, skillful behaviors in daily living. The skills instructor focuses on fostering the individual's internal motivation and commitment to maintain skillful behavior. The following activities are a few home study options that can be assigned by the instructor and/or utilized by the individual for independent study.

Homework Assignments

The primary homework assignments within the Skills System are to practice specific and/or nonspecific skills use. In addition, the instructor may assign worksheets or practice exercises (from the *Skills System Workbook,* online, or created by the instructor) as homework. The individual may complete these sheets independently or with support. The focus of these assignments is not the reading and writing, but the content of the worksheet. It is not critical that the individual fill out the paper. When homework assignments are given, each individual makes a plan about how to accomplish the assignment. The Skills System homework assignments are generally simple, so that a person can be successful. The instructor may give special homework assignments to particular group members for individualized study.

Skills Cards

Skills cards are a fun home study and group activity. Skills flash cards help an individual (or group) learn the components of each skill and the System Tools. Cards give the individual a chance to engage physically to learn names, numbers, and pictures associated with the skills. An individual or group can put the skills cards in order on a large table or on the floor. The cards can be put together in skills chains to represent skills that were or could be used in a scenario. In group, an instructor can also ask quiz questions and the individual can search the skills cards for the correct answer. Making practice fun enhances skills elaboration and generalization.

The individual can do partnership activities with family members, friends, and/or support providers to enhance skills capacities of both people. The Skills System can create a common skills language, as well as promote a reciprocal relationship between the individual and the other person. As the individual teaches the people around him, he fosters a sense of mastery and self-efficacy.

Skills Games

Skills games are a great way to practice skills. Many games can be adapted as a skills game. Who Wants to Be a Skillionaire or Skills Jeopardy are fun skills trivia activities. The instructor or participants develop skills questions and create a game show format. Many other games can be turned into skills activities by setting a rule that to take a move or receive a token, for example, the participant must correctly answer a skills question.

Skills Journaling

The person may choose to write in a journal. Focusing on exploring self-awareness, self-expression, and descriptive skills can be advantageous. Ruminating on past issues or current problems may be less helpful than highlighting a problem and writing about possible skills that could be used to manage the difficulty effectively.

Phone Consultation and Skills Coaching

When the Skills System is used in conjunction with DBT, phone skills coaching by the individual therapist is integrated into the treatment model (Linehan, 1993a). This mode of treatment facilitates generalization of skills in the natural environment. It is important to establish and follow mutually agreed-upon rules for skills coaching calls.

TRANSITION TO CHAPTER 7

Chapter 7 is a worked example of a 12-week curriculum. The skills instructor should read the entire section through, prior to starting a group. Each week, the instructor focuses on the week's materials, integrating information from Chapters 5 and 6, to create effective teaching plans for skills groups.

CHAPTER 7

Skills System 12-Week-Cycle Curriculum

Chapter 7 contains a sample 12-week-cycle curriculum. Each week of this framework includes a detailed teaching plan and options for future cycles through the material. The instructor will notice that instructions and explanations are presented as quotes. This format is intended to provide a worked example for instructors rather than to prescribe language. All Skills System visual aid materials are contained in the *Skills System Workbook* (sold separately).

It is impossible to predict whether the group will complete a teaching plan. Different settings have varying time frames for group sessions. Additionally, the instructor must remember that the academic abilities of group members are unique. This curriculum is a general guide for an instructor. It is unlikely that all planned activities will be completed during the time frames that are available to the group.

There is a Lesson Planning worked example and worksheet in the Appendix of this book. The Lesson Planning worksheet lists different elements of a group and has space for the instructor to write down activities he may want to do with the group to fulfill each element. While it is important to be flexible, making adjustments to the plan and having a list of ideas can reduce cognitive load for the instructor.

Creativity is an important feature of effective instruction. Instructors are encouraged to develop various skills exercises, games, and practice activities that reflect the capacities, interests, and contexts of the group members. It is important to remember that a creative intervention does not necessarily need to be complex. Keeping an activity simple and clear can often facilitate more learning while maintaining a lower cognitive load. Overcomplicating interventions may not only increase cognitive load but also muddy the key points you are trying to make. The DBT term "one-mindfully" or "one thing in the moment" (Linehan, 2025a, p. 447) helps the instructor remember to have the individual focus on a single element to reap maximum benefit from the experience.

In the event that the group does not complete the outlined material, instructors must determine whether to return to that week's materials during the next group or move on. If the group continues on, the remainder of the previous week's lessons can be addressed when the group returns to those topics in the following cycle through the curriculum. It is challenging to leave material unfinished, yet it may be the best long-term alternative. It is vital that an individual develop a broad understanding of the Skills System, so that she can deepen awareness within the full range of Skills System topics. Focusing on a few elements in depth may increase understanding of those topics, yet hinder development of overall emotion regulation capacities and generalization of Skills System concepts. Although it is difficult, it is recommended that the group leave unfinished topics and progress to the following week's teaching. Do what you can and keep marching forward. As you gain a fuller understanding of the Skills System and the skills group, it will be easier to create realistic and effective teaching plans.

The 12-week-cycle curriculum presents detailed teaching suggestions. Participants will have a wide variety of responses to the activities and discussion questions. Although the script presented below assumes compliance and participation, the realities may be very different in a skills instruction session. For example, the instructor may encounter silence, partial answers, irreverent attitudes, belligerence, and/or dissociation all at the same time! It may be necessary for the instructor to use his skills during group to remain on-track to the learning goals. The following suggestions may help the skills instructor when the group is not going well.

HELPFUL HINTS FOR THE INSTRUCTOR

We offer some strategies for the instructor when one or more group members are not engaged, but are not harming themself, others, or property.

- The instructor can take a few breaths and get a Clear Picture of the present moment.
- The instructor can self-reflect as to whether her mindset, tone, and interventions are on-track. An agitated, judgmental, or impatient instructor can trigger problematic transactions and resistance from the group. Check It, Turn It Up, and Cheerleading may be useful to try. A more careful chain analysis after group may help the instructor make changes in tactics for future groups.
- Utilizing the Quick Step Assessment to evaluate and adjust interventions can help the instructor assess whether one or more group members are experiencing high cognitive load. Cognitive overload can have myriad presentations that disrupt harmony in group. The instructor makes necessary adjustments to simplify and/or break down topics further—for example, asking questions or framing points in alternative ways to prompt engagement.
- The instructor may consider offering skills coaching to an individual experiencing stress. The instructor may ask questions to elicit Clear Picture and On-Track Thinking as the first steps; if the person is more dysregulated, the instructor may help the individual take an On-Track Action. Reminding the individual about her goals, capacities, and skills can help her get back on-track. To help normalize the experience, it may be useful to acknowledge that learning new things can be a challenging experience.
- Initiating a brief breathing exercise may help the participants and instructors improve focus. Shifting to a game form can Switch Tracks as well. The instructor needs to be mindful of behavioral principles, in that having off-track group members control the group lesson plan on a long-term basis is not in anyone's best interest.

- If a participant is experiencing a Level 3 or higher feeling, Safety Planning may be warranted. It may be helpful for the person to do a Solo New-Me Activity while remaining in group, move to a different area in the room, or leave the group. The individual could do a Focus New-Me Activity in the waiting area (e.g., puzzle or card sorting) and return when she is more on-track.
- If the individual refuses to leave the area, the group may have to evacuate the room. It is essential that the skills instructor notice the early warning signs for an individual who is likely to demonstrate violent behaviors. Taking precautions and intervening efficiently is necessary to protect the well-being of the other group members. Having two exits in a group room is optimal. After a problematic event in group, it may be helpful to debrief the other group members to discuss skills that the participants used to manage the event.
- The instructor may need to be cautious about using significant group time to do skills coaching if it is not pertinent for the topic. It may be necessary to ask a participant who does not regain control to step into the waiting area to do Safety Planning with his support staff. Following the group, the instructor may want to review the event and work with the individual to create an On-Track Action Plan for group.

Facilitating any type of therapeutic group can be challenging. It is impossible to know how each individual is going to react. It may be helpful to have co-leaders or other staff members as resources in case there are difficulties. If the instructor is alone, it may be difficult for him to monitor individuals that leave group in a dysregulated state. If there are risk issues such as these, it is important to have procedures in place to manage dangerous situations.

The following sections present options for leading skills groups. A newer skills instructor will want to review this information prior to group and organize a teaching plan. The instructor may make a copy of that week's curriculum, highlighting key points and handouts to review. An instructor working with a stable group may decide to follow the curriculum in the book, reading teaching points; this could be a more collaborative learning approach. More experienced instructors who know the Skills System concepts well may have more unplanned, organic approaches. Generally speaking, the 12-week-curriculum lesson plans in the following sections are merely a guide and should not be followed verbatim if they do not fit for the individual or group. The handouts, worked examples, and worksheets used in this curriculum are in the *Skills System Workbook.* Worked examples specifically designed for the developmental level of elementary school-age children and high school-age youth are available on the workbook's companion website.

WEEK 1: THE SKILLS LIST

Preparing for Group

Handouts Needed

✓ Learning Skills, System Tools Review Questions (p. 47 of *Skills System Workbook*)
✓ Learning Skills, Skills List Handout 1 (p. 23)
✓ Learning Skills, Skills List Handout 2 (p. 24)

E-Spiral Phase 1. Exploring Existing Knowledge Base (Review)

➡ ***Welcome group.*** "Hello, everyone! How are you all doing today? [Wait for response.] OK, it is wonderful to see you all; I am very excited about beginning a skills group with you. Are we ready to get to know each other? We are going to jump in with our first On-Track Action by introducing ourselves. If you are feeling a little shy, notice that feeling and tell us your name anyway! Who is really brave and would like to start?"

Note: Skills instructors may want to consider entering the group and greeting participants in a friendly and positive way. Engaging in chitchat is an opportunity for the skills instructor to better understand who the individual is, what is important to her, and how she currently regulates feelings. Instructors can use the information to begin the process of doing a Quick Step Assessment in group for each member.

When the group is beginning or new members join, participants should introduce themselves to each other. Instructors may begin by having group members share their names. The group leader may also have group members share a piece of fun personal information—for example: "What is your favorite kind of pizza?" or "What is your favorite TV show?" If the group members are already familiar with each other, the leader may request that each person respond to questions such as "What are you hoping to learn from this group?" or "What is one of your goals?" The leader is trying to create a comfortable and safe therapeutic environment. Validating the challenges of starting a new group may be helpful.

After reviewing names, it is important that the group members talk about the goal of the group. The leader asks a few simple questions, such as "What do we study in this group?" or "Why do we do that?" Not all group members may know why they are there. Additionally, they may not be there voluntarily. The instructor may want to validate challenges of joining a group and communicate enthusiasm about helping group members reach their personal goals.

➡ ***Orient to the mindfulness activity: noticing the breath.*** "OK, is everyone ready to learn some skills? Great, let's get started. We are going to begin by noticing our breathing."

Note: After introductions, group leaders want to orient the group to the first group activity. Instructors are prepared to deal with a client saying "no" to invitations; keep invitations open and move on to interact with an individual who is actively participating. It may be helpful to check in with the nonparticipating person after group to do problem solving, if necessary. Additionally, as mentioned in the previous chapter, this curriculum uses a Tibetan singing bowl or chime in mindfulness activities. The auditory cue helps the participants begin and end tasks. Adjust the instructions as needed to accommodate not using a bowl or chime.

Instructions for the mindfulness exercise. "We begin every group by doing a mindfulness practice. Today we will start with a simple breathing exercise. When we focus our attention on our breathing, we are being mindful. We are using our minds to pay attention to our breath, as it is, without changing it. Unfortunately, our minds are not always easy to control. That's why we have to practice being mindful. The cool thing is that when we are mindful, we are very focused on what is happening right now. Noticing our breath is actually a really important skill, and it is so simple. When we notice our breathing, it helps us be aware and focused, even in stressful and emotional situations. Are you ready to hear about what we have to do? Are you ready to give 100% when we do this exercise? OK, first, please sit in a comfortable position with your eyes open. Then I will ring the bowl six times [involves tapping the bowl with a small wooden striker]. When you hear the first ring, begin to notice your breathing. Notice how your body feels as the air goes in and out. Notice whether you breathe through your mouth or your nose. Usually our minds try to wander to other things. Sometimes we think of the past or the future. Notice where your mind goes and gently bring your mind back to noticing your breath. You may notice feelings inside of you; notice your feelings and bring your attention back to your breathing. One of our goals is to learn to control and shift our attention; this activity helps us practice that. Do you have any questions?"

Note: Careful and detailed instructions about the tasks and how to reorient are important. After the exercise, the group members review the mindfulness activity and share details describing what they noticed. The instructor may want to write down the observations on the board. It is important to reinforce effort and participation. This exercise is intended to teach awareness of attention and the action of reorienting attention to the breath.

Describe questions. Perhaps choose a few questions to ask: "Were you breathing through you nose or mouth?"; "Where did you feel the breath in your body?"; "Did you notice it in different places: your nose, chest, or belly?"; "Did your breathing change at all?"; "Did you notice the bell sound?"; "Did you notice your attention drifting away?"; "What did you do to bring your attention back?"

➡ ***Orient to Skills System review.*** "Great describing and sharing. After doing our mindfulness practice each week, we will review the Skills List and other important Skills System information. Since it is our first week, we will jump right into new learning. Next week, we will review our skills at this time in group."

Note: In other cycles through Week 1, the skills review can include either answering the Skills System Review Questions (*Skills System Workbook,* p. 47) or doing a creative skills review activity that prompts recall of the names and numbers of each skill, along with the basics of the Feelings Rating Scale, Categories of Skills, and Recipe for Skills. The instructor uses the review process to evaluate how participants are integrating the information. The weekly assessment helps the instructor shape and expand each participant's skills knowledge base.

➡ ***Orient to skills practice.*** "Great job! Not only do we have to remember the names and numbers of the skills, but we practice using our skills at home. Each week we will share with each other about a time when we used our skills during the week. So our homework every week is to use our skills and to be willing to talk about it at the next group. The more skills we use the better! Sound OK? Great."

Disclosure questions. "I bet folks are using some skills to handle tough situations. Who would like to tell us about a challenging time this week that they were able to manage? What did you do that was helpful?"

Note: In the first week of Cycle 1, the group discusses existing coping skills that the members used during the week. The leader then can label the skill using the Skills System names. For example, if the individual labels a feeling, the instructor can say, "That's a good Clear Picture."

The activity of labeling existing skills can help the individual understand that she already has basic capacities that will be enhanced. Otherwise, in later groups, the instructor will say more specifically, "Let's talk about how we used Clear Picture this week," depending on the assignment from the week before.

➡ ***Orient to new skills topic.*** "I think many of you are already using some of the skills, and you don't know it! Today we are going to talk together about different ways we handle stressful situations. You might feel shy, but it is great to jump in with both feet and share your ideas and opinions. Ready?"

Note: Questions that are provided are samples. The instructor can choose one, none, or all to discuss. Each group marches through the material differently, the instructor capitalizing on available teachable moments.

Discuss existing knowledge about the new topic.

Assessment questions. "What is stress?"; "What are feelings?"; "What is it like when feelings go high?"

Relevant context questions. "What kinds of situations stress us out?"; "Is it sometimes hard for people to do things that are helpful in these situations"; "Why do you think that is?"

➡ ***Orient to relevant context of the new topic.*** "Great discussion—thank you all. It seems as if all of us have seen or done both helpful and not helpful things when we are in tough situations. Life is very difficult sometimes for all of us. [Cite specific examples given previously in the group.] As we have heard, our thoughts and our feelings can be overwhelming and hard to handle. The Skills System can help us stay on-track even when life gets stressful. We have already learned an important skill today: noticing our breath. It can help in stressful situations. We are already on our way to learning skills!"

E-Spiral Phase 2. Encoding: New Learning

➡ ***Orient to new learning: Skills List.*** "The Skills System helps us learn how to control our behaviors so that we can reach our goals. These nine skills help us do things that help us feel better and get what we need. Right now we are going to learn the names, numbers, and pictures of the nine skills in the Skills System. How many skills are there in the Skills System?" [Group: "Nine!"; Instructor: "All together, how many?"; Group: "NINE!"] Great, see, you are already getting it! I knew you could do this! Are you ready to learn more about how to handle things well? Great."

Instructions for the encoding activity. "Let's all find Learning Skills, Skills List Handout 1. It is on page 23 and it looks like this. [Hold up the page and be sure each participant has the page before continuing.] Would someone like to read, or would you like me to? We are going to read the number and name of each skill. We are also going to discuss each skill picture and what it means. Any questions?"

Note: After reading each skill, the group talks about each skill picture. They discuss the skill and the relevance of the picture to the skill. If a group member reads and the communication is unclear, the instructor repeats the section so that each group member clearly understands the information. The group moves through the teaching material; leaders may have to limit group reading if it hinders progression through the information.

➡ ***Orient to reviewing Learning Skills, Skills List Handout 2.*** "OK, fantastic. Now we have to read Learning Skills, Skills List Handout 2: How Our Skills Help Us. It is on page 24 and looks like this. Would anyone like to read?"

Note: This handout is used as an overview to introduce group members to the function of each skill. This handout is not intended to be used as an in-depth teaching tool. A brief explanation about each skill as time allows is useful.

➡ ***Orient to the end of the Encoding Phase.*** "Does anyone have any questions about that handout? Great, now we are going to practice some of what we have learned."

E-Spiral Phase 3. Elaboration: Practice and Linking

➡ ***Orient to the elaboration activity.*** "So, we have gone over the Skills List once, and now we are going to practice it more, so that we can learn and remember the information. The more we go over this, the easier it is to remember the skills when we need them."

Instructions for the elaboration exercise. Note: Sample exercises A–G are listed below; choose one exercise per cycle. Elaboration exercises ask participants to practice recognition and recall of skills material in a noncontextual format. This phase focuses on having participants expand their capacities effectively to demonstrate the tasks with increasingly less support.

The activities listed below can be completed with or without visual aid materials. The group can begin using handouts as a worked example, then shift away from using the cues as confidence builds. The instructor may allow each individual to make a personal decision as to whether she wants to look at the sheet, although prompting the individual to stretch and try to close the book may be helpful at some point.

The exercises below become progressively more difficult; thus, during initial cycles through the curriculum, easier exercises minimize cognitive load demands. Be sure to explain the exercise so that the group members clearly understand the activity. Leaders and groups can invent fun ways to practice the numbers and names of skills that fit the learning needs of the participants.

Options for Basic Review Exercises

A. The skills instructor says a number from 1 to 9 and the group reads the skill name from the handout. The group members try to get quicker and more accurate as the exercise progresses.

B. Using handouts to guide them, the group members put the skills cards representing the numbers, pictures, initials, and skills names in order on a large table or the floor.

C. The leader creates a competition between individuals or teams. She holds up one of the skills cards and asks a question about another element of the skill. For example, if she holds up a card with a "2," the group may have to say the associated skill name, describe the skill picture, or tell the initials. The team that gets it correct gets a point.

D. The group members close their books. A group leader writes 1–9 on the board. The group members try to fill in the blank spaces.

E. With no visual aids, a leader asks the group to say the nine skills in order.

F. With no visual aids, a group leader says a number, and the group members say the skill.

G. A group leader has a group member say the first skill, and the next person says the second, and so on.

Describe question. "How was that exercise for you?"

➡ ***Orient to discussion.*** "I think you all did a great job with that exercise. Now, we are going to talk together about skills, so that we can begin to understand them a little better."

Note: The goal of an elaboration-oriented discussion is to begin the process of linking, personalizing, and expanding the participants' semantic knowledge related to the new learning; connecting past and present learning increases integration of the material.

Linking question. "Have any of you used skills like these in the past?"

Disclosure question. "Can you tell us about a time in the past when you had problems handling thoughts or feelings?"

Expansion questions. "Has anyone else had a similar experience?"; "Do you think that there are times when knowing skills would help you reach your goals?"

Note: These discussions are not intended to delve into traumatic memory material or detailed accounts of events. The instructor listens to the specific point that is being made, then creates a general statement that applies to all participants. For example, "That situation with your coworker sounds difficult. So, are coworker relationships situations in which we need to use our skills? Has anyone else had challenges with coworkers?"

➡ ***Orient to the end of the Elaboration Phase.*** "I can't believe how much you all know about skills already. We are going to do very well with the Skills System."

E-Spiral Phase 4. Efficacy: Bridge to Real Life

➡ ***Orient to efficacy activities.*** "It is important to have fun while we are learning, so that we will like doing it. Right now we are going to play a game."

Note: It is important to have group members participate in activities. During the first cycle through the Skills System curriculum, games, worksheets, and role plays are simple and brief. Over time, leaders can design more complex, lengthy activities that foster generalization of skills information.

Instructions for efficacy activities. "I am going to ask the group some questions. Raise your hand if you think you know the answer. If you want to look at your handouts, that's OK. Ready?"

"What is the name of the skill that helps us fix our problems?"

"What skill helps me know what is going on inside and outside of me?"

"What skill is it when I enjoy a cup of tea and have a snack?"

"What skill is it when I do something to get back on-track?"

"What skill is it when I tell someone how I feel?"

"What skill is it when I think about how to handle a situation?"

"What skill is it when I try to get what I want?"

"What skill helps me handle risky situations?"

"What skill is it when I show my friend that I care about them?"

Note: This activity is intended to elicit correct answers. When the individual guesses incorrectly, the skills instructor may say, "Close," "Almost," or "Try one more time," rather than "No, that's wrong." It may be necessary for a leader to give hints so that the group gets the correct answer. These questions are suggestions; instructors may adapt questions to ensure success for the participants.

Review questions. "How do you think that game went?"; "Was it hard to remember the skills?"

➡ ***Orient to discussion.*** "I thought you all did really well. We are going to take a few minutes to chat together before we leave for the day."

Note: The goal of these efficacy-oriented questions is to help the individual understand realistic challenges related to the topic. The discussion offers an opportunity for self-reflection about the learning. Participants are invited to make a personal commitment and plan for integrating the skill into their lives.

Barrier question. "So far, what is difficult for you about learning the Skills System?"

Wisdom question. "Do you think that it is important for you to learn skills?"

Commitment questions. Asking one or more of these commitment questions can help increase motivation: "Are you willing to face the challenge of trying new things?"; "Are you willing to learn and practice skills in group and in your life?"; "Are you willing to do some homework for group?"

Coaching question. "How can you coach yourself to learn and practice skills?"

➡ ***Orient to home study.*** "We can see that learning skills is challenging. It also sounds as if we all know that practice will help us get better at skills. We may not love doing homework, so it is a good thing that we have our On-Track Action skill to help us jump into our practicing!

This week for homework, we are going to start learning our skills. Perhaps look over your skills handouts. Next week in group, we will review our skills. Also, notice your breath this week as many times as you can. We will talk about when you noticed your breathing and what you noticed about it. Do you have any questions?

"If anyone would like to study skills at home this week, you can go to the Learning Skills section of the *Skills System Workbook* and do the Skills List Worksheets 1 or 2 (pp. 25–26). You could also review today's handouts. Going over the (Week 2) System Tools Review Questions on page 47 is very helpful. Perhaps you can go over this sheet with staff members. As staff members learn skills, they are able to be skills coaches for us. Talk to me after group if you would like to go over these."

Note: Be sure the group members are clear about the locations of materials. Skills List Worksheets 1, 2, or 3 (pp. 25, 26, or 27, respectively) and the (Week 2) System Tools Review Questions (p. 47) can be found in the Learning Skills section of the *Skills System Workbook* and completed as self-study or as homework in later cycles through the material. Following group, meet with any individuals to make a plan for completing the worksheets.

➡ ***Orient to group ending.*** "We ring the bowl six times at the end of group. It is a chance to notice our breathing. We take a moment to focus our minds as we go back to our activities. Who would like to ring the bell today?"

Skills System Component Handouts to Review in Future Cycles or for Home Study

✓ Learning Skills, Skills List Worksheet 1 (p. 25)

☆ *Teaching point.* This worksheet helps the individual recall the names of the nine core skills, using the icons as cue pictures.

✓ Learning Skills, Skills List Worksheet 2 (p. 26)

☆ *Teaching point.* This worksheet helps the individual associate the initials of each skill with the picture.

✓ Learning Skills, Skills List Worksheet 3 (p. 27)

☆ *Teaching point.* This worksheet helps the individual recall the names of the nine core skills by number without the pictures.

WEEK 2: SYSTEM TOOLS

Preparing for Group

Handouts Needed

✓ Learning Skills, System Tools Review Questions (p. 47)
✓ Learning Skills, System Tools Handout 1 (p. 31)

✓ Learning Skills, System Tools Handout 2 (p. 32)
✓ Learning Skills, System Tools Handout 4 (p. 36)
✓ Learning Skills, System Tools Handout 5 (p. 41)
✓ Learning Skills, System Tools Worked Example 4 (p. 45)
✓ Learning Skills, System Tools Worksheet 7 (p. 46)

E-Spiral Phase 1. Exploring Existing Knowledge Base (Review)

➡ ***Welcome group.*** "It is great to see everybody. How are you all doing? Are we ready to learn about skills?"

➡ ***Orient to the mindfulness activity: noticing the air going in and out of our noses.*** "What do we do first in group? You are right; we ring the bell. Why do we do that? Very good, because we want to focus our minds. OK, today we are going to learn more about breathing. We are going to notice the air going in and out of our noses as we breathe."

Instructions for mindfulness exercise. "Last week we rang the bell and noticed our breathing. Today we are going to ring the bell six times and notice our breathing again. This time we are going to notice the air going in and out of our noses. Our job is to bring 100% of our attention and focus to our noses. Sometimes our minds act like puppies; they jump all around. We have to be the boss of our minds so that our attention goes where we tell it. So, if your attention drifts to things other than your nose, reel it in [makes a gesture of a fishing reel] and notice the air going in and out of your nose. You may notice other thoughts and feelings, too; notice them, allow them to pass, and bring your attention to your nose. This is important to us, because we have to be able to control our attention; we have to direct our minds to what is helpful to us. We have to get our puppies to listen and mind. Any questions? I will ring the bell, and we will start."

Describe questions. "What did you notice about the air going in and out of your nose?"; "Where else did your attention go?"; "Did you bring your focus back to your breathing?"; "How did you bring your attention back?"

Note: The group shares details about what they noticed. The leader may want to write observations on the board.

➡ ***Orient to Skills System review.*** "Good job! Now we are going to review the Skills List and the System Tools."

Note: The instructor can choose one of the review exercises A–G in Week 1 (see pp. 134–135).

➡ ***Orient to skills practice.*** "OK, great job. You are really starting to learn skills! Let's shift gears and go over our Skills Practice for this week. Your homework was to practice noticing your breath."

Disclosure questions related to the breath. "Who can tell us about when you noticed your breath this week?"; "What did you notice?"

Disclosure questions related to studying skills. "Who had a chance to practice learning their skills?"; "Did any of you look at your notebook?"

Note: Starting with volunteers is helpful, because it gets the discussion started. Low self-efficacy can hinder volunteering. As an individual shares, leaders can include a less participatory group member by asking one or more simple, direct questions, which may reduce the barriers for volunteering: "Bill, did you notice your breathing at all during the week?"; "Great, when was that?"; "OK, what did you notice?"

➡ ***Orient to new skills topic.*** "Great! I am going to ask a few questions that will help us talk about what we already know about handling strong feelings. OK?"

Discuss existing knowledge about the new topic.

Assessment questions. "How does stress or strong feelings affect people?"; "How do strong feelings affect our actions?"

Relevant context question. "Do you think that people ever feel so confused that they just react without thinking?"

Clarifying questions. "Have you ever seen that happen?"; "How did it work out for the person?"

➡ ***Orient to relevant context of the new topic.*** "Today we are going to learn about three important Skills System tools. First is the Feelings Rating Scale. Second is the Categories of Skills. Third is the Recipe for Skills."

E-Spiral Phase 2. Encoding: New Learning

➡ ***Orient to new learning: System Tools.*** "We use the Feelings Rating Scale, Categories of Skills, and Recipe for Skills to know which skills to use in every situation. Having these three tools can help us handle even very stressful and confusing situations! Life can be confusing for all of us. Being able to focus our attention and shift our attention helps us be in control of ourselves and our lives. When we know what is going on, we can be on-track. When we are unfocused, often we go off-track. Being focused helps us use our skills well."

Instructions for the encoding activity. "Does that sound OK?"; "Great. We are going to look at four different handouts in the Learning Skills section of the *Skills System Workbook*. Please raise your hand if you have a question or feel lost. How about we turn to System Tools Handout 1 on page 31. What is our plan for reading this handout?"

Note: Instructors have many options about how to progress through the handouts, worked examples, and worksheets. This teaching plan reviews four basic handouts that serve as a preliminary introduction to the System Tools. There are worked examples and worksheets listed below that offer expansions of the concepts in these introductory handouts. The supplemental materials can be used in future cycles of the Skills System curriculum. How the leader decides to utilize these materials depends on the status of the group.

There are four handouts to review in this section. The information in the teaching points below is intended as learning tools for instructors, more so than as scripts to be read in group. As the leaders understand the skill concepts, briefer descriptions can be utilized in group that hit main points without being boring.

➡ ***Orient to reviewing System Tools Handout 1.*** "Now if you are ready, let's turn to page 31 in the Learning Skills sections of the *Skills System Workbook,* the System Tools Handout 1; it looks like this."

☆ *Section A teaching points.* "The first System Tool is the Feelings Rating Scale. It helps us rate how strong our feelings are. At 0–3 feelings, you can think clearly and talk and listen with others. When you have strong feelings and have a fuzzy mind, you are at a Level 4. If the feeling is overwhelming and you hurt yourself, someone else, or destroy property, the feeling would be rated a 5. We will learn more about the Feelings Rating Scale in the next handout. Any questions?"

☆ *Section B teaching points.* "The second System Tool is the Categories of Skills. Skills 1, 2, 3, 4, and 5 are our All-the-Time skills. We can use them any time, at any level of feeling rated 0–5. Skills 6, 7, 8, and 9 are Calm-Only skills. We use Calm-Only skills *only* when we are calm. This means we cannot use skills 6, 7, 8, and 9 when we are over feelings Level 3. We will learn when we can use each skill and when we need to wait to use a skill until we are a little calmer. We will learn more about this on System Tools Handout 4 (p. 36). Any questions?"

☆ *Section C teaching points.* "It is important that we link skills together in skills chains, one after another, especially when we have strong feelings. The Recipe for Skills helps us remember to link together more skills when we are more emotional. We should use even more skills than the Recipe for Skills tells us to! The more skills we use, the more on-track to our goals we are. Any questions?"

➡ ***Orient to System Tools Handout 2.*** "Good job! Now we are going to take a few minutes to learn more about the Feelings Rating Scale. Please turn to page 32 in the *Skills System Workbook.* This is System Tools Handout 2."

☆ *System Tools Handout 2 teaching points.*

- "When we are at a Level 0, we are not having that feeling. For example, Level 0 sadness means that the person is not sad at that time."
- "A Level 1 is a tiny feeling. We have a Level 1 feeling when we have a tiny reaction to something. For example, if I have Level 1 sadness, I might feel an empty sensation in my chest or feel like looking at the ground."
- "A Level 2 is a small feeling. We may notice different body sensations that a Level 2 feeling causes. At Level 2 sadness, I might notice my face changing, and my smile disappears; my

shoulders may drop because I feel a heaviness. My heart may begin to pound more, and my breathing may be affected. A Level 2 may be a little uncomfortable, if it is a painful feeling."

- "A Level 3 is a medium feeling. A Level 3 will cause body sensations. For example, I might have a stomachache, feel the urge to pace, and feel muscle tension at Level 3 sadness. I am able to talk and listen and be on-track. It is more difficult to be focused when at a Level 3 feeling, and I may have more off-track urges, but I am able to let them pass and stay focused on doing what works to reach my goal. We can still use All-the-Time and Calm-Only skills at a Level 3 feeling, but it is important to be careful in case the level increases. If the feeling is even a tiny bit over a Level 3, then we use only All-the-Time skills, *not* Calm-Only ones."

- "A Level 4 is a strong feeling. If it is a painful feeling, we will be very uncomfortable. For example, I would cry at Level 4 sadness. I also might want to get angry about what is making me sad. I might have urges to scream, swear, and storm around. At this level, it is difficult to focus, and action urges will be strong. At a Level 4 feeling, we do not use Calm-Only skills, even though we may have the urge to do so. We wait until we are below a Level 3 feeling."

- "A Level 5 is an overwhelming feeling. At Level 5, we harm ourselves, others, or property. At Level 5, we have to use All-the-Time skills to get back in control. Any questions?"

Content questions. "What might make you have a Level 1 feeling?"; "What would the feeling be?"; "How would your body feel?"; "What might make you have a Level 2 feeling?"; "What would the feeling be?"; "How would your body feel?"; "What might make you have a Level 3 feeling?"; "What would the feeling be?"; "How would your body feel?"; "What might make you have a Level 4 feeling?"; "What would the feeling be?"; "How would your body feel?"; "What might make you have a Level 5 feeling?"; "What would the feeling be?"; "How would your body feel?"

➡ ***Orient to System Tools Handout 4.*** "The Feelings Rating Scale might seem harder than it really is; you will get it! Now we are going to learn more about Categories of Skills from the System Tools Handout 4 on page 36 of the *Skills System Workbook.* It looks like this. All set?"

☆ *System Tools Handout 4 teaching points.* "There are two Categories of Skills. Skills 1, 2, 3, 4, and 5 are called All-the-Time skills. [Perhaps ask the group what skills 1–5 are.] These skills can be used at any level of feeling: 0, 1, 2, 3, 4, and even 5. The other Category of Skills, Calm-Only, can *only* be used when we are having feelings between Levels 0 and 3. If we are even a tiny bit over Level 3, we do not use Calm-Only skills! Any questions?"

Assessment questions. "What is it like when we use Expressing Myself at a Level 4?", "What kinds of behaviors do we have at a Level 4 when we try to solve our problems?"

➡ ***Orient to System Tools Handout 5.*** "The last handout reviewed here is on page 41 of the *Skills System Workbook.* System Tools Handout 5 looks like this. Everyone ready?"

☆ *System Tools Handout 5 teaching points.* "The Recipe for Skills tells us how many skills at least we need to use in a situation. We add at least one skill to our skills chain for every level of feeling, including Level 0. At Level 0 we are using Clear Picture to know what is going on. At a Level 1, we have to link at least two skills. At Level 1, we will use Clear Picture and On-Track Thinking. This is a 12 skills chain. At a Level 2 feeling, we have to use at least three skills. Again, we use Clear Picture, On-Track Thinking, then take some kind of On-Track Action. This is a 123 skills chain. At a Level 3, we link at least four skills. Once again, we use Clear Picture, On-Track Thinking, On-Track Action, and at least one more skill that we think will help us reach our goals. If we are at a Level 4 feeling, we use at least five skills. These five skills have to be skills 1–5, because we cannot use any Calm-Only skills at a Level 4 feeling. At a Level 5, we have to use at least six skills. Once again, at Level 5, we cannot use Calm-Only skills, so all six skills have to be All-the-Time skills. Often we double up on On-Track Actions or New-Me Activities to help us focus and feel better. Any questions?"

Content questions. "At a Level 1, how many skills do we need?"; "At a Level 2?"; "At a Level 3?"; "At a Level 4?"; "At a Level 5?"

➡ ***Orient to the end of the Encoding Phase.*** "We have learned a lot today. We learned how to put our skills together. It takes time to understand how to use these tools. Practicing is very important."

E-Spiral Phase 3. Elaboration: Practice and Linking

➡ ***Orient to the elaboration activity.*** "If it is OK, let's turn to page 45 of the *Skills System Workbook,* which says System Tools Worked Example 4: Week 2 Practice Activity on the top and looks like this. All set? We will read through this together. [The group reads through the worked example together.] Next we are going to complete System Tools Worksheet 7, the Week 2 Practice Activity worksheet (p. 46), together. Who is willing to share a stressful situation that happened this week that we can use as an example?"

Note: The instructor decides on a topic. The topic needs to be interesting enough to hold the group's attention, yet not so intense that it cognitively overloads anyone in group.

Describe question. "How was that exercise for you?"

➡ ***Orient to discussion.*** "I thought that was fun. Working together like that is what skill? Right—Relationship Care! Now we are going to have a discussion before we finish for the day."

Linking question. "Is using the Skills System different from how you have handled feelings in the past?"

Disclosure questions. "Have there been times in the past when you were confused about what to do in a stressful situation?"; "What did you do?"; "How did it work?"

Expansion question. "How can the Feelings Rating Scale, Categories of Skills, and Recipe for Skills help you when you are upset or confused?"

➡ ***Orient to the end of the Elaboration Phase.*** "Great discussion. I think we are ready to move on to another activity. OK?"

E-Spiral Phase 4. Efficacy: Bridge to Real Life

➡ ***Orient to the efficacy activity.*** "Now we will play a game to practice using the Feelings Rating Scale, Categories of Skills, and the Recipe for Skills.

"I will say a feeling and the level. For example, Mad Level 3. We will then figure out together which skills we can use. At Mad Level 3, we can use both our All-the-Time and Calm-Only skills, right? Then we are going to figure out how many skills we have to use, at least, in that situation using the Recipe for Skills. So at a Level 3 feeling, we have to use four skills, right? OK, Sad Level 2?"

Note: The instructor continues to generate different feelings and rating levels, so that the group members can practice deciding whether all nine skills are available or only the All-the-Time skills, and how many skills are needed. The group members can also generate questions for other participants to answer. Depending on the cognitive abilities of the group, the instructor may want to write the Categories of Skills on the board or prompt more vulnerable learners to look at their handouts.

Review question. "How was that exercise for you?"

➡ ***Orient to discussion.*** "Wonderful job—that isn't easy! We are going to talk now about some of the challenges we face when we use skills like these. OK?"

Barrier question. "So far, what is hard about using the Feelings Rating Scale, the Categories of Skills, and the Recipe for Skills?"

Wisdom question. "Do you want to be able to use these tools?"

Commitment questions. "Are you willing to learn and practice using these tools?"; "When are you going to use these tools in your life?"

Coaching question. "How can you coach yourself to practice using these tools?"

➡ ***Orient to home study.*** "That was a good discussion—thank you. That helps me understand what is challenging for you. Our homework this week will be to practice using the Feelings Rating Scale, the Categories of Skills, and the Recipe for Skills. Whenever you think of it, label and rate what you are feeling. Think about whether you are over or under a Level 3 feeling. Ask yourself if you are able to talk and listen, and to be on-track. Try to remember which category of skills you can use and how many skills would be helpful. Any questions?

"Also, if anyone is interested in doing home study this week, you can look at the handouts that we have gone over. You could look over the worked examples in the Learning Skills, System Tools section of the *Skills System Workbook*. You could also do the worksheets. Check in with me after group if you need to make a plan for home study."

➡ ***Orient to group ending.*** "I thought you all did well. We ring the bell six times at the end of group. It is a chance to notice our breathing. We take a moment to focus our minds as we go back to our activities. Who would like to ring the bell today?"

System Tools Handouts to Review in Future Cycles or for Home Study

✓ Learning Skills, System Tools Handout 3 (p. 33)

☆ *Teaching points.* This handout is a home-study tool for participants and staff to review the Feelings Rating Scale. Understanding the Feelings Rating Scale helps the individual become more organized and more able to integrate skills at lower levels of emotional arousal. It is critical that the individual learn the difference between Feelings Levels 4 and 5. At Level 4, the person may feel horrible, yet she is not acting in an out-of-control way. At Level 5, she is taking actions that harm herself, others, or property. A participant may say that she is at a 4.5 level to express being nearly out of control. If the person is in the group and states that she is currently at Level 5, the leaders can ask, "Are you hurting yourself, others, or property right now?" The person can then adjust the rating to a Level 4, if she is extremely uncomfortable, yet she is not taking abusive actions.

✓ Learning Skills, System Tools Worked Example 1 (p. 34)

☆ *Teaching points.* The group reviews this worked example, which shows how the events prompted different levels of feeling. This sheet is presented using a scenario that links all of the answers to help the individual learn how feelings and situations can interact in escalating patterns.

✓ Learning Skills, System Tools Worksheet 1 (p. 35)

☆ *Teaching points.* This worksheet is intended to have the individual practice associating events with levels of feeling. System Tools Worksheet 1 does not have to describe a specific situation, as did the previous worked example. The participant can list events that would lead to levels of feeling that are not associated with each other. For example, losing keys might be a Level 2 frustration, and losing a child would be Level 5 sadness.

✓ Learning Skills, System Tools Worksheet 2 (p. 37)

☆ *Teaching points.* This worksheet asks the individual to fill in the names and categories of the skills.

✓ Learning Skills, System Tools Worked Example 2 (p. 38)

☆ *Teaching points.* This worked example shows the Categories of Skills that may be used at different levels of feeling.

✓ Learning Skills, System Tools Worksheet 3 (p. 39)

☆ *Teaching points.* This worksheet lists feelings and ratings and asks the individual to circle the Categories of Skills that may be used at different levels of feelings.

✓ Learning Skills, System Tools Worksheet 4 (p. 40)

☆ *Teaching points.* This worksheet asks the participant to write in a feeling and a rating level. The person then circles which Categories of Skills may be used in that situation.

✓ Learning Skills, System Tools Worked Example 3 (p. 42)

☆ *Teaching points.* This worked example shows how many skills are needed at different levels of feelings. Sometimes we feel halfway between one rating level and another. For example, we are more than a Level 2 feeling and less than a 3, so we rate this a 2.5. In these cases, we round up to the next level of feeling (Level 3 in this example), so we are sure to use enough skills.

✓ Learning Skills, System Tools Worksheet 5 (p. 43)

☆ *Teaching points.* This worksheet lists feelings and ratings; the individual circles the number of skills that are necessary.

✓ Learning Skills, System Tools Worksheet 6 (p. 44)

☆ *Teaching points.* This worksheet requests that the participant write down feelings and ratings. The individual then circles how many skills are necessary at that level of emotional escalation.

WEEK 3: CLEAR PICTURE

Preparing for Group

Handouts Needed

✓ Learning Skills, System Tools Review Questions (p. 47)
✓ Learning Skills, Clear Picture Handout 1 (p. 52)
✓ Learning Skills, Clear Picture Worked Example 1 (p. 53)
✓ Learning Skills, Clear Picture Worksheet 1 (p. 54)

E-Spiral Phase 1. Exploring Existing Knowledge Base (Review)

➡ ***Welcome group.*** "Hi, everybody; how is it going today? Are we ready to learn about skills? Does anyone remember what we do to start group? [Wait for answer.] You are right; we ring the bell. Why do we do that? [Wait for answer.] Very good—because we want to focus our minds. We are going to learn even more about breathing today!"

➡ ***Orient to the mindfulness activity: noticing air filling our chests.*** "Last week we noticed our breathing. We learned how to turn our attention to the air going in and out of our noses."

Instructions for the mindfulness exercise. "Today we are going to pay attention to our breath in our chests—just as it is. We will notice the air going in and out of our lungs. As the air goes in, we may feel our chests expand. You might notice your shoulders rise up as your lungs get full. As the air goes out, your lungs will empty and your chest will go down. Putting your hand on your chest might help you focus attention there. How about we try it a few times before we ring the bell? [Observes each participant.] That looks good. If your attention drifts away from your breathing, try to bring your focus back to the air in your chest. If you notice feelings, gently bring your attention back to your breathing. If you notice other thoughts, gently bring your focus back to . . . ? [Wait for response.] Right, your chest! Let's try to keep our puppies in control. We want to practice being the boss of our minds. All set? Any questions?"

Note: Leaders observe the participants and provide individual instruction to those who have difficulty performing the breathing task. Additionally, it may be helpful for the leader to use the gesture of two hands turning a car steering wheel when he refers to turning attention. The metaphor can be expanded to include acting as though the steering wheel is hard to turn (rusty or lacking power steering), exemplifying times when our attention is difficult to shift.

Describe questions. "What did you notice about the air filling your lungs?"; "Where else did your attention go?"; "Did you bring your focus back to your chest rising and falling?"; "How did you bring your attention back?"

Note: The group members share details about what they noticed. The leader may choose to write observations on the board.

➡ ***Orient to Skills System review.*** "Every week, we will review the Skills List, the Feelings Rating Scale, the Categories of Skills, and the Recipe for Skills. It is important that we learn these things inside and out, backward and forward."

Note: Group leaders can utilize the System Tools Review Questions (p. 47 in the *Skills System Workbook*) or create another way to review this material. The goal is to practice recalling the information, so that the terms and concepts become learned and automatic. A basic review of exercises (A–G) (pp. 134–135) addresses the names and numbers of the nine skills. The list below is a more inclusive list of options that incorporate the skills names and the System Tools. The instructor and/or the group can choose which review activities best suit the needs of the group.

Examples of Advanced Review Activities.

- The instructor asks the group the System Tools Review Questions (p. 47).
- The instructor asks the group to list the names, numbers, initials, categories, and functions of each skill.
- The instructor names a feeling and a rating level. The group says which Categories of Skills can be used and the minimum number of skills needed according to the Recipe for Skills.
- The group sorts the laminated skills cards to put them in order using the Categories of Skills cards and subsets of skills (i.e., placing the six Clear Picture Do's cards under the Clear Picture card).
- The instructor has the group look at the Skills Plan Map (in the Learning Skills, Using Skills in My Life section on p. 219 of the *Skills System Workbook*) and asks different skills questions related to making skills chains.

➡ ***Orient to skills practice.*** "I think we are doing well; it does take time. The more we practice, the easier it will be to remember these things. This week's homework was to practice using the Feelings Rating Scale, the Categories of Skills, and the Recipe for Skills. Right?"

Disclosure questions. "Who can talk to us about what it was like to use the Feelings Rating Scale?"; "Who can tell us about practicing using the Categories of Skills?"; "Who can tell us about using the Recipe for Skills?"

➡ ***Orient to new skills topic.*** "Great! Let's see what we already know about getting a Clear Picture."

Discuss existing knowledge about the new topic.

Assessment question. "When we are focused, are our minds clear or fuzzy?"

Relevant context questions. "How do people handle things when they are in clear mind?"; "How do people handle things when they are in fuzzy mind?"; "What happens to our feelings when we are in fuzzy mind?"

Clarifying questions. "How does clear mind help people get to their goals?"; "How does fuzzy mind keep people from reaching their goals?"; "What does it mean to be in emotional mind?"; "What is our thinking like in emotional mind?"; "How do you think noticing your breathing can help you handle feelings?"; "How can noticing our breathing help us manage off-track thoughts?"

➡ ***Orient to relevant context of the new topic.*** "From our discussion, it sounds like we agree that feelings and thoughts can become overwhelming. Sometimes we block or avoid feelings. Unfortunately, that makes things worse. Noticing feelings and thoughts helps us know what is really happening inside and outside of us. When we are clear, we can see where we are going; when we are fuzzy, we cannot. Clear information about ourselves and our situation helps us make decisions that lead us to our goals. Our Clear Picture skills will help us get a clear mind, so that we can take actions that help us reach our goals. Any questions?"

E-Spiral Phase 2. Encoding: New Learning

➡ ***Orient to new learning: Clear Picture.*** "Today we are going to learn about the first skill in the Skills System. Skill 1 is Clear Picture. You can tell by the name of the skill that we will be learning how to have a clear mind."

Instructions for encoding activity. "If you are ready, let's turn to page 52 of the *Skills System Workbook.* This is the Learning Skills, Clear Picture Handout 1. [Holds up the page.] This is what it looks like. OK, what is our plan for reviewing this? Would anyone like to read?"

Note: When group members read, it is important that the leader restate terms so that the group is very clear about the information.

➡ ***Review Learning Skills, Clear Picture Handout 1***

☆ *Teaching points.* "When we get a Clear Picture, we focus 100% on what is happening inside and outside of us right now. We pay attention to what is happening so that we understand the facts of the situation. When we are clear about the facts, we can make skills plans to reach our goals. When we are fuzzy or try to change the facts, we end up off-track.

"We get a Clear Picture by going through the Clear Picture Do's. These are things we do to become aware of what is happening inside and outside of us in the moment. We take a Breath,

Notice our Surroundings, do a Body Check, Label and Rate Feelings using the 6-point (0–5) scale, Notice Thoughts, and Notice Urges. When we go through the Do's, it is like taking a picture of what is happening right now. It is like taking a snapshot. [Snaps fingers to show how quickly and easily this can be done.]

"It is important to have a Clear Picture of situations, so we can figure out how to do what works. It helps us make strong Skills Plans. If we have a fuzzy picture, we usually do what does not work. We need a Clear Picture of ourselves, others, and the situation to make on-track choices that help us reach our goals."

➡ ***Orient to Learning Skills, Clear Picture Worked Example 1.*** "Does anyone have any questions about that handout? OK, now we are going to learn more about getting a Clear Picture. Let's turn to page 53 of the *Skills System Workbook.* This is the Clear Picture Worked Example 1. It looks like this. [Holds the page up.] Would anyone like to read?"

➡ ***Review Learning Skills, Clear Picture Worked Example 1.*** The group reviews the worked example. If this worked example is not relevant to the population being treated, skills instructors can create a worked example on a copy of Learning Skills, Clear Picture Worksheet 1 (p. 54). The group leader tries to explain each concept, so the participants understand each step of the Clear Picture. It is not necessary that the participant be able to recall each concept initially; that knowledge base will build as the person is exposed to Clear Picture repeatedly.

➡ ***Orient to ending Encoding Phase.*** "Does anyone have questions about Clear Picture so far? OK, are we ready to practice some of the things we have learned?"

E-Spiral Phase 3. Elaboration: Practice and Linking

➡ ***Orient to the elaboration activity.*** "Great, let's practice getting a Clear Picture!"

Instructions for the practice exercise. "I am going to say one of the Clear Picture Do's and then I will ring the bell. When I ring the bell, I would like you to do the Do. For example, when I say, 'Notice the Breath,' we will all listen to the bell and pay attention to our breathing. Then I will ring the bell and say, 'Notice Surroundings.' As the bell ring fades, we will all notice what is happening around us. We will do this for Body Check, Label and Rate Feelings, Notice Thoughts, and Notice Urges. Together we will listen to six rings, and we will do all six Clear Picture Do's. If you get lost, notice what getting lost is like and try to follow along at the next bell ring. Any questions? [Wait for response.] Great, here we go."

Describe questions. "What did you notice about your breath?"; "What did you notice when you noticed surroundings?"; "What did you notice during the Body Check?"; "What feeling did you notice, and how strong was it?"; "What thoughts did you notice?"; "What urges did you notice?"

➡ ***Orient to discussion.*** "Good job. Now we are going to take a few minutes to talk a little more about what it is like to get a Clear Picture."

Linking questions. "Have you ever had a Clear Picture in the past?"; "What actions did you take?"; "Have you been in emotional mind?"; "What actions did you take?"

Disclosure questions. "What is it like to be more aware of things inside and outside of you?"; "Can it be difficult to see how things really are?"; "What do you do when it is hard to face what is really happening?"

Expansion questions. "What other skills do we use with Clear Picture?"; "How can having a Clear Picture help you reach your goals?"; "Does a fuzzy or clear picture help you reach your goals?"; "Why?"

➡ ***Orient to the end of the Elaboration Phase.*** "That was a good discussion. I was thinking that it would be helpful to read a story that teaches us more about how we use Clear Picture in our lives."

E-Spiral Phase 4. Efficacy: Bridge to Real Life

➡ ***Orient to efficacy activities: reading a story.*** "I will read this story, and we will answer some questions when we are done. Is everyone all set?"

Instructions for the efficacy activity. Story: "There is a man named Robert, and he is 22 years old. Robert works in a grocery store, stocking shelves. One day at work, Robert was kneeling and putting cans on a bottom shelf. Suddenly an older lady pushed her cart into him when he was working. He did not see the woman coming toward him; he only felt the cart hitting him. Robert did a Body Check and noticed a sharp pain in his back. Right away, he knew he had to get a Clear Picture, because he was feeling confused at a Level 4. He noticed an urge to scream, 'Look out! What are you doing? Didn't you see me working here?' As he stood up to see what had happened, he took a few breaths. He checked around him and saw the old woman looking the other way at some spaghetti sauce. He noticed the thought, *I don't think she knows that she ran into me.* Robert did another Body Check, and the pain in his back was nearly gone."

Review questions.

"Do you think Robert had a Clear Picture of the situation?"

"Can you point out the six Clear Picture Do's?" (Write them in the order in which they happened on the board.)

"When did he think to take a breath?"

"How long did it take for Robert to do the Clear Picture Do's?"

"Do you think Robert ended up screaming at the woman?"

"What do you think he did next?"

"What would have happened if he had yelled at that old woman?"

"Do you think Clear Picture helped Robert reach his goals?"

➡ ***Orient to discussion.*** "It sounds like Robert is learning skills! Before we finish for the day, we are going to have a brief discussion. OK?"

Barrier questions. "What is hard about taking a few seconds to get a Clear Picture?"; "We have to use Clear Picture all day. What is difficult about that for you?"

Wisdom questions. "Would the Clear Picture Do's help you?"; "Do you think you want to use Clear Picture?"

Commitment question. "When will you use Clear Picture?"

Coaching question. "How can you coach yourself to use Clear Picture every day, all day?"

➡ ***Orient to home study.*** "This week our homework will be to jump in with both feet to practice Clear Picture. As many times as you can, take a few seconds to notice your breathing, surroundings, body, feelings, thoughts, and urges. You might find that the more you practice, the more quickly you can do the Do's. We can learn to do it in a snap! [Snaps fingers.] At first it might be hard to remember all six Clear Picture Do's. Try to take a few seconds to be aware of what is happening inside and outside of you before you take action. Good luck; we will talk about it next week. Also, if you want to study skills at home, review all the handouts we have gone over so far. You can also do Clear Picture Worksheet 1 (p. 54), in which you list what you notice in the moment. Ask someone to help you write if you need to."

➡ ***Orient to group ending.*** "As you know, we ring the bell six times at the end of group. We do one ring for each of the Clear Picture Do's. It is a chance to notice what is happening inside and outside of us right now. We take a moment to get a Clear Picture as we go back to our activities. Who would like to ring to bell today?"

Clear Picture Handouts to Review in Future Cycles or for Home Study

Note: Skills instructors use these handouts, worked examples, and worksheets to develop teaching plans in future cycles through the Skills System curriculum. Orienting, questions, exercise, and skills practice are created to teach expanded material through subsequent cycles.

✓ Learning Skills, Clear Picture Summary Sheet (p. 51)

☆ *Teaching points.* The summary sheet can be used during the encoding phase to explain concepts as teaching points. It may be too boring to read in group but having different group members read different sections can break it up. Summary sheets are helpful for home study and for teaching skills to skills coaches.

✓ Learning Skills, Clear Picture Worksheet 1 (p. 54)

☆ *Teaching points.* This worksheet is helpful for participants to use in the moment at home. The pictures prompt the individual to Take a Breath, Notice Surroundings, do a Body Check, Label and Rate Feelings, Notice Thoughts, and Notice Urges. This is a useful activity for the person to do when he needs to get a Clear Picture.

✓ Learning Skills, Clear Picture Worksheet 2 (p. 55)

☆ *Teaching points.* This worksheet guides the participant to focus attention on breathing to tolerate distress. It shifts the person's focus from the stressful situation to awareness of breathing. The awareness of breathing shifts from being aware of current breathing to doing diaphragmatic or belly breaths. Belly breathing can help the individual remain regulated so that she can think things through. The last step is to practice patterned breathing by counting to four on the inhalation and to four on the exhalation.

✓ Learning Skills, Clear Picture Handout 2 (p. 56)

☆ *Teaching points.* This handout helps the participant understand how we observe our surroundings. Practice exercises can include sensory awareness activities.

✓ Learning Skills, Clear Picture Worked Example 2 (p. 57)

☆ *Teaching points.* This worked example shows how to get a Clear Picture of our surroundings.

✓ Learning Skills, Clear Picture Worksheet 3 (p. 58)

☆ *Teaching points.* This worksheet helps the participant understand how to get a Clear Picture of their surroundings.

✓ Learning Skills, Clear Picture Worked Example 3 (p. 59)

☆ *Teaching points.* This worked example describes different sensations that an individual may feel in different parts of the body.

✓ Learning Skills, Clear Picture Worksheet 4 (p. 60)

☆ *Teaching points.* This worksheet is used by the individual to describe what is observed in different parts of her body in different situations.

✓ Learning Skills, Clear Picture Worked Example 4 (p. 61)

☆ *Teaching points.* This worked example reviews possible body sensations at different levels of anger.

✓ Learning Skills, Clear Picture Worksheet 5 (p. 62)

☆ *Teaching points.* This worksheet helps the participant associate body sensations with a feeling. Increasing awareness can help assist the individual in Labeling and Rating Feelings.

✓ Learning Skills, Clear Picture Handout 3 (p. 63)

☆ *Teaching points.* This handout introduces nine different feelings. These labels serve as a starting point to describe many other feelings that people experience; it is fun to have the group brainstorm a list of all different feelings.

✓ Learning Skills, Clear Picture Handout 4 (p. 64)

☆ *Teaching points.* This handout teaches the participant how feelings function. The participant comes to understand that events prompt feelings. The person learns that chemical changes happen in the body when feelings happen. People communicate what is happening inside of them through their facial expressions and body language. Awareness of these factors can help individuals understand themselves and other people better. It is important for the participant to understand that feelings create action urges. This would be an opportunity to educate the group about "fight–flight–freeze" responses. By being aware of these forces, the participant is better able to observe them, describe them, and make decisions versus reacting quickly without thought.

✓ Learning Skills, Clear Picture Worked Example 5 (p. 65)

☆ *Teaching points.* This worked example lists events that may elicit various responses.

✓ Learning Skills, Clear Picture Worksheet 6 (p. 66)

☆ *Teaching points.* This worksheet asks participants to list situations that elicit specific feelings. This activity helps individuals understand links between prompting events and their responses.

✓ Learning Skills, Clear Picture Handout 5 (p. 67)

☆ *Teaching points.* This handout on noticing thoughts teaches participants that thoughts are continually produced by the brain. It is important that the individual understand that some thoughts are helpful, and others are not. The goal is for the person to observe thoughts and allow unhelpful thoughts, or off-track thoughts, to pass without taking action. The metaphor of thoughts being like city buses can be helpful because the individual only gets on a bus that is heading to the desired destination. Getting on the wrong bus, or responding to off-track thoughts, will hinder the individual from reaching goals.

✓ Learning Skills, Clear Picture Worked Example 6 (p. 68)

☆ *Teaching points.* This worked example offers a sample of situations that generate thoughts.

✓ Learning Skills, Clear Picture Worksheet 7 (p. 69)

☆ *Teaching points.* This worksheet gives the individual an opportunity to list multiple situations that generate thoughts.

✓ Learning Skills, Clear Picture Worked Example 7 (p. 70)

☆ *Teaching points.* This worked example highlights thoughts that can elicit certain feelings. It is important that the individual understands how thinking patterns can affect emotional status.

✓ Learning Skills, Clear Picture Worksheet 8 (p. 71)

☆ *Teaching points.* This worksheet gives the individual an opportunity to list thoughts that may elicit specific feelings.

✓ Learning Skills, Clear Picture Worked Example 8 (p. 72)

☆ *Teaching points.* This worked example highlights how situations create thoughts and feelings that lead to action urges.

✓ Learning Skills, Clear Picture Worksheet 9 (p. 73)

☆ *Teaching points.* This worksheet asks the individual to write down a situation, a thought, a feeling, and the possible action urge that might result.

✓ Learning Skills, Clear Picture Worked Example 9 (p. 74)

☆ *Teaching points.* This worked example outlines examples of urges that a person may experience when having specific feelings.

✓ Learning Skills, Clear Picture Worksheet 10 (p. 75)

☆ *Teaching points.* This worksheet asks the individual to list urges she notices when experiencing certain feelings. Increasing awareness of feelings and action urges facilitates management of action urges.

✓ Learning Skills, Clear Picture Worked Example 10 (p. 76)

☆ *Teaching points.* This worked example demonstrates how action urges intensify as a feeling strengthens.

✓ Learning Skills, Clear Picture Worksheet 11 (p. 77)

☆ *Teaching points.* This worksheet asks the individual to observe action urges that occur at increasing levels of feeling. This activity helps the participant improve awareness of affective experiences; enhanced awareness during preliminary escalation can result in proactive skill use.

✓ Learning Skills, Clear Picture Worked Example 11 (p. 78)

☆ *Teaching points.* This worked example offers a sample of situations that generate urges.

✓ Learning Skills, Clear Picture Worksheet 12 (p. 79)

☆ *Teaching points.* This worksheet gives the individual an opportunity to list multiple situations that generate urges.

✓ Learning Skills, Clear Picture Worked Example 12 (p. 80)

☆ *Teaching points.* This worked example offers a sample of how when we Label and Rate Feelings, Notice Thoughts, and Notice Urges we can get a clearer picture of a situation.

✓ Learning Skills, Clear Picture Worksheet 13 (p. 81)

☆ *Teaching points.* This worksheet gives the individual an opportunity to Label and Rate Feelings, Notice Thoughts, and Notice Urges to get a clearer picture of situations.

WEEK 4: ON-TRACK THINKING

Preparing for Group

Handouts Needed

✓ Learning Skills, On-Track Thinking Handout 1 (p. 86)
✓ Learning Skills, On-Track Thinking Worked Example 1 (p. 87)
✓ Learning Skills, On-Track Thinking Worksheet 2 (p. 89)
✓ Learning Skills, On-Track Thinking Worked Example 2 (p. 90)
✓ Learning Skills, On-Track Thinking Worksheet 3 (p. 91)
✓ Learning Skills, On-Track Thinking Worksheet 4 (p. 93)

E-Spiral Phase 1. Exploring Existing Knowledge Base (Review)

➡ ***Welcome group.*** "Hello, everybody! It is wonderful to see you all! How are you doing today?"

➡ ***Orient to the mindfulness activity: paying attention to our bellies as we breathe.*** "Are we ready to get started with our mindful breathing?"

Instructions for the mindfulness exercise. "Today we are going to pay attention to our breath in our bellies. We will breathe and notice the air going into our diaphragm, which is near our belly. When we do belly breathing, our tummies may get bigger. Putting your hand on your belly might help you focus attention there. You might notice your pants or your belt getting tighter as your belly fills with air. How about we try it a few times before we ring the bell? [Observes each participant.] That looks good. So, I will ring the bell six times. We all will bring our attention to our belly breathing. If your attention drifts away from your belly breathing, try to bring your focus back to the belly breaths. If you notice feelings, gently bring your attention back to your breathing. If you notice other thoughts, gently bring your focus back to . . . ? [Wait for response.] Right, your belly breathing! Let's try to keep our puppies in control. We want to practice being the boss of our minds. All set? Any questions?"

Describe questions. "What was that like?"; "Were you able to notice the breath in your belly?"; "What was challenging about that?"; "Were you able to bring your attention back to your breath and the bell if it wandered?"

➡ ***Orient to Skills System review.*** "You are all really doing well. Learning about breathing is an important skill. The cool thing is that we always have our breath with us. If we need to focus, all we have to do is bring our attention to our breathing. It is time for our skills review."

Note: The skills instructor can choose a Basic Review Exercise from Week 1 (pp. 134–135) or an Advanced Review Activity from Week 3 on page 146 or create a new one.

➡ ***Orient to skills practice.*** "Very good—I think we are doing well. OK, let's talk about how we did practicing Clear Picture this week."

Disclosure questions. Choosing one or more of these questions can help participants review the use of Clear Picture: "Who used Clear Picture?"; "Could you tell us how it went?"; "Which of the Clear Picture Do's did you do?"; "Which of the Clear Picture Do's didn't you do?"; "Did you find that Clear Picture was helpful?"

➡ ***Orient to new skills topic.*** "It sounds as if using our skills helps us focus more and feel better. It also sounds as if we can feel pretty out of control and uncomfortable when we don't use our skills. Unfortunately, it is really hard to reach goals when we are off-track. I am going to ask a few questions that will help us share what we already know about thinking things through."

Discuss existing knowledge about the new topic.

Assessment questions. "What is it like to be confused?"; "What kinds of situations make people confused?" [Brainstorm this list on the board.]

Relevant context questions. "What kinds of plans do we make when we are confused?"; "What kinds of actions do we take when we are in fuzzy mind?"; "What kinds of plans do we make when we are in clear mind?"; "What kinds of actions do we take when we are focused?"

Clarifying questions. "When we take actions when we are fuzzy or unfocused, how does it usually turn out?"; "When we take actions when we are focused and clear, how does it usually turn out?"

➡ ***Orient to relevant context of the new topic.*** "It is important to use On-Track Thinking because, as we know, life can be confusing. We experience stress and strong feelings every day. It is difficult to reach goals when we are upside down or out of our minds. So, to reach our goals, we have to be in our minds and make good plans. Getting organized helps us handle stressful situations. On-Track Thinking helps us think clearly so that we can handle what is happening inside and outside of us to reach our goals. Any questions?"

E-Spiral Phase 2. Encoding: New Learning

➡ ***Orient to new learning: On-Track Thinking.*** "OK, today we are going to learn about Skill 2, On-Track Thinking. We use On-Track Thinking after we get a Clear Picture. On-Track Thinking helps us check our urges, create on-track thoughts, and use skills plans to handle every situation."

Instructions for the encoding activity. "Now we are going to learn about the different parts of On-Track Thinking. Please turn to page 86 of your *Skills System Workbook.* This is Learning Skills, On-Track Thinking Handout 1."

➡ ***Review Learning Skills, On-Track Thinking Handout 1.***

☆ *Teaching points.* "When we do Clear Picture, we are finding out what is happening inside and outside of us in a situation. We do On-Track Thinking before we take any actions; we have to be sure to have an on-track skills plan before we move ahead. When we notice an urge to take action, first we stop and Check It. We take a few seconds and Check It to see whether the urge is helpful or not helpful to us. We ask ourselves, "If I do this, will it help me reach my goals?" We give helpful thoughts a thumbs-up and unhelpful thoughts a thumbs-down. When we notice that an urge is not helpful, we create a Turn It thought. Turn It thoughts are ones that coach us not to take the off-track action. I may Turn It by thinking about all the negative things that will happen in my life if I do the off-track action. Turn It could also be when I coach myself to be New-Me. We do not want to get on the off-track city bus, because it is not going where we want to go! We Check It, Turn It to thumbs-up thinking, and Cheerlead. It is hard to stay on track sometimes, and off-track thoughts sneak back into our minds. So we use lots of Cheerleading to help us keep working toward our goals.

"Making lemonade out of lemons is an important type of On-Track Thinking. This means that when life gives us something difficult (sour lemons), we add sugar and look on the bright side. We have a Clear Picture that the situation is difficult, and we try to see it in a positive way. Making lemonade can help us deal with tough situations in ways that make us feel better.

"Once we have checked it and turned it to On-Track Thinking, we make a Skills Plan. This is when we think about what skills will help us in this situation. First, we check to see whether we can use Calm-Only skills at this time using the Category of Skills. If we are over a Level 3 feeling, we use All-the-Time skills. [Asks the group to list verbally the All-the-Time skills and the Calm-Only skills.] Then, using the Recipe for Skills, we figure out how many skills to use. We have to be sure to use enough skills. Then, we decide what other skills will help us reach our goals. We think about whether we need to use a Safety Plan. Safety Plans help us handle risky situations. Maybe doing a New-Me Activity would be helpful. It may help us keep busy and focused. If we are under a Level 3 feeling, we might want to use Problem Solving to fix problems, Expressing Myself to communicate, Getting It Right to get what we want, and Relationship Care to balance relationships. We keep Cheerleading ourselves to be sure we stay on-track! Any questions?"

Content question. "What are the different steps in On-Track Thinking?"

➡ ***Orient to Learning Skills, On-Track Thinking Worked Example 1.*** "There is a lot to learn about On-Track Thinking. Let's go through On-Track Thinking Worked Example 1 on page 87 of the *Skills System Workbook* together. It looks like this."

Note: The On-Track Thinking Worked Example 1 is self-explanatory. Skills instructors read through the worksheet with the group.

➡ ***Orient to Learning Skills, On-Track Thinking Worked Example 2.*** "Let's look a little closer at how we use Check It, Turn It, and Cheerleading to help us reach our goals. Please turn to the On-Track Thinking Worked Example 2 on page 90 together. It looks like this."

Note: The group members discuss how taking action on the urge works against the goal. They may also talk about how the Turn It thought helps them move toward the goal, and how Cheerleading helps them stay on track.

➡ ***Orient to the end of the Encoding Phase.*** "Excellent job! Any questions about On-Track Thinking so far?"

E-Spiral Phase 3. Elaboration: Practice and Linking

➡ ***Orient to Learning Skills, On-Track Thinking Worksheet 2.*** "Great, are we ready to practice On-Track Thinking? Now we are going to fill out On-Track Thinking Worksheet 2 together. Turn to page 89 of the *Skills System Workbook*. This is what it looks like."

Instructions for filling out the worksheet. "This worksheet helps you to practice checking urges. I will read a list of eight urges. You will think about each one and decide whether the urge would be helpful or unhelpful for you in this moment. If it is helpful, circle the thumb that goes up. If the urge is not helpful, circle the thumb that goes down. If you have a hard time reading, you can get the person next to you to help, or you can just show the group a thumbs-up or thumbs-down for your answer. Any questions?"

☆ *Teaching points.* "Each of us has to decide what is on-track and off-track for ourselves. No one can tell you what is right for you; we have to search within ourselves to find those answers. This worksheet is a chance to practice looking inside to see if an urge is helpful or unhelpful. Our goals change, so we have to be sure to check within our hearts to find out whether something is helpful or unhelpful in this moment. Every situation is different. So it is best to check urges each time you use On-Track Thinking. Any questions?"

Note: If time allows, choose a relevant situation and complete On-Track Thinking Worksheet 2 (p. 89) as a group activity.

Disclosure questions. "What were these exercises like for you?"; "How did you decide whether the urge was helpful or unhelpful?" and "How long did it take for you to check the urge?"; "Have you used Turn It and Cheerleading before?"; "Can it be difficult?"

➡ ***Orient to discussion.*** "You all did really well with that. We are going to talk together for a few moments about using On-Track Thinking."

Linking question. "How is On-Track Thinking different from how you have thought in the past?"

Disclosure questions. "Have you ever just reacted quickly without thinking things through?"; "How did that work?"

Expansion questions. "What other skills do you use with On-Track Thinking?"; "When can On-Track Thinking help you in your life?"

➡ ***Orient to the end of Elaboration Phase.*** "Now that we know a little more about On-Track Thinking, are we ready to read a story together?"

E-Spiral Phase 4. Efficacy: Bridge to Real Life

➡ ***Orient to Learning Skills, Worked Example 3."We are going to go through a scenario for a practice activity to see how Clear Picture and On-Track Thinking go together.*** Let's turn to On-Track Thinking, Worked Example 3 (p. 91)."

Instructions for the efficacy activity. "We will read through this worked example and see how the person in the example manages a situation when she feels hurt by a friend. We will discuss her responses and share some of our own ideas."

Describe question. "Did you have any thoughts about how this person used her skills?"; "Do you have any other ideas that could help her?"

➡ ***Orient to discussion.*** "I thought you all did an awesome job. We have worked with lots of handouts today, and you all really did a good job hanging in there. It isn't easy to use skills, but you will find it gets easier and easier with practice. On-Track Thinking is one of the toughest skills! Let's talk for a few minutes about some of the challenges of using skills before we finish for today."

Barrier question. "What is difficult about using On-Track Thinking for you?"

Wisdom question. "Do you think it is important for you to use On-Track Thinking?"

Commitment question. "Are you going to use On-Track Thinking?"

Coaching question. "How can you get yourself to use On-Track Thinking?"

➡ ***Orient to home study.*** "It sounds as if we know it is hard, and we still have to use skills. When we understand this, we really are on our way to learning skills. To know skills, we have to practice them outside of group. So this week we will work on using On-Track Thinking. Practice whenever you have a chance to do Clear Picture and On-Track Thinking. Good luck!

"Also, if you want to study skills at home, review all the handouts we have gone over so far. You can also do Learning Skills, On-Track Thinking Worksheet 1 (p. 88). Choose a situation and fill out the worksheet. You can do it by yourself or ask a staff member to help. Any questions?"

➡ ***Orient to group ending.*** "As you know, we ring the bell six times at the end of group. We do one ring for each of the Clear Picture Do's. It is a chance to notice what is happening inside and outside of us right now. We take a moment to get a Clear Picture as we go back to our activities. Who would like to ring the bell today?"

On-Track Thinking Handouts to Review in Future Cycles or for Home Study

✓ Learning Skills, On-Track Thinking Summary Sheet (p. 85).

☆ *Teaching points.* The summary sheet can be used during the encoding phase to explain concepts as teaching points. It may be too boring to read in group, but having different group members read different sections can break it up. Summary sheets are helpful for home study and for teaching the skills to skills coaches.

✓ Learning Skills, On-Track Thinking Worksheet 1 (p. 88).

☆ *Teaching points.* The individual chooses a situation to review and completes each of the questions.

✓ Learning Skills, On-Track Thinking Worked Example 4 (p. 94)

☆ *Teaching points.* This worked example offers samples of multiple Cheerleading statements that can encourage the individual to be on-track to his goals. If the individual gets overwhelmed by off-track thoughts, Cheerleading: Blast It could be helpful.

✓ Learning Skills, On-Track Thinking Worksheet 5 (p. 95)

☆ *Teaching points.* This worksheet provides an opportunity for the individual to name a situation and list several Cheerleading statements that will help her be on-track to her goals.

✓ Learning Skills, On-Track Thinking Worked Example 5 (p. 96)

☆ *Teaching points.* The Skills in My Life worked example shows how each skill can be used in a person's life. These processes help with creating skills plans.

✓ Learning Skills, On-Track Thinking Worksheet 6 (p. 97)

☆ *Teaching points.* This worksheet offers the individual an opportunity to identify situations in his life when he can use skills.

✓ Learning Skills, On-Track Thinking Worked Example 6 (p. 98)

☆ *Teaching points.* This worked example weighs the pros and cons of using skills in different situations.

✓ Learning Skills, On-Track Thinking Worksheet 7 (p. 99)

☆ *Teaching points.* This worksheet allows the individual to practice weighing the pros and cons of using skills in different situations in her life.

WEEK 5: ON-TRACK ACTIONS

Preparing for Group

Handouts Needed

✓ Learning Skills, On-Track Action Handout 1 (p. 104)
✓ Learning Skills, On-Track Action Handout 2 (p. 105)
✓ Learning Skills, On-Track Action Handout 3 (p. 106)
✓ Learning Skills, On-Track Action Handout 4 (p. 109)
✓ Learning Skills, On-Track Action Handout 5 (p. 112)
✓ Learning Skills, On-Track Action Handout 6 (p. 118)
✓ Learning Skills, On-Track Action Handout 7 (p. 119)
✓ Learning Skills, On-Track Action Worked Example 1 (p. 107)
✓ Learning Skills, On-Track Action Worksheet 1 (p. 108)

E-Spiral Phase 1. Exploring Existing Knowledge Base (Review)

➡ ***Welcome group.*** "How is everyone doing today? OK, ready to learn some skills? Great! What activity do we do to start group? [Pause for response.] Exactly—we ring the bell. All set?"

➡ ***Orient to the mindfulness activity: noticing surroundings.*** "Are you ready to do our mindfulness exercise? [Wait for response.] Great!"

Instructions for the mindfulness exercise. "OK, as I ring the bell, please bring your attention to your surroundings. Notice Surroundings is one of the Clear Picture Do's. We use our five senses to notice what is happening around us. We look to see different things where we are. We listen to hear any sounds. We notice tastes in our mouths and smells in the air. We notice anything we are touching, like our feet on the floor or where our bodies are touching the chair. If your mind drifts to something other than surroundings, gently bring your mind back. Getting a Clear Picture about what is happening around us helps us make on-track choices. Having a fuzzy picture about what is happening around us can help us go off-track. I will ring the bell five times and ask you to notice each of your five senses: see, hear, taste, smell, and touch."

Describe questions. "What did you notice during this exercise?"; "Did your mind drift?"; "Were you able to bring your mind back?"

➡ ***Orient to Skills System review.*** "Fantastic! How about we go through our Skills System review?"

Note: The skills instructor can choose a Basic Review Exercise from Week 1 (pp. 134–135), an Advanced Review Activity from Week 3 (p. 146), or create a new one.

➡ ***Orient to skills practice.*** "Great! It is getting a little easier, isn't it? OK, let's go over our homework. This week we were going to practice using Clear Picture and On-Track Thinking."

Disclosure questions. "Who would like to share about how they used Clear Picture and On-Track Thinking this week?"; "How did it work?"; "Do you wish you had done anything differently?"

➡ ***Orient to new skills topic.*** "That is a good start. Shall we talk about taking On-Track Actions?"

Discuss existing knowledge about the new topic.

Assessment questions. "Are there times when people have urges to go off-track?"; "What kinds of things make us want to go off-track?"; "Do people feel out of control sometimes?"; "Why do you think that happens?"; "What is wisdom?"

Relevant context questions. "What is it like to be off-track?"; "Do you ever feel as if you are stuck off-track, and you can't get back on-track?"; "Do you ever want to get back on-track but don't do anything to make that happen?"

Clarifying questions. "Do off-track actions help us reach our goals?"; "Where do off-track actions take us?"; "Do On-Track Actions help us reach our goals? How?"

Note: It is helpful to orient participants to the possible short-term benefits of off-track actions to validate the urge. Then, highlighting the long-term results can help participants make an informed decision.

➡ ***Orient to relevant context of the new topic.*** "From our discussion, it is clear that we all have off-track urges. It sounds like it is hard to stay on-track. We have to use Clear Picture and On-Track Thinking to stay on-track. Thinking about being on-track must be followed by action. Taking action means that we do something on-track."

E-Spiral Phase 2. Encoding: New Learning

➡ ***Orient to new learning: On-Track Action.*** "Great discussion. Today we are going to learn about On-Track Actions. We will learn about how we get a Clear Picture, use On-Track Thinking, and take an On-Track Action reaching toward our goal. This is a 123 skills chain. When we use skills 123, it helps us act in Wise Mind. Let's turn to page 104 of the *Skills System Workbook.* We are going to work on Learning Skills, On-Track Action Handout 1. It looks like this. All set?"

Instructions for encoding activity. "Great, we are going to go through the handout together. I will talk a little about each main point; then we will have a discussion, OK?"

☆ *Teaching points.* "Clear Picture and On-Track Thinking help us do On-Track Actions. First, we use Skill 1, Clear Picture, to know what is happening inside and outside of us. We check our feelings, thoughts, and urges and Turn It to Skill 2, On-Track Thinking. Then we make a Skills Plan and figure out what our On-Track Actions, Skill 3, will be to reach our goal. When we start with Skills 1, 2, and 3, we can usually stay on-track to our goals. [Points to the line that leads to the star.] Using Skills 123 together helps us be in Wise Mind. In Wise Mind we are balancing having feelings *and* thinking clearly to be on-track. Sometimes we are in emotional mind and have a fuzzy picture. Often when we are out-of-balance with our feelings, we have off-track thinking that leads to off-track actions. [Points to the line that leads to the crash site.] The good news is that once we are off-track, we can get back on-track by doing 1, 2, 3 Wise Mind! What are Skills 1, 2, 3? Right: Clear Picture, On-Track Thinking, and On-Track Action! Staying on-track is as easy as . . . [Says '1, 2, 3' with everyone at once.] Right: 1, 2, 3! Any questions?"

➡ ***Orient to Learning Skills, On-Track Action Handout 2.*** "OK, let's learn more about On-Track Actions. Turn to page 105 in the *Skills System Workbook.* Learning Skills, On-Track Action Handout 2 looks like this. Ready?"

☆ *Teaching points.*

1. "There are lots of different kinds of On-Track Actions. An On-Track Action is the first step toward our goals. For example, if we want to learn skills, practicing at home is an On-Track

Action. Practicing will help us learn skills. Throwing our skills book in the garbage would probably be an off-track action in that situation." (Optional: Refer to Learning Skills, On-Track Action Handout 3 on p. 106.)

2. "Sometimes we need to do the On-Track Action of Switch Tracks when we are heading off-track. It might be helpful to do an On-Track Action that is opposite of our off-track urges to Switch Tracks. When we do the opposite of our urge, we are doing Opposite Action."

Assessment question. "What does the word 'opposite' mean?"

"For example, if we want new friends, and we are standing in the corner at a party, we may need to take actions to be very friendly and introduce ourselves to people rather than hiding in the corner. Our urge may be to hide, yet we take an Opposite Action and jump into the social situation with both feet. Doing the opposite may be a great idea to help us reach our goal." (Optional: Refer to Learning Skills, On-Track Action Handout 4 on p. 109.)

3. "It is often helpful to make an On-Track Action Plan. Doing on-track things every day that make us healthy and happy can help us feel good and make on-track choices. For example, if we eat well, exercise, and sleep in balanced ways, we are less grumpy and moody. When we feel good, we are more able to be on-track." (Optional: Refer to Learning Skills, On-Track Action Handout 5 on p. 112.)

4. "There are times when we need to Accept the Situation. Sometimes we have done everything we can in a situation, and we just have to accept what is happening. We may not like it, but we have to realize that it must be accepted. The great thing is that we have skills to deal with waiting for things to get better! When we know skills, we learn to make the best of a bad situation or make lemonade when life gives us lemons." (Optional: Refer to Learning Skills, On-Track Action Handout 6 on p. 118.)

5. "There are times when we need to Turn the Page. For example, if we broke a favorite mug, we can be sad for a while, but at some point, we are dwelling on problems. When we dwell on problems for too long, it can make us more emotional. We have to learn when enough is enough for ourselves. We may have the urge to get stuck on certain things, but getting stuck can keep us from our goals. Any questions?" (Optional: Refer to Learning Skills, On-Track Action Handout 7 on p. 119.)

Note: If time allows, try to review the On-Track Action Handouts (3–7).

☆ *Teaching points for Learning Skills, On-Track Action Handout 3 (p. 106).* This handout explores the first type of On-Track Action—Take a Step toward My Goal. The group reviews the handout to see that the individual in the picture does Clear Picture, On-Track Thinking, and takes an On-Track Action of doing a Safety Plan—Move Away to reach his goal. After that his On-Track Action is to do a New-Me Activity (playing solitaire), which helps him focus. The boxes above him show what skills he can choose as On-Track Actions at 0–5 and 0–3 feelings.

☆ *Teaching points for Learning Skills, On-Track Action Handout 4 (p. 109).* The group reviews this handout that explains On-Track Action—Switch Tracks. The example is self-explanatory. Giving examples for jumping in with both feet and acting opposite to the urge will be helpful.

☆ *Teaching Points for Learning Skills, On-Track Action Handout 5 (p. 112).* This handout outlines different components of an individual's On-Track Action Plan. It is important to focus on the concept of balance versus absolute rules. The individual needs to be able to make adjustments as her life changes.

☆ *Teaching Points for Learning Skills, On-Track Action Handout 6 (p. 118).* This handout describes when we may consider practicing acceptance. The group members go through each instance and discuss examples.

☆ *Teaching Points for Learning Skills, On-Track Action Handout 7 (p. 119).* The group members review this handout and discuss the process and challenges associated with turning the page.

➡ ***Orient to the end of the Encoding Phase.*** "On-Track Actions are our friends! They keep us on-track! Are we ready to practice On-Track Actions?"

➡ ***Orient to Learning Skills, On-Track Action Handout 3.*** "OK, let's learn more about On-Track Actions, First Step to My Goal. Turn to page 106 in the *Skills System Workbook.* On-Track Action Handout 3 looks like this. Ready?"

☆ *Teaching points.* This handout describes how we take an On-Track Action of the first step toward our goal in Wise Mind. We first get a Clear Picture, do On-Track Thinking, and then take On-Track Actions toward our goals. When we are at Levels 0–3, we can use all our skills—All-the-Time and Calm-Only. If we are at a Level 4 or 5, it is best to use our All-the-Time skills, because using our Calm Only skills over a Level 3 may lead us off-track.

E-Spiral Phase 3. Elaboration: Practice and Linking

➡ ***Orient to Learning Skills, On-Track Action Worked Example 1 and Worksheet 1.*** "OK, we are going to fill out a worksheet together (p. 108 of the *Skills System Workbook*), but first let's look at a completed one (p. 107) to get an idea about how to do it."

Note: The group can read the answers on the worked example and discuss whether they agree that each is an On-Track Action. Then the group can generate different goals and On-Track Actions that would support the goal.

Disclosure question. "How did that exercise go for you?"

➡ ***Orient to discussion.*** "OK, let's talk a little more about On-Track Actions."

Linking questions. "This is a 123 skills chain: What does this mean?"; "How is this different from what you have done in the past?"

Disclosure questions. "When was a time when it was difficult to do an On-Track Action?"; "What was going on that made it difficult?"

Expansion questions. "What are other skills we use with On-Track Action?"; "Could On-Track Action help you in your life?"; "At home?"; "At work?"; "In your relationships?"; "When you deal with family members?"

➡ ***Orient to the end of the Elaboration Phase.*** "Great discussion. It is important for us to understand how to use our skills in difficult situations. In tough situations, it is easy to go off-track and hard to reach goals."

E-Spiral Phase 4. Efficacy: Bridge to Real Life

➡ ***Orient to efficacy activities: role playing a scenario.*** "So, now we are going to do a role play. We are going to have a little, tiny argument! I am actually going to irritate you on purpose, so that you can practice Clear Picture, On-Track Thinking, and On-Track Action. Who would like to start?"

Instructions for the efficacy activity. "I am going to walk up to you and accuse you of stealing my video game. As I am talking, I would like you to quickly get a Clear Picture and do On-Track Thinking. I am not going to keep talking too much, because I want you to have time to figure out what to do. Once you make a Skills Plan, take an On-Track Action. You can ask the group for help whenever you need to. Now, group members, if you have suggestions, raise your hand. Our volunteer may point to you, and you can give the advice. He can ask for volunteers or try to handle it on his own. We are going to do this slowly to practice putting these skills together. Any questions?"

Note: It is helpful for the skills instructor to stop and prompt the group members to help the participant through the Clear Picture Do's, On-Track Thinking, and figuring out an On-Track Action that fits for the participant. If a psychodrama format was used, different group members could offer coaching on specific skills (e.g., Clear Picture and On-Track Thinking). Depending on the group's level of skills knowledge, the instructor gauges how much depth to go into, as well as how much support to offer.

Disclosure questions. "Did you get a Clear Picture?" [review each of the Clear Picture Do's]; "Did you use Check It?"; "Turn It?"; "Cheerleading?"; "What was your skills plan?"; "Did you take an On-Track Action?"; "Were you in Wise Mind?"

➡ ***Orient to discussion.*** "Great job on the role play. Before we finish, would it be OK if we have a brief discussion about some of the challenges involved in taking On-Track Actions?"

Barrier question. "What is difficult about using On-Track Action?"

Wisdom question. "Do you feel it is important for you to use On-Track Action in your life?"

Commitment question. "When will you use On-Track Action?"

Coaching question. "How can you coach yourself to use On-Track Action when you feel stuck?"

➡ ***Orient to home study.*** "Good discussion about On-Track Actions. Homework time! This week we are going to practice using On-Track Actions. Let's try to take actions that are Taking a Step to My Goal. Also, please practice Switching Tracks when you have off-track urges. If you want to study skills at home, you can review all the handouts we have gone over so far. You can look at the On-Track Action Worked Examples and complete the Worksheets (see below). Perhaps find someone to help you, if you need it. Any questions?"

➡ ***Orient to group ending.*** "As you know, we ring the bell six times at the end of group. We do one ring for each of the Clear Picture Do's. It is a chance to notice what is happening inside and outside of us right now. We take a moment to get a Clear Picture as we go back to our activities. Who would like to ring the bell today?"

On-Track Action Handouts to Review in Future Cycles or for Home Study

✓ Learning Skills, On-Track Action Summary Sheet (p. 103).

☆ *Teaching points.* The summary sheet can be used during the encoding phase to explain concepts as teaching points. It may be too boring to read in group, but having different group members read different sections can break it up. Summary sheets are helpful for home study and for teaching skills to skills coaches.

✓ Learning Skills, On-Track Action Handouts 3–7 (pp. 106, 109, 112, 118, 119).

☆ *Teaching points.* If the group was not able to review On-Track Action Handouts 3–7, the individual can complete these in future cycles, during individual therapy, or while at home.

✓ Learning Skills, On-Track Action Worksheet 1 (p. 108)

☆ *Teaching points.* This worksheet offers an opportunity for the individual to list On-Track Actions that will help her reach her goals.

✓ Learning Skills, On-Track Action Worked Example 2 (p. 110)

☆ *Teaching points.* This worked example helps the individual see how off-track actions can be switched to On-Track Actions.

✓ Learning Skills, On-Track Action Worksheet 2 (p. 111)

☆ *Teaching points.* This worksheet offers an opportunity for the individual to list her off-track actions that can be switched to On-Track Actions.

✓ Learning Skills, On-Track Action Worked Example 3 (p. 113)

☆ *Teaching points.* This worked example is a sample of a person's On-Track Action Plan.

✓ Learning Skills, On-Track Action Worksheet 3 (p. 114).

☆ *Teaching points.* This worksheet is used by the individual to create his own On-Track Action Plan.

✓ Learning Skills, On-Track Action Worksheet 4 (p. 115)

☆ *Teaching points.* This worksheet offers an opportunity for the individual to list different aspects of her life that she needs to balance.

✓ Learning Skills, On-Track Action Worksheet 5 (p. 117)

☆ *Teaching points.* This worksheet offers an opportunity for the individual to list On-Track Actions that allow him to balance different aspects of his life.

✓ Learning Skills, On-Track Action Worked Example 5 (p. 120)

☆ *Teaching points.* This worked example shows how to do Clear Picture, On-Track Thinking, and take On-Track Actions—Accepting the Situation and Turning the Page.

✓ Learning Skills, On-Track Action Worksheet 6 (p. 121)

☆ *Teaching points.* This worksheet helps the individual do Clear Picture, On-Track Thinking, and take On-Track Actions—Accepting the Situation and Turning the Page.

✓ Learning Skills, On-Track Action Worked Example 6 (p. 122)

☆ *Teaching points.* This worked example provides examples of the five types of On-Track Actions and On-Track Actions for skills 4–9.

✓ Learning Skills, On-Track Action Worksheet 7 (p. 123)

☆ *Teaching points.* This worksheet offers an opportunity for the individual to write in On-Track Actions for the five types of On-Track Actions and skills 4–9.

✓ Learning Skills, On-Track Action Worksheet 8 (p. 124)

☆ *Teaching points.* This worksheet is a practice linking different On-Track Actions in skills chains.

WEEK 6: SAFETY PLANS

Preparing for Group

Handouts Needed

✓ Learning Skills, Safety Plan Handout 1 (p. 128)
✓ Learning Skills, Safety Plan Worked Example 1 (p. 129)
✓ Learning Skills, Safety Plan Handout 2 (p. 131)
✓ Learning Skills, Safety Plan Worked Example 2 (p. 132)
✓ Learning Skills, Safety Plan Handout 3 (p. 134)
✓ Learning Skills, Safety Plan Handout 4 (p. 135)
✓ Learning Skills, Safety Plan Worked Example 3 (p. 137)
✓ Learning Skills, Safety Plan Worksheet 4 (p. 138)

E-Spiral Phase 1. Exploring Existing Knowledge Base (Review)

➡ ***Welcome group.*** "Welcome back! How is everyone doing today? Well, how about we get started?"

➡ ***Orient to the mindfulness activity: Body Check.*** "Are you ready to do our mindfulness exercise? [Wait for response.] Great!"

Instructions for the mindfulness activity. "Today we are going to notice the breath and then do a Body Check. Practicing a Body Check can help us be more self-aware. The more we notice what is happening inside us, the clearer we are. It helps us label and rate our feelings when we notice how our body is reacting to a situation.

"As I ring the bell, please bring your attention to body sensations you feel. You may notice aches, pains, or muscle tightness. You may notice muscle relaxation and calmness in your body. You might notice sensations where your body is touching things around you like the table, chair, and floor. Notice whatever is happening in your body—*as it is, without changing it.* If your mind drifts away from doing the Body Check, gently bring your mind back to your body. I will ring the bell six times and you will notice different sensations in your body. Any questions?"

Describe questions. "What did you notice during your Body Check?"; "Did you stay focused on your body check?"; "What was difficult about this exercise?"

Note: It may be helpful to write the different observations on the board.

➡ ***Orient to Skills System review.*** "Good observations. Now, how about we do our Skills System review?"

Note: The skills instructor can choose a Basic Review Exercise from Week 1 (pp. 134–135), an Advanced Review Activity from Week 3 (p. 146), or create a new one.

➡ ***Orient to skills practice.*** "Great job—we are getting there! Now, we are going to review our skills practice. We were practicing doing On-Track Actions this week. Let's not forget how we also use Clear Picture and On-Track Thinking to do what works."

Disclosure questions. "Who would like to share about how they used On-Track Actions this week?"; "What were some of the positive things people did as an On-Track Action?"; "Did anyone Switch Tracks?"; "What did we do that was opposite of Off-Track Urges?"; "Who used 123 Wise Mind?"; "What things did you have to accept this week?"; "Did anyone Turn the Page on something this week?"

➡ ***Orient to new skills topic.*** "Excellent! Before we get started on our new skill for this week, can we talk about what we already know about keeping ourselves safe?"

Discuss existing knowledge about the new topic.

Assessment questions. "What does the word 'risk' mean?"; "What is a risky situation?"

Relevant context questions. "What are some examples of risky situations that you have noticed?"; "How do we know when a situation is not safe?"; "What are some situations that may be helpful to avoid?"

Clarifying questions. "What can happen if we move toward risky situations?"; "What happens if we move away from risky situations?"

➡ ***Orient to relevant context of new topic.*** "Sometimes there are difficult situations in life. Much of the time, it is best that we face challenging situations so that we learn how to deal with them. Sometimes, avoiding can make things worse. Other times, situations should be avoided, because there is risk that can cause us problems. In these situations, we use our Safety Plan. We use our Clear Picture and On-Track Thinking to make these important decisions."

E-Spiral Phase 2. Encoding: New Learning

➡ ***Orient to new learning: Safety Plan.*** "The Safety Plan is the fourth skill in the Skills System. Safety Plans help us handle risky situations. We are going to go over several handouts today; it seems like a lot! I do not expect us to learn all about Safety Plans today, but we will review the three types of Safety Plans, the three Levels of Risk, and the three things we can do when we notice risk."

Instructions for the encoding activity. "Let's get started by turning to page 128 in the *Skills System Workbook.* Learning Skills, Safety Plan Handout 1 looks like this. All set?"

☆ *Teaching points.* "Safety Plans help us handle risks that come from both inside and outside of us. Inside risks are ones that happen inside our bodies. When we have TUFFs [off-track Thoughts, Urges, Feelings, and Fantasies], we need to use Safety Plans. TUFFs make it more difficult for us to stay on-track.

"Things, such as people, places, or things, can be outside risks. Certain people, places, or things can cause us problems. These outside risks can make us have off-track thoughts, urges, feelings, and fantasies that make the situation dangerous for us or other people. Any questions?"

➡ ***Orient to Learning Skills, Safety Plan Worked Example 1.*** "Let's turn to the Safety Plan Worked Example 1 on page 129. It looks like this."

☆ *Teaching point.* "Let's read through this worked example together to learn more about inside and outside risks."

➡ ***Orient to Learning Skills, Safety Plan Handout 2.*** "OK, good start. Now let's learn about the three levels of risk. Please turn to page 131 in the *Skills System Workbook.* Safety Plan Handout 2 looks like this."

Note: The leader reads through the handout with the group.

☆ *Teaching points.* "There are three Levels of Risk: low, medium, and high. To identify risk, we ask ourselves (1) How much damage can the risk cause? and (2) How close is it to us?

In a high-risk situation, either there is a chance for serious damage or the thing is very close to us. In a medium-risk situation, the risk can cause us problems or is in our area. In low-risk situations, the risk may cause stress or is far away from us. So, the more damage something can cause, the higher the risk. The closer the risk is to us, the higher the risk. For example, if a rattlesnake is next to us, it is high risk. If the snake is 100 feet away, the risk is lower. Any questions?"

➡ ***Orient to Learning Skills, Safety Plan Worked Example 2.*** "OK, let's look at the example on page 132 of the *Skills System Workbook;* it looks like this."

➡ ***Orient to Learning Skills, Safety Plan Handout 3.*** "Great! I know there is a lot to learn about Safety Plans. It will take some time learn it; we take one step at a time. OK, let's turn to page 134 to see the three types of Safety Plans."

☆ *Teaching points.* "Let's read this together to learn about the three types of Safety Plans. We have to do more safety planning as the situation becomes more risky. For example, in a low-risk situation, it might be all right to just do a Thinking Safety Plan. In a medium-risk situation, it is usually best to do a Thinking and Talking Safety Plans. In a high-risk situation, it is helpful to do Thinking, Talking, and Written Safety Plans to be sure the danger is managed well."

Note: The leader or group reads through the handout with the group.

➡ ***Orient to Learning Skills, Safety Plan Handout 4.*** "So far we have learned about low, medium, and high risks. We have also learned about Written, Talking, and Thinking Safety Plans. Next we are going to learn about what we do in these situations to handle risk. Please turn to page 135 of the *Skills System Workbook.* The Safety Plan Handout 4 looks like this."

Note: The leader or group reads through the handout with the group.

☆ *Teaching points.* "When there is a low risk, it may be possible to focus on the New-Me Activity that we are doing at the time. For example, if I notice a small issue far away, I can just focus on my activity. I am not ignoring the problem; I am choosing to focus on something helpful. Next, if there is a risk that is closer or will cause me problems, I move away to get distance between me and the risk. For example, I may move my seat in a room if someone is bothering me, then continue focusing on my New-Me Activity. If there is a high-risk situation, I will want to leave the area completely. I want to be sure I cannot hear, see, talk to, or touch the risk. For example, I would go to my room and close the door."

Content questions. "Why is it dangerous to be able to see, hear, talk to, or touch the risk?"; "How do we know where to go when we have to move or leave an area?"; "Why is it good to do a New-Me Activity?"; "What New-Me Activities are helpful to focus on?"; "How far away do we need to go when we move away?"; "How do we focus our attention on our activity when there is a low risk?"; "How do we know when we should do a Safety Plan to avoid a situation and when it is best to try to face a difficult situation?"

➡ ***Orient to end of the Encoding Phase.*** "There are many parts of the Safety Plan skill: levels of risk, types of Safety Plans, and actions that we take to handle risky situations. How about we move on to practice safety planning?"

E-Spiral Phase 3. Elaboration: Practice and Linking

➡ ***Orient to Learning Skills, Safety Plan Worked Example 3.*** "OK, we are going to put all of these new things together into a Written Safety Plan. Please turn to page 137 of the *Skills System Workbook.* The Safety Plan Worked Example 3 looks like this."

Instruction for practice exercise. "We are going to read through this Safety Plan together and talk about it."

Disclosure question. "What are your thoughts about Safety Plans?"

➡ ***Orient to discussion.*** "OK, I know you have done Safety Plans in the past; let's talk about that a little bit."

Linking questions. "What does it mean that this is a 1234 skills chain?"; "What is it like to do a Safety Plan in Wise Mind?"; "How is Safety Plan different from what you have done in the past?"

Disclosure questions. "Were there times when you did not use a Safety Plan and wish you had?"; "What happened?"

Expansion questions. "What are other skills we use with Safety Plans?"; "Are there times in your life that you could use a Safety Plan?"; "At work?"; "At home?"; "With family?"; "With friends?"

➡ ***Orient to the end of the Elaboration Phase.*** "It sounds like there are times when we need to use Safety Plans. I'm glad we are learning this today!"

E-Spiral Phase 4. Efficacy: Bridge to Real Life

➡ ***Orient to efficacy activities: Learning Skills, Safety Plan Worksheet 3.*** "OK, I think we are ready to do a Safety Plan together. Let's turn to page 136 of the *Skills System Workbook.* The Safety Plan Worksheet 3 looks like this. Who would like to share a risky situation that happened this week that we could go through and do a Safety Plan for? [Wait for response.] Very brave, thank you!"

Note: It is important to pick a scenario that is interesting, yet not highly arousing for the volunteer or the group. A medium- or low-risk situation is best to review.

Instructions for the efficacy activity. The instructor leads the person through the Safety Plan. The instructor focuses on moving through the Safety Plan rather than stopping to do Expressing Myself or Problem Solving about the situation. The group is encouraged to participate. The instructor and group ask questions to foster thinking about different options and check the fit of each. Together the instructor, the volunteer, and the group make the Safety Plan.

Disclosure questions. "How do you think this Safety Planning went?"; "Do you think the Safety Plan would have helped?"; "Do you have any questions about Safety Plans?"

➡ ***Orient to discussion.*** "That was very good; everyone was helpful. Before we finish up today, I would like us to talk together about some of the challenges of doing Safety Plans."

Barrier questions. "What is difficult about using a Safety Plan?"; "What is it like to have to walk away from situations, especially ones that we enjoy but know are risky?"; "What is it like to have to stop doing something we like because of someone else?"

Wisdom question. "Do you think Safety Plans are important for you to use?"

Commitment question. "When can you use Safety Plans in your life?"

Coaching question. "How can you coach yourself to use Safety Plans?"

➡ ***Orient to home study.*** "Great job today! There is a lot to learn about Safety Plans. Practice can really help. So, this week, please practice noticing risky situations. Think about whether the risk is low, medium, or high. Think about whether you should do a Thinking, Talking, and/or Written Safety Plan. Also, decide whether it is best to refocus, move away, or leave the area completely. Are there any questions? [Wait for response.] Good luck!

"Also, if you want to study skills at home, review all the handouts we have gone over so far. You can also do Learning Skills, Safety Plan Worksheets 1, 2, 3, and 4."

➡ ***Orient to group ending.*** "As you know, we ring the bell six times at the end of group. We do one ring for each of the Clear Picture Do's. It is a chance to notice what is happening inside and outside of us right now. We take a moment to get a Clear Picture as we go back to our activities. Who would like to ring the bell today?"

Safety Plan Handouts to Review in Future Cycles or for Home Study

✓ Learning Skills, Safety Plan Summary Sheet (p. 127)

☆ *Teaching points.* The summary sheet can be used during the encoding phase to explain concepts as teaching points. It may be too boring to read in group, but having different group members read different sections can break it up. Summary sheets are helpful for home study and for teaching the skills to skills coaches.

✓ Learning Skills, Safety Plan Worksheet 1 (p. 130)

☆ *Teaching points.* The individual lists on this worksheet specific inside and outside risks that he experiences.

✓ Learning Skills, Safety Plan Worksheet 2 (p. 133)

☆ *Teaching points.* The individual lists specific low, medium, and high risks on this worksheet.

✓ Learning Skills, Safety Plan Worksheet 3 (p. 136)

☆ *Teaching points.* The individual thinks of a different situation that happened to her and circles the type of risk, level of risk, type of Safety Plan, and how she would handle the risk.

✓ Learning Skills, Safety Plan Worksheet 4 (p. 138)

☆ *Teaching points.* The individual writes down (or has assistance in writing) information about a risky situation. He then determines the level of risk and on-track ways to manage the situation.

✓ Learning Skills, Safety Plan Worked Example 3 (p. 137)

☆ *Teaching points.* This is a more detailed Written Safety Plan. Review the Worked Example and discuss information about a risky situation (urges and actions), level of risk, types of Safety Plans, how to handle risks, and actions the individual will take to manage the risks.

✓ Learning Skills, Safety Plan Worksheet 5 (p. 140)

☆ *Teaching points.* On this more detailed Written Safety Plan, the individual writes down (or has assistance in writing) information about a risky situation (urges and actions), level of risk, types of Safety Plans, how to handle risks, and actions she will take to manage the risks.

WEEK 7: NEW-ME ACTIVITIES

Preparing for Group

Handouts Needed

✓ Learning Skills, New-Me Activities Handout 1 (p. 144)
✓ Learning Skills, New-Me Activities Handout 2 (p. 145)
✓ Learning Skills, New-Me Activities Handout 3 (p. 146)
✓ Learning Skills, New-Me Activities Handout 4 (p. 149)
✓ Learning Skills, New-Me Activities Handout 5 (p. 151)
✓ Learning Skills, New-Me Activities Handout 6 (p. 153)

E-Spiral Phase 1. Exploring Existing Knowledge Base (Review)

➡ ***Welcome group.*** "Hi, everybody. How are we doing today? Ready for some mindfulness?"

➡ ***Orient to the mindfulness activity: noticing feelings.*** "Today we are going to notice our feelings."

Instructions for the mindfulness exercise. "As I ring the bell, please bring your attention to noticing any feelings you are having. You may notice comfortable feelings. You may notice uncomfortable feelings. Notice the feelings just as they are without changing them. Notice the sensations and then label what feeling it is. If your mind starts to wander to other things, gently bring your mind back to the feeling. Notice the feelings come and let them go without needing to act on them or make them stronger by focusing on the issues. Learning to turn our minds to and from feelings helps us manage them. OK, here goes; let's focus on feelings. Any questions?"

Describe questions. "How was that for you?"; "What feelings did you notice?"; "Did your mind drift?"; "Did you notice urges to take actions?"; "Were you able to bring your mind back to your feelings?"

➡ ***Orient to Skills System review.*** "Great job with Clear Picture. OK, how about we review our skills, System Tools, and the Clear Picture Do's."

Note: The skills instructor can choose a Basic Review Exercise from Week 1 (pp. 134–135), an Advanced Review Activity from Week 3 (p. 146), or create a new one.

➡ ***Orient to skills practice.*** "Great, on to homework! How did we do this week practicing Safety Plans?"

Disclosure questions. "Who would like to tell us about a Thinking Safety Plan they did this week?"; "Who can tell us about doing a Talking Safety Plan this week?"; "Who can tell us about doing a Written Safety Plan this week?"; "Did any of you wish you had used a Safety Plan this week?"

➡ ***Orient to new skills topic.*** "Good start. Safety Plans take time to learn; you all will get it. Now, let's talk about what we know about doing New-Me Activities."

Discuss existing knowledge about the new topic.

Assessment questions. "What do you think 'new-me' means?"; "What do you think 'old-me' means?"; "What are some activities that help you stay on-track?"

Relevant context questions. "What is the difference between an on-track activity and an off-track activity?"; "How do we decide if an activity is helpful or not helpful?"

Clarifying questions. "Why do people choose New-Me Activities?"; "Why do people choose off-track activities?"

➡ ***Orient to relevant context of the new topic.*** "New-Me Activities help us in many ways. We are going to learn about how to choose the right activities at the right time to help us reach our goals."

E-Spiral Phase 2. Encoding: New Learning

➡ ***Orient to new learning: New-Me Activities Handout 1.*** "We are going to learn about New-Me Activities today! We are going to read through five New-Me Activities handouts. Let's turn to page 144 of the *Skills System Workbook.* The New-Me Activities Handout 1 looks like this."

Instructions for the encoding activity. The group reads through the New-Me Activities handout and discusses different activities. "Would anyone like to read or should I?"

☆ *Teaching points.* "This handout introduces the four different types of New-Me Activities. Different activities help us do different things. Some help us focus, feel better, distract us, and are fun. We have to learn to do many different New-Me Activities and to choose the one that helps most in the moment. Handouts 2–5 go into detail about each kind."

➡ ***Orient to Learning Skills, New-Me Activities Handout 2.*** "Now let's learn more about Solo and Partnership New-Me Activities. Please turn to page 145 in the *Skills System Workbook*. The New-Me Activities Handout 2 looks like this."

☆ *Teaching points.* "Solo New-Me Activities are activities we do by ourselves. We can do Solo New-Me Activities at any level of feeling: 0, 1, 2, 3, 4, or 5. Partnership New-Me Activities are activities we do with other people. When we interact with others we are doing Relationship Care, which is a Calm-Only skill. Because other people are involved when we are doing Partnership New-Me Activities, we need to be at a Level 0–3 of feeling.

➡ ***Orient to Learning Skills, New-Me Activities Handout 3.*** "Now let's learn more about Focus New-Me Activities. Please turn to page 146. The New-Me Activities Handout 3 looks like this."

☆ *Teaching points.* "Focus New-Me Activities help us focus our attention. We have to concentrate and pay attention carefully when we do these activities. Let's brainstorm a list on the board of each kind of activity on the handout."

Note: It is particularly important that each individual has accessible activities that fit his means and logistical situation.

Content questions. "What are different things we can organize and sort?"; "What kind of things can you clean?"; "When is it helpful to use Focus New-Me Activities?"

➡ ***Orienting to Learning Skills, New-Me Activities Handout 4.*** "Now we are going to look at page 149 in the *Skills System Workbook*. It is the New-Me Activities Handout 4 that shows us Feel Good New-Me Activities. It looks like this."

☆ *Teaching points.* "Feel Good New-Me Activities use our senses to make us feel more comfortable and happy. When we are feeling stressed or upset, it can help to do an activity that soothes and makes us feel better. Let's read these and brainstorm on the board a list of activities that utilize each of our senses that help us feel good."

Content questions. "What do you enjoy looking at?"; "What are things that you enjoy listening to?"; "What do you enjoy touching?"; "What do you enjoy smelling?"; "What do you enjoy tasting?"; "When is it helpful to use Feel Good New-Me Activities?"

➡ ***Orient to Learning Skills, New-Me Activities Handout 5.*** "On to Distraction New-Me Activities Handout 5. It is on page 151, and it looks like this."

☆ *Teaching points.* "Sometimes, we are overwhelmed and need to chill out and take a break. If we have done everything we can to fix a situation, there are times when it is best to distract our minds and/or distract our bodies. When we distract, we are switching our focus from one situation to another. We are focused on the new activity and Turning the Page from the one that is bothering us.

"It is important that we use Distract New-Me Activities when we have used all necessary skills in a situation and we need to wait, relax, or get our mind off of the situation. We don't want to distract if we need to deal with the situation. Distracting ourselves when we need to focus may lead us off-track. Knowing when and how to distract your mind and distract your body is important. We have to use Clear Picture and On-Track Thinking to figure out whether a Distraction New-Me Activity is an On-Track Action. Let's brainstorm a list on the board of activities that are useful to distract us."

Content questions. "What are things that help you get your mind off of your problems?"; "When is it helpful to distract ourselves?"; "When is it not helpful to distract ourselves?"

➡ ***Orient to Learning Skills, New-Me Activities Handout 6.*** "Fun New-Me Activities are next! Please turn to page 153. The New-Me Activities Handout 6 looks like this."

☆ *Teaching points.* "It is important to do activities that are fun. Doing activities that we enjoy helps us have a higher quality of life. If we do not do things that give us joy, we tend to get depressed. Let's brainstorm on the board a list of activities that people find fun."

Content questions. "What sports do you like to watch?"; "What hobbies do you enjoy?"; "What kind of crafts do you like to make?"

Note: It is important that the group discusses realistic options, so that the participants can readily integrate the activities into their lives.

➡ ***Orient to the end of the Encoding Phase.*** "We have come up with many great new ideas today. It's time to practice!"

E-Spiral Phase 3. Elaboration: Practice and Linking

➡ ***Orient to the elaboration activity.*** "We are going to do a New-Me Activity right now! Today we are going to do some drawing. Here are some markers and paper. We are going to draw for a few minutes."

Instructions for the practice exercise. "We are going to draw something, anything you wish. It can be a house, a person, a car, a tree, a boat, mountains—anything. It does not have to be fancy. The activity is to use your skills to jump into this activity with both feet! I know that not everyone is going to love this New-Me Activity. So for those of you who think you can't draw or are embarrassed, we are going to do an On-Track Action and give 100% effort to drawing. As we are drawing, we may notice our minds starting to insult our drawings or ourselves; we have to allow those off-track thoughts to pass and gently bring our attention back to our picture. Does this sound similar to how we control our attention when we ring the bell? It does to me! We want to stay focused on our picture, not on off-track thoughts or feelings. If we say nice things to other people about their drawings, what skill is that? [Wait for response.] Right—Relationship Care! If we say nice things to others, they might say our drawing is good. That might make us feel better! You can draw anything you want for 5 minutes. If you want to share the picture and even a story about what it is, great. Sharing our pictures might be stressful, so we may have to do another On-Track Action to make ourselves give 100% to this activity. Does everyone have something to draw on and to draw with? Any questions?"

Note: The instructor may want to offer verbal praise evenly across the group for effort, skill use, and drawings.

Disclosure questions. "Did you use Clear Picture and On-Track Thinking while you were drawing?"; "How was that activity for people?"; "What was helpful about it?"; "What was difficult about it?"; "Did you have to do an On-Track Action?"; "Were you able to jump in with both feet?"

➡ ***Orient to discussion.*** "Great, we are going to talk for a few minutes about doing New-Me Activities."

Linking questions. "New-Me Activities are a 1235 skills chain; what does this mean?"; "What is it like when we do a New-Me Activity in Wise Mind?"; "What is a 12345 skills chain?"; "In the past, have you ever been bored because you did not do enough New-Me Activities?"; "What was that like?"

Disclosure questions. "Did you use skills 1235 during this activity?"; "Who can describe a time when using a New-Me Activity really helped you feel better?"; "Who can describe a time when you had to do an On-Track Action because you didn't feel like doing anything?"; "Who can describe a time when you chose the wrong New-Me Activity to do?"; "What happened?"; "How can you tell when your New-Me Activities are in balance?"

Expansion questions. "What other skills do we use with New-Me Activities?"; "How can New-Me Activities help you reach your goals?"

➡ ***Orient to the end of the Elaboration Phase.*** "That was a great discussion. Guess what? We are going to practice a New-Me Activity again!"

E-Spiral Phase 4. Efficacy: Bridge to Real Life

➡ ***Orient to efficacy activities: group game.*** "Some of us like games and others may need to do some On-Track Thinking to help us jump in and play. What is some On-Track Thinking that can help us fully participate. Any ideas?"

Note: The skills instructor presents a game that will be fun for the group. This is an opportunity for the group leader to be creative. The instructor can make up an activity or bring in some kind of game that fits the ability level of the group members. The game should be simple, short, and fun. The goal is for all members to participate and to experience joy. It can be a skills game, such as Skills Person (similar to hangman, but each correct answer adds a body part to a person standing rather than a person hanging). In Skills Person someone draws a number of blank spaces that represent skills terms, and the group guesses the letters and ultimately the term. Team skills Jeopardy can be fun; the instructor or group members generate questions.

Instructions for the efficacy activity. The skills instructor gives clear, step-by-step directions. Be sure all participants are ready prior to beginning.

Disclosure questions. "Was this activity a Focus, Feel Good, Distraction, and/or Fun New-Me Activity?"; "Did you use 1235?"; "How was that activity for you?"; "Did you have fun?"; "Was there anything challenging about it?"

➡ ***Orient to discussion.*** "Let's talk a little more about some of the challenges we face when we do New-Me Activities."

Barrier questions. "What is difficult about doing New-Me Activities?"; "Is it difficult to ask people to join you?"; "How can we deal with that?"

Wisdom questions. "Are New-Me Activities important for you to do?"; "Do you need to do more New-Me Activities?"

Commitment question. "What new New-Me Activities will you try?"

Coaching question. "How can you coach yourself to do different New-Me Activities?"

➡ ***Orient to home study.*** "Great group today. Now it is homework time! This week we are going to practice doing all four kinds of New-Me Activities. We will do at least one Focus New-Me Activity, one Feel Good New-Me Activity, one Distraction New-Me Activity, and one Fun New-Me Activity. Also, please go over the Learning Skills, Problem Solving Summary Sheet on page 159 for next week. Any questions?

"Also, if you want to study skills at home, review all the handouts we have gone over so far. You can also do Learning Skills, New-Me Activities Worksheets 1–5."

➡ ***Orient to group ending.*** "As you know, we ring the bell six times at the end of group. We do one ring for each of the Clear Picture Do's. It is a chance to notice what is happening inside and outside of us right now. We take a moment to get a Clear Picture as we go back to our activities. Who would like to ring the bell today?"

New-Me Activities Handouts to Review in Future Cycles or for Home Study

✓ Learning Skills, New-Me Activities Summary Sheet (p. 143).

☆ *Teaching points.* The summary sheet can be used during the encoding phase to explain concepts as teaching points. It may be too boring to read in group, but having different group members read different sections can break it up. Summary sheets are helpful for home study and for teaching skills coaches the skills.

✓ Learning Skills, New-Me Activities Worksheet 1 (p. 147)

☆ *Teaching points.* In this worksheet, the individual lists New-Me Activities that help her focus attention.

Learning Skills, New-Me Activities Exercise 1 (p. 148)

☆ *Teaching points.* When we get stressed, our bodies can get tight and tense. Doing a progressive relaxation, can help. Starting at your feet, tighten and loosen all the parts of your body on this worksheet. This Focus New-Me Activity might make you feel like a New-Me!

✓ Learning Skills, New-Me Activities Worksheet 2 (p. 150)

☆ *Teaching points.* For this worksheet, the participant writes down New-Me Activities that help the body feel good.

✓ Learning Skills, New-Me Activities Worksheet 3 (p. 152)

☆ *Teaching points.* For this worksheet, the individual lists New-Me Activities that help provide distraction.

✓ Learning Skills, New-Me Activities Worksheet 4 (p. 154)

☆ *Teaching points.* For this worksheet, the individual writes down Fun New-Me Activities that the individual likes to do.

✓ Learning Skills, New-Me Activities Worked Example 1 (p. 155)

☆ *Teaching points.* Combining Solo New-Me Activities and Self Care can be very beneficial. Not only do the activities often increase focus, they help us take care of tasks that help us be on-track.

✓ Learning Skills, New-Me Activities Worksheet 5 (p. 156)

☆ *Teaching points.* This worksheet provides the opportunity for the individual to list several self-care Solo New-Me Activities and check off whether the activities help her focus, feel good, be distracted from situations that are increasing feelings, or have fun. Different kinds of activities can help us in multiple ways!

WEEK 8: PROBLEM SOLVING

Preparing for Group

Handouts Needed

✓ Learning Skills, Problem Solving Summary Sheet (p. 159)
✓ Learning Skills, Problem Solving Worked Example 1 (p. 160)

- ✓ Learning Skills, Problem Solving Worksheet 1 (p. 161)
- ✓ Learning Skills, Problem Solving Handout 1 (p. 162)
- ✓ Learning Skills, Problem Solving Worked Example 2A (p. 163)
- ✓ Learning Skills, Problem Solving Worked Example 2B (p. 165)
- ✓ Learning Skills, Problem Solving Worked Example 2C (p. 167)

E-Spiral Phase 1. Exploring Existing Knowledge Base (Review)

➡ ***Welcome group.*** "Welcome back! How is everybody today? Ready to go?"

➡ ***Orient to the mindfulness activity: breathing and rating feelings.*** "Last week, we noticed feelings when we rang the bell. This week we are going to notice feelings again, and this time we are going to rate the feelings."

Instructions for the mindfulness exercise. "As I ring the bell, please bring your attention to one feeling you have and rate how strong it is using the Feelings Rating Scale. If you feel like you can focus, the feeling may be between a Level 1 and 3 feeling. If you have a fuzzy mind it may be a Level 4. Label and rate any other feelings you notice. During this exercise we notice the feelings as they are; we don't change them. We label and rate feelings and let them pass. If your mind drifts to things in the past or future, bring your mind back to the feelings you have right now. It is important to be able to focus your attention on a task. It is also important to be able to notice, label, rate, and allow feelings to pass like clouds in the sky. Any questions?"

Describe questions. "How was that exercise?"; "What did you notice about rating your feelings?"; "Where did your attention go during this exercise?"

➡ ***Orient to Skills System review.*** "It is time for us to review our skills, System Tools, and the Clear Picture Do's."

Note: The skills instructor can choose a Basic Review Exercise from Week 1 (pp. 134–135), an Advanced Review Activity from Week 3 (p. 146), or create a new one.

➡ ***Orient to skills practice.*** "Great, let's talk about how our practice of New-Me Activities went this week."

Disclosure questions. "Who can tell us about the Focus New-Me Activities they did?"; "Who can tell us about the Feel Good New-Me Activities they did?"; "Who can tell us about the Distraction New-Me Activities they did?"; "Who can tell us about the Fun New-Me Activities they did?"

➡ ***Orient to new skills topic.*** "Sounds as if we did a lot of interesting things this week. Would it be OK if you talked a little about what we already know about Problem Solving?"

Discuss existing knowledge about the new topic.

Assessment questions. "How do we know when we have a problem?"; "What is it like to solve problems when we are in emotional mind? Fuzzy mind? Wise Mind?"

Relevant context questions. "What are some examples of on-track Problem Solving?"; "What are some examples of off-track Problem Solving?"

Clarifying questions. "What happens when people try to do Problem Solving when they are upset?"; "How does that usually work out?"; "What happens if we do Problem Solving when we are clear and calm?"; "How does that usually work out?"

➡ ***Orient to relevant context of the new topic.*** "Knowing how and when to fix problems is important. Life gives us challenges all the time. If we try to fix problems at the wrong time, we can make things worse. If we don't know how to solve problems, we can also make things worse. The goal of our skills is to make our lives better and to reach our goals."

E-Spiral Phase 2. Encoding: New Learning

➡ ***Orient to new learning.*** "We are going to learn about Problem Solving today. Problem Solving, Skill 6, is a Calm-Only skill. This means that we, and anyone we are talking to, have to be at or below a Level 3 feeling when we are solving problems. Problem Solving helps us fix problems, so we can reach our goals. Knowing when and how to fix problems is important. I hope you had a chance to review the Problem Solving Summary Sheet (p. 159) during the week."

➡ ***Orient to Learning Skills, Problem Solving Worked Example 1.*** "Let's start by going over Problem Solving Worked Example 1 on page 160. This is what it looks like. We can do a Quick Fix when the situation is simple and clear. When situations are confusing, it is better to do all the steps in Problem Solving. We will go over those steps after we see how to do a Quick Fix."

Note: The instructor goes through the Quick Fix example and the group discusses the concepts and the scenario. The group can refer to Learning Skills, Problem Solving Summary Sheet (p. 159) for explanations of specific concepts as needed.

E-Spiral Phase 3. Elaboration: Practice and Linking

➡ ***Orient to Learning Skills, Problem Solving Handout 1.*** "Now we are going to learn about how to do Problem Solving when we have medium and large problems. Let's turn to page 162 to Problem Solving Handout 1. It looks like this."

☆ *Teaching points.* "There are three basic steps to Problem Solving. First we get a Clear Picture of the problem. Second, we fast-forward and Check All Options that we have for fixing the problem. Third, we make Plans A, B, and C for solving the problem. Ready to learn more?"

➡ ***Orient to Learning Skills, Problem Solving Worked Example 2A.*** "Let's turn to page 163, so we can learn more about getting a Clear Picture of the problems by turning to Problem Solving Worked Example 2A. It looks like this. Everyone all set?"

☆ *Teaching points.* "There are four steps to do when we get a Clear Picture of the problem. First, we think about what we want to happen. Second, we think about what is in our way. Third, we focus on the one part of the situation that we want to fix. Fourth, it is helpful to think about how big the problem is. Some problems are more serious than others. Small problems are often not too serious and cause low-level feelings. Medium problems cause higher-level feelings (Levels 3 and 4) and take more steps and time to fix. Large or overwhelming problems are very serious and often cause us to have Level 4 or 5 feelings, may take weeks/months/years to fix, and change our lives in serious ways. In this situation, the person wants to buy sneakers and there isn't enough money. Is this a small, medium, or large problem? If we react like the sneakers are a large problem, what might happen to our actions?"

➡ ***Orient to Learning Skills, Problem Solving Worked Example 2B.*** "Great, we know what we want and what the problem is. Now we move on to Check All Options. Turn to page 165 of the *Skills System Workbook,* to Problem Solving Worked Example 2B. It looks like this."

Note: The instructor or group reads through the worked example to explore options, fast-forwarding to determine the pros and cons of each option.

☆ *Teaching points.* "When we Check All Options, we think of many different ways to solve a problem. For each option, we fast-forward to see what the pros and cons are. The pros of an option are helpful results. [Makes the thumbs-up gesture.] The cons of an option are the unhelpful results. [Makes the thumbs-down gesture.] Once we look at several options, we check the fit to choose the best option for us.

"Problem Solving takes a lot of thinking and focus. It takes time and energy to fast-forward each idea to see what might happen if we make that choice. This is why it is a Calm-Only skill. When we are calm, we can think of options, pros, and cons. When we are upset, we rush to solutions that make us feel better in the moment. We don't take time to think clearly. In fuzzy mind, we have a hard time focusing on what is good in the long term."

Note: Some group members may understand pros and cons quickly. Other participants will comprehend the concepts when the worked example is reviewed.

Content questions. "Can you think of any other options?"; "What would be the pros of your ideas?"; "What would be the cons of your ideas?"; "Which option do you think is the best?"; "What does it mean for something to fit in the short term but not the long term?"

➡ ***Orient to Learning Skills, Problem Solving Worked Example 2C.*** "It will help us to go through an example of this. Please turn to page 167, the Problem Solving Worked Example 2C. It looks like this. We have gotten a clear picture of the problem, checked all the options, and found the best option. Now we are ready to make Plans A, B, and C."

☆ *Teaching points.* "Once we figure out our best option, we have to make plans. We use Clear Picture, On-Track Thinking, and On-Track Actions to help us do Problem Solving. We call our favorite idea Plan A. Usually we need to take several steps to fix problems well. We determine who we need to talk to. We plan what we are going to say and how we are going to say it. We focus on doing what works to fix our problem.

"Sometimes we start Plan A and find out that our favorite plan will not work. It can be upsetting. We come up with a Plan B, so that we are prepared when things go wrong with Plan A. Plan B is a backup plan; it may help us get part of what we want. It may make sense even to make a fallback plan, Plan C, in case Plans A and B do not work. Plan C will help us stay on-track. Any questions?"

➡ ***Orient to discussion.*** "If it is OK with you, I would like to ask a few questions that will help us understand Problem Solving even better."

Linking questions. "Problem Solving is skills chain 1236; what does that mean?"; "What is it like to solve problems in Wise Mind?"

Disclosure questions. "Who can describe a time when you did on-track Problem Solving in the past?"; "Who can describe a time when you did off-track Problem Solving in the past?"

Expansion question. "What do we do if we notice we are doing off-track Problem Solving?"

➡ ***Orient to the end of the Elaboration Phase.*** "Very interesting discussion. Problem Solving can be pretty complicated. That is why we must be at or below a Level 3 feeling. We need to take time to carefully solve problems. We also may need to talk to our friends, coaches, and therapist to help us think things through. OK, let's step it up another notch. How about solving one of our own problems?"

E-Spiral Phase 4. Efficacy: Bridge to Real Life

➡ ***Orient to efficacy activities: Learning Skills, Problem Solving Worksheet 1.*** "We are going to practice doing a Quick Fix of a group member's problem now. Please turn to page 161 of the *Skills System Workbook;* it looks like this. Who would like to tell us a simple problem that the group can use to practice doing a Quick Fix?"

Note: The instructor leads the group through the Quick Fix using an example provided by a group member. It is important that the group understand when a Quick Fix will work (e.g., when the solution is fairly clear) and when the expanded version of Problem Solving is needed.

Describe question. "What did you learn about Problem Solving in that exercise?"

➡ ***Orient to discussion.*** "We are just about done for today, but first, how about chatting for a few minutes about the challenges of Problem Solving?"

Barrier questions. "What is difficult about doing a Quick Fix?"; "What is difficult about going through all the steps of Problem Solving?"; "Is it hard to tell the difference between when we do a Quick Fix and full Problem Solving?"

Wisdom question. "Is it important for you to know how to solve problems?"

Commitment question. "Are you going to use Problem Solving?"

Coaching question. "How can you coach yourself to use Problem Solving?"

➡ ***Orient to home study.*** "Great group; homework time! This week we are going to practice doing Problem Solving. Please also read or have someone read to you the Learning Skills, Expressing Myself Summary Sheet on page 173 of your *Skills System Workbook.* Any questions?

"Also, if you want to study skills at home, review all the handouts we have gone over so far. You can also do Learning Skills, Problem Solving Worksheets 1, 2A, 2B, 2C, and 3, if you like."

➡ ***Orient to group ending.*** "As you know, we ring the bell six times at the end of group. We do one ring for each of the Clear Picture Do's. It is a chance to notice what is happening inside and outside of us right now. We take a moment to get a Clear Picture as we go back to our activities. Who would like to ring the bell today?"

Problem Solving Handouts to Review in Future Cycles or for Home Study

✓ Learning Skills, Problem Solving Summary Sheet (p. 159)

☆ *Teaching points.* The summary sheet can be used during the encoding phase to explain concepts as teaching points. It may be too boring to read in group, but having different group members read different sections can break it up. Summary sheets are helpful for home study and for teaching the skills to skills coaches.

✓ Learning Skills, Problem Solving Worksheet 1 (p. 161)

☆ *Teaching points.* This worksheet can help the individual solve small problems and/or assist her to better understand factors involved with larger dilemmas.

✓ Learning Skills, Problem Solving Worksheet 2A (p. 164)

☆ *Teaching points.* This worksheet can help the individual get a Clear Picture of a problem in his life.

✓ Learning Skills, Problem Solving Worksheet 2B (p. 166)

☆ *Teaching points.* This worksheet can help the individual Check All Options that may solve the problem.

✓ Learning Skills, Problem Solving Worksheet 2C (p. 168)

☆ *Teaching points.* This worksheet guides the individual to make Plans A, B, and C to solve the problem.

✓ Learning Skills, Problem Solving Worked Example 3 (p. 169)

☆ *Teaching points.* Read through and discuss this Worked Example of the parts of Problem Solving.

✓ Learning Skills, Problem Solving Worksheet 3 (p. 170)

☆ *Teaching points.* This worksheet leads the individual through all of the parts of Problem Solving.

WEEK 9: EXPRESSING MYSELF

Preparing for Group

Handouts Needed

✓ Learning Skills, Expressing Myself Summary Sheet (p. 173)
✓ Learning Skills, Expressing Myself Handout 1 (p. 174)
✓ Learning Skills, Expressing Myself Worked Example 1 (p. 175)
✓ Learning Skills, Expressing Myself Handout 2 (p. 177)
✓ Learning Skills, Expressing Myself Handout 3 (p. 178)
✓ Learning Skills, Expressing Myself Handout 4 (p. 179)
✓ Learning Skills, Expressing Myself Worksheet 2 (p. 180)
✓ Learning Skills, Expressing Myself Worked Example 2 (p. 181)
✓ Learning Skills, Expressing Myself Worksheet 3 (p. 182)

E-Spiral Phase 1. Exploring Existing Knowledge Base (Review)

➡ ***Welcome group.*** "Hi, everyone! How are we doing today? Are we ready to get started? [Wait for response.] Great, it is time to ring the bell."

➡ ***Orient to the mindfulness activity: noticing thoughts.*** "Last week we did a mindfulness activity of noticing and rating our feelings. Today we are going to practice the next Clear Picture Do, Notice Thoughts. Are we ready?"

Instructions for the mindfulness exercise. "OK, as I ring the bell, please Notice Thoughts that go through your mind. Notice a thought in your mind and let it go. When you notice a thought, watch it pass like a city bus driving by. We are only going to watch thoughts as they are. We will practice allowing thoughts to pass without thinking more about that thought or taking action. We will let the bus pass by and look for the next bus that comes by. If our attention drifts from noticing thoughts, we will gently bring our minds back to our thoughts. The practice of Notice Thoughts is helpful. There are many times when we need to watch thoughts and not take actions. Any questions?"

Describe questions. "What was it like to watch thoughts?"; "Did your mind drift at all?"; "Were you able to bring your attention back to Notice Thoughts and allow them to pass?"

➡ ***Orient to Skills System review.*** "Great job. It is time to review our skills."

Note: The skills instructor can choose a Basic Review Exercise from Week 1 (pp. 134–135), an Advanced Review Activity from Week 3 (p. 146), or create a new one.

➡ ***Orient to skills practice.*** "We are really getting good at this! How about we review how we used Problem Solving this week?"

Disclosure questions. "Who would like to share how the Problem Solving went this week?"; "Did anyone do a Quick Fix?"; "Did anyone do Problem Solving?"

➡ ***Orient to new skills topic.*** "The skill we are going to learn about today often helps us with Problem Solving, Getting It Right, and Relationship Care. Let's spend a few minutes talking about what we know about Expressing Myself."

Discuss existing knowledge about the new topic.

Assessment questions. "What does it mean when someone is expressing herself?"; "Why do we express ourselves?"; "How do we express ourselves?"; "When do we express ourselves?"; "How does it go when we express ourselves when we are in emotional mind?"

Relevant context questions. "Did you have to express yourself to anyone when you were trying to solve problems this week?"; "Are there on-track ways to express ourselves?"; "Are there off-track ways to express ourselves?"

Clarifying questions. "What happens to our relationships when we do on-track expressing?"; "Do we reach our goals?"; "What happens when we use off-track expressing?"; "Do we reach our goals?"

➡ ***Orient to relevant context of the new topic.*** "Expressing Myself helps us communicate well with other people. Having clear communication helps us feel better about ourselves, our lives, and relationships. It helps us solve problems, get what we want, and keep our relationships in balance."

E-Spiral Phase 2. Encoding: New Learning

➡ ***Orient to new learning.*** "We are going to learn what 'Expressing Myself' is, why it is helpful, how we can do it well, and when is best to use it. It is important to remember that Expressing Myself is a Calm-Only skill and can be used *only* when we are at a Level 0–3 feeling. Are we ready to get started?"

➡ ***Instructions for Learning Skills, Expressing Myself Handout 1.*** "Let's begin by turning to page 174 in the *Skills System Workbook.* Learning Skills, Expressing Myself Handout 1 looks like this."

☆ *Teaching points.* "This handout will help us begin to understand more about what 'Expressing Myself' is. Let's read through it and discuss the points; perhaps we can add some things to it, as well."

➡ ***Orient to Learning Skills, Expressing Myself Worked Example 1.*** "We are now going to turn to Learning Skills, Expressing Myself Worked Example 1 on page 175. It looks like this. Let's read through it and discuss it together."

➡ ***Orient to Learning Skills, Expressing Myself Handout 2.*** "Good start. Let's check out Learning Skills, Expressing Myself Handout 2 on page 177. It teaches us why we use Expressing Myself. It looks like this. All set?"

➡ ***Orient to Learning Skills, Expressing Myself Handout 3.*** "OK, so now we are going to learn more about how we use Expressing Myself by reading through this handout and discussing the points. Let's turn to Learning Skills, Expressing Myself Handout 3 on page 178."

➡ ***Orient to Learning Skills, Expressing Myself Handout 4.*** "Next, we are going to learn about when we use Expressing Myself. Let's turn to page 179. We will read through and discuss the points."

➡ ***Orient to the end of the Encoding Phase.*** "Great discussion about all these parts of Expressing Myself planning. Are we ready to practice putting all the parts together to practice Expressing Myself?"

E-Spiral Phase 3. Elaboration: Practice and Linking

➡ ***Orient to the elaboration activity.*** "Now we are going to use a worksheet to help us practice expressing what is in our minds and in our hearts. Let's turn to Learning Skills, Expressing Myself Worksheet 1 on page 176 of your *Skills System Workbook.* Each of us will practice how we would share a thought, a concern, a need, a feeling, a like, a dislike, a hope, and a dream. Please tell the group who in your life you would say this to and demonstrate how you would say it."

Note: Writing is optimal in this exercise. The instructor can either fill in this worksheet as a group activity listing each person's responses on the board (if the individuals in the group are unable to write) or each group member can take a few minutes to write down responses, then verbally express them to the group.

Disclosure questions. "What was it like to use Expressing Myself?"; "Were any responses more difficult to express?"

➡ ***Orient to discussion.*** "Great, I feel like I know you all a little better! Would it be all right if I asked you a few more questions that will help us understand Expressing Myself better?"

Linking questions. "Expressing Myself is skills chain 1237; what does that mean?"; "Who can describe a time in the past when you did on-track Expressing Myself?"; "What is Expressing Myself like in Wise Mind?"; "Who can describe a time when you did off-track Expressing Myself?"

Disclosure questions. "What happened when you used on-track Expressing Myself?"; "How did it make you feel about yourself and your life?"; "What happened when you did off-track Expressing Myself?"; "How did it make you feel about yourself and your life?"

Expansion questions. "What other skills do we use with Expressing Myself?"; "What do you do if you notice you are doing off-track Expressing Myself?"; "What can you do instead?"; "In what parts of your life can Expressing Myself help you?"; "At work?"; "At home?"; "With family?"; "With friends?"

➡ ***Orient to the end of the Elaboration Phase.*** "Good discussion. It sounds as if Expressing Myself is an important skill."

E-Spiral Phase 4. Efficacy: Bridge to Real Life

➡ ***Orient to efficacy activities: Learning Skills, Expressing Myself Worked Example 2.*** "Great, I think we are ready to use Expressing Myself in our lives. We are going to make plans to use the Expressing Myself skill this week. Let's turn to the Expressing Myself Worked Example 2 on page 181."

Instructions for the efficacy activity. "We are going to read through the worked example that shows us how to make an Expressing Myself Plan. Making a plan can help us prepare for communicating with people, so that it goes well. Once we read through this worked example, we are each going to make an Expressing Myself plan."

Note: The group members can do this activity verbally or by writing on the sheet. Going through each step of the plan with each group member is ideal, but time may not allow it. Having a few people complete it verbally may be helpful. The group may have previously practiced what is important to say to someone in the elaboration exercise, so perhaps choosing which of those are most important to share could be a way to save time. This worksheet can be assigned for homework.

Disclosure questions. "How was it to make an Expressing Myself Plan?"; "Do you think it will help you express yourself?"

➡ ***Orient to discussion.*** "Before we finish up for today, we are going to talk about some of the challenges we face when we use Expressing Myself. OK?"

Barrier question. "What is difficult about using Expressing Myself?"

Wisdom question. "Do you want to learn how to use Expressing Myself?"

Commitment question. "When are you going to use Expressing Myself?"

Coaching question. "How can you coach yourself to use Expressing Myself when you need it?"

➡ ***Orient to home study.*** "Good discussion! Time for homework! This week we are going to practice using Expressing Myself. We are going to practice communicating what we think and feel. Remember, Expressing Myself is a Calm-Only skill, so when can we use it? [Wait for response.] Right—when *both* people are at or below a Level 3 feeling! Good luck! Also, if you want to study skills at home, review all the handouts we have gone over so far."

➡ ***Orient to group ending.*** "As you know, we ring the bell six times at the end of group. We do one ring for each of the Clear Picture Do's. It is a chance to notice what is happening inside and outside of us right now. We take a moment to get a Clear Picture as we go back to our activities. Who would like to ring the bell today?"

Expressing Myself Handouts to Review in Future Cycles or for Home Study

✓ Learning Skills, Expressing Myself Summary Sheet (p. 173)

☆ *Teaching points.* The Summary Sheet explains how we can effectively use Expressing Myself. This sheet can be used with the individual and skills coaches.

✓ Learning Skills, Expressing Myself Worksheet 1 (p. 176)

☆ *Teaching points.* This worksheet can help us practice expressing as if we were telling someone about our thoughts, concerns, needs, feelings, likes and dislikes, and hopes and dreams. Write down examples of each of these.

✓ Learning Skills, Expressing Myself Worksheet 2 (p. 180)

☆ *Teaching points.* This worksheet can help the individual think through whether it is on-track or off-track to Express Myself.

✓ Learning Skills, Expressing Myself Worksheet 3 (p. 182)

☆ *Teaching points.* This worksheet can help the individual create a plan to express what is in her mind or heart.

WEEK 10: GETTING IT RIGHT

Preparing for Group

Handouts Needed

✓ Learning Skills, Getting It Right Summary Sheet (p. 185)
✓ Learning Skills, Getting It Right Handout 1 (p. 186)
✓ Learning Skills, Getting It Right Handout 2 (p. 187)
✓ Learning Skills, Getting It Right Handout 3 (p. 189)
✓ Learning Skills, Getting It Right Handout 4 (p. 190)
✓ Learning Skills, Getting It Right Handout 5 (p. 191)
✓ Learning Skills, Getting It Right Handout 6 (p. 192)
✓ Learning Skills, Getting It Right Worksheet 1 (p. 188)
✓ Learning Skills, Getting It Right Worked Example 1 (p. 193)
✓ Learning Skills, Getting It Right Worksheet 2 (p. 194)

E-Spiral Phase 1. Exploring Existing Knowledge Base (Review)

➡ ***Welcome group.*** "Hi, everyone. How are we doing today? Ready to build some skills? [Wait for response.] Excellent! How about we start with mindfulness?"

➡ ***Orient to mindfulness activity: noticing urges.*** "Last week we worked on noticing our thoughts. Today we are going to practice the Clear Picture Do, Notice Urges. OK?"

Instructions for the mindfulness exercise. "Great. As I ring the bell, please notice any urges you are having. An urge is a feeling inside of us that makes us want to do something or to take an action. You might feel the urge to have a snack. You may feel the urge to sleep. You might feel the urge to fidget. Just notice the urge as it is. We will notice the urge and allow it to pass, without taking action. If your mind drifts to something other than noticing urges, gently bring your mind back to the bell and the urges. We have to be able to experience an urge and not take action until we Check It. Any questions?"

Describe questions. "What urges did you notice?"; "How did you handle the urge?"; "Did your mind drift?"; "Were you able to bring your attention back to Notice Urges?"

➡ ***Orient to Skills System review.*** "Handling urges is very important; all of us have urges that make us want to go off-track. Noticing the off-track urges and allowing them to pass is difficult *and* important! Let's review our skills so they are fresh in our minds."

Note: The skills instructor can choose a Basic Review Exercise from Week 1 (pp. 134–135), an Advanced Review Activity from Week 3 (p. 146), or create a new one.

➡ ***Orient to skills practice.*** "OK, how about we talk about our skills practice for the week? Who would like to share about using Expressing Myself this week?"

Disclosure questions. "What different ways did you use Expressing Myself?"; "When did you use it?"; "How did it work out for you?"

➡ ***Orient to new skills topic.*** "Great job. Today we are going to talk about getting things that we need from people. Let's talk for a little bit about what we already know about getting people to give us what we need and want."

Discuss existing knowledge about the new topic.

Assessment questions. "Has anyone ever asked you for something in an on-track way?"; "What happened?"; "Has anyone ever asked you for something in an off-track way?"; "What happened?"

Relevant context questions. "How does it work when people want to help us?"; "Do people want to help us when we are on-track or off-track?"; "Why is that?"

Clarifying questions. "How do we feel when people help us?"; "How do we feel when people refuse to help us?"

➡ ***Orient to relevant context of the new topic.*** "It sounds like Problem Solving, Expressing Myself, and Getting It Right are important skills to help us make our lives happier. Knowing what to say and how to say it really helps us reach our goals. Getting It Right can give us more joy; getting it wrong can lead us off-track!"

E-Spiral Phase 2. Encoding: New Learning

➡ ***Orient to new learning.*** "We are going to learn about Getting It Right today; it is Skill 8 in the Skills System. Ready to get started? Let's turn to page 186. Learning Skills, Getting It Right Handout 1 looks like this. Got it?"

Instructions for the encoding activity. The skills instructor reads through the handout. This handout functions as an introduction.

➡ ***Orient to Learning Skills, Getting It Right Handout 1.*** "Getting It Right is how we get what we want from other people. We will go through five handouts to learn how to Get It Right."

☆ *Teaching points.* "Getting It Right is a Calm-Only skill. This means that we have to be at or below a Level 3 feeling if we are going to use it. We have to remember that the person we are talking to has to be at or below a Level 3 feeling, too. So, if we notice that the person is starting to get upset or overly excited, we should step back and get a Clear Picture of the situation. We will want to do On-Track Thinking to decide what to do. We have to be careful, because when we want things, we can become nervous and impatient. These feelings can make us want to rush. Rushing Getting It Right usually makes it turn out wrong."

➡ ***Orient to Learning Skills, Getting It Right Handout 2.*** "Let's start with being in the Right Mind. Please turn to page 187. Learning Skills, Getting It Right Handout 2 looks like this. Has everyone found the page?"

Note: The group discusses each of the points about Right Mind. The individual must understand that being in the Right Mind is critical to reaching goals.

➡ ***Orient to Learning Skills, Getting It Right Handout 3.*** "OK, let's keep going. Please turn to page 189 in the *Skills System Workbook.* Learning Skills, Getting It Right Handout 3 looks like this. We are going to learn about talking to the Right Person now. All set?"

Note: The group members or the instructor read through this handout. A discussion about who people go to for particular issues is helpful. Support teams can be complex systems; an individual with significant cognitive disabilities may not have a clear understanding of who to talk to about certain issues.

➡ ***Orient to Learning Skills, Getting It Right Handout 4.*** "Great! Not only do we have to be in the Right Mind and talk to the Right Person, we have to choose the Right Time and Place. Let's turn to page 190. Learning Skills, Getting It Right Handout 4 looks like this. Ready?"

Note: The group and/or skills instructor reads through this handout. The group discusses the reasoning for each of the points.

➡ ***Orient to Learning Skills, Getting It Right Handout 5.*** "Awesome! Now let's learn about using the Right Tone. Please turn to page 191 in the *Skills System Workbook.* Getting It Right Handout 5 looks like this. Did you find it?"

Note: The group and/or instructor reads through this handout. The group discusses the reasoning for the each of the points.

➡ ***Orient to Learning Skills, Getting It Right Handout 6.*** "Almost there—one more handout to review. We are going to learn about the Right Words: SEALS. SEALS stands for Sugar, Explain, Ask, Listen, and Seal the Deal. Let's turn to page 192. Getting It Right Handout 6 looks like this. All set?"

Note: The group and/or instructor reads through this handout. The group members discuss the reasoning for each of the points.

➡ ***Orient to the end of the Encoding Phase.*** "OK, let's learn more about how to Get It Right."

E-Spiral Phase 3. Elaboration: Practicing and Linking

➡ ***Orient to the elaboration activity.*** "OK, we are going to practice Getting It Right. Let's turn to the Learning Skills, Getting It Right Worked Example 1 on page 193 first. Let's read through this example, then work as a group to complete a Getting It Right Plan together."

Note: Once the group members review the worked example, they choose a scenario to use that is relevant to making a Getting It Right Plan, Learning Skills, Getting It Right Worksheet 2 (p. 194). After this plan is complete, this scenario may be used in a role play instead of the scenario in the worked example. Ideas: Asking a coworker, housemate, friend, or family member for something or to stop doing something. Choosing highly emotional topics will increase cognitive load demands, decreasing integration of the concepts. The key is to pick something interesting/fun but not dysregulating.

Instructions for the worksheet. "First you have to figure out what you want before you can make a plan. So, perhaps you can think about things you need from people in your life. We will make a Getting It Right Plan and role-play after that. Who needs something from someone that we can use as an example? Any questions?"

Note: The instructor and group choose the broadest topic that is salient for the group and suitable for a role-play exercise. The group members work together with the individual to address each aspect on the Getting It Right Plan.

➡ ***Orient to discussion.*** "Let's talk a little more about getting what we want from people."

Linking questions. "The skills chain for Getting It Right is 1238; what does that mean?"; "Have you ever gotten something from someone in the past?"; "What worked?"; "What is Getting It Right like in Wise Mind?"; "Have you ever used getting it wrong and not gotten what you wanted?"; "What happened?"

Disclosure questions. "What parts of Getting It Right are you good at?"; "What parts of Getting It Right do you need to work on?"

Expansion questions. "What other skills do we use with Getting It Right?"; "How can Getting It Right help you in your life?"; "What is something that you need or want in the future?"; "How are you planning to get it?"

➡ ***Orient to the end of the Elaboration Phase.*** "It is great when we know how to get what we want; let's practice Getting It Right some more!"

E-Spiral Phase 4. Efficacy: Bridge to Real Life

➡ ***Orient to efficacy activities: role play.*** "Ready for a role play? We can choose the topic of the role play. We can use the scenario in the worked example of the person asking for more hours, or we can use the scenario for which we just made a plan. Any thoughts about which we should do? A volunteer to begin?"

Note: Once the group decides on the topic, the instructor sets up the role play. The following instructions apply when the group chooses the worked example option.

Instructions for the efficacy activity. "You are going to talk to your boss about adding another day to your work schedule. I will play the boss to start with and may have someone else jump into that role once we get going. The situation is that you work 2 days a week now, and you would like to work 3 days a week in the future. Are you in the Right Mind? Are you over a Level 3 feeling? Am I the Right Person? Is this the Right Time and Place? Did you call me ahead of time to set up a meeting? Are you just showing up at my office? Where is this role play taking place so that you get more hours from me? Think about the tone and words you want to use. Remember SEALS: <u>S</u>ugar, <u>E</u>xplain, <u>A</u>sk, <u>L</u>isten, and <u>S</u>eal a Deal. You can do this."

Note: Skills instructors will adjust the boss's responses for each participant. Hitting the "pause" button can give the group a chance to chat about what is happening and to offer feedback and coaching. Helping the individual shape behaviors to be effective is the goal.

Disclosure questions. "How was that role play for you?"; "What did you learn about Getting It Right?"

➡ ***Orient to discussion.*** "Before we head home, let's talk about some of the challenges of using Getting It Right."

Barrier questions. "What is difficult about Getting It Right?"; "What do you do if you think you have all the steps right and the person still says no?"

Wisdom question. "Do you think that Getting It Right is important for you?"

Commitment question. "When are you going to try to use Getting It Right?"

Coaching question. "How are you going to coach yourself to use Getting It Right?"

➡ ***Orient to home study.*** "Homework time already! This week we are going to practice Getting It Right. What are the parts of Getting It Right? [Allows the group to answer.] That is correct: Right Mind, Right Person, Right Place, Right Time, Right Tone, and Right Words. You remembered that after only one day. Very good!

"Also, if you want to study skills at home, review all the handouts we have gone over so far. You can also do Learning Skills, Getting It Right Worksheet 1 on page 188. This is a great worksheet to use if you want to make a good plan to Get It Right."

➡ ***Orient to group ending.*** "As you know, we ring the bell six times at the end of group. We do one ring for each of the Clear Picture Do's. It is a chance to notice what is happening inside and outside of us right now. We take a moment to get a Clear Picture as we go back to our activities. Who would like to ring the bell today?"

Getting It Right Handouts to Review in Future Cycles or for Home Study

✓ Learning Skills, Getting It Right Summary Sheet (p. 185)

☆ *Teaching points.* The summary sheet can be used during the encoding phase to explain concepts as teaching points. It may be too boring to read in group, but having different group members read different sections can break it up. Summary sheets are helpful for home study and for teaching the skills to skills coaches.

Learning Skills, Getting It Right Worksheet 1 (p. 188)

☆ *Teaching points.* This worksheet helps the individual evaluate whether she is in Right Mind or not prior to doing Getting It Right.

✓ Learning Skills, Getting It Right Worksheet 2 (p. 194)

☆ *Teaching points.* This worksheet helps the individual plan ahead to do Getting It Right successfully. The individual can complete this sheet independently or with support.

WEEK 11: RELATIONSHIP CARE

Preparing for Group

Handouts Needed

✓ Learning Skills, Relationship Care Handout 1 (p. 199)
✓ Learning Skills, Relationship Care Handout 2 (p. 200)
✓ Learning Skills, Relationship Care Handout 3 (p. 202)

- ✓ Learning Skills, Relationship Care Handout 4 (p. 203)
- ✓ Learning Skills, Relationship Care Handout 5 (p. 204)
- ✓ Learning Skills, Relationship Care Handout 6 (p. 206)
- ✓ Learning Skills, Relationship Care Handout 7 (p. 209)
- ✓ Learning Skills, Relationship Care Handout 8 (p. 212)
- ✓ Learning Skills, Relationship Care Worked Example 2 (p. 210)
- ✓ Learning Skills, Relationship Care Worksheet 4 (p. 211)

E-Spiral Phase 1. Exploring Existing Knowledge Base (Review)

➡ ***Welcome group.*** "Welcome, everyone! How are we doing today?"

➡ ***Orient to the mindfulness activity.*** "We are going to learn about Skill 9, Relationship Care, today! Are we ready to get started with mindfulness?"

Instructions for the mindfulness exercise. "As I ring the bell, please follow my instructions to do the Clear Picture Do's. I will say, 'Notice the Breath,' and ring the bell. Please bring your attention to your breath, noticing it as it is. Then I will say, 'Body Check,' and ring the bell. As the bell rings, please do a Body Check. Then I will say, 'Notice Surroundings,' and ring the bell. You will shift your attention to notice your surroundings. Next I will say, 'Label and Rate Feelings.' I will ring the bell and you will notice and rate your feelings using the Feelings Rating Scale. Then I will say, 'Notice Thoughts,' and I will ring the bell. You will Notice Thoughts that are in your minds. Last, I will say, 'Notice Urges.' I will ring the bell, and we will all Notice Urges. If you feel your mind drifting off, gently bring your mind back to following the directions. This exercise helps us pay attention, shift our focus, and practice Clear Picture. Any questions?"

Describe questions. "How was that exercise for you?"; "Were you able to follow the instructions?"

➡ ***Orient to Skills System review.*** "Ready to review our skills?"

Note: The skills instructor can choose a Basic Review Exercise from Week 1 (pp. 134–135), an Advanced Review Activity from Week 3 (p. 146), or create a new one.

➡ ***Orient to skills practice.*** "OK, time to review our skills practice for the week. We were working on Getting It Right."

Disclosure questions. "Who can tell us about using Getting It Right?"; "Did anyone get it wrong?"

➡ ***Orient to new skills topic.*** "As we have learned, relationships are an important part of our lives. Let's take a few minutes to talk about what we know about Relationship Care."

Discuss existing knowledge about the new topic.

Assessment questions. "What does the word 'relationship' mean?"; "What does the word 'care' mean?"; "What does it mean to balance a relationship?"

Relevant context questions. "What do people do to keep relationships in balance, or on-track?"; "What are things that make relationships go off-track?"

Clarifying questions. "How does it feel when our relationships are on-track?"; "What is it like when our relationships are off-track?"; "What happens to our relationships when we are in Wise Mind?"

➡ ***Orient to relevant context of the new topic.*** "Relationships can be wonderful when they are on-track and stressful when they are off-track. Relationship care can help us manage our relationships so they add to the quality of our lives."

Note: Relationship Care is a complex skill that integrates several other skills. The instructor has to decide what elements are most important to address for a group. The teaching notes for all eight handouts are below; some are lengthy due to the complexity of relationships. The E-Spiral Elaboration and Efficacy phase activities depend on which Relationship Care handouts are covered. The tactic presented here reviews the first six handouts, with brief discussions on points during the Encoding phase and focus on Finding Middle Ground during the Elaboration and Efficacy phases.

E-Spiral Phase 2. Encoding: New Learning

➡ ***Orient to new learning: Learning Skills, Relationship Care Handout 1.*** "Ready to get started learning about Relationship Care? Let's turn to page 199 in the *Skills System Workbook.* Relationship Care Handout 1 looks like this."

Instructions for the encoding activity. Note: The skills instructor can decide how best to read through the material in all of the Relationship Care handouts. This handout is an overview of the different parts of Relationship Care.

☆ *Teaching points.* "There are three types of Relationship Care that we are going to learn. First, we will learn about building on-track relationships with ourselves and other people. Second, we will learn how to balance on-track relationships by having One-Way- and Two-Way-Street relationships. Third, we will learn how to change off-track relationships using Finding Middle Ground and Steps of Responsibility."

➡ ***Orient to Learning Skills, Relationship Care Handout 2.*** "Let's turn to page 200, the Relationship Care Handout 2. It looks like this."

☆ *Teaching points.* "We build on-track relationships with ourselves as we learn skills that help us become more self-aware. We are able to understand what is happening inside and outside of us. When we start being self-aware, we also learn to accept ourselves. The more we find out about ourselves, other people, and life, the clearer it becomes that life is hard for us all sometimes. We realize that we are as perfect as the next person; we are all perfectly human. We learn to accept that we are doing the best we can. As we become self-aware and self-accepting, we begin to value things about ourselves. We realize we have strengths. We have resources that we can rely on. We start believing in our resources, abilities, and skills—we lean on them to support us. As we build our strength, we try new things and meet new people. As we keep practicing skills every day, all day, we begin to trust that we can handle most anything that comes our way. We know how to get a Clear Picture, and we stop and think things through. We learn that deep in our hearts we will be OK—no matter what. So, as we practice skills and Relationship Care with ourselves, we learn to be self-aware, self-accepting, self-valuing, and self-trusting.

"We also learn how to be aware of, accept, value, and trust other people. We use Clear Picture and On-Track Thinking to decide when a relationship is on-track or off-track. We use Safety Plans to be sure we keep relationships safe. We use On-Track Actions to help us handle off-track urges that can harm relationships. New-Me Activities help people in relationships share experiences. Problem Solving helps people work together to fix problems between them and in the world around them. Expressing Myself helps people know how other people think and feel. All these skills are important parts of having on-track relationships. Relationship Care makes us aware of all the things we do to keep our relationships on-track. Any questions?"

➡ ***Orient to Learning Skills, Relationship Care Handout 3.*** "There are many different types of relationships. Let's turn to page 202, Relationship Care Handout 3, to see about some of the different kinds. It looks like this."

Note: The group discusses these options and adds more to a brainstormed list on the board. The goal is to teach participants about how different relationships are and the need to be flexible and adaptive in each different situation.

➡ ***Orient to Learning Skills, Relationship Care Handout 4.*** "Great, how about we move on to Learning Skills, Relationship Care Handout 4? This helps us learn different things we can do to make relationships closer and more distant as we need to. It is on page 203 of the *Skills System Workbook* and it looks like this."

Note: The skills instructor can lead a discussion about the points, emphasizing the need to make decisions in the moment that reflect the person's wisdom. Other options can be added on the board.

➡ ***Orient to Learning Skills, Relationship Care Handout 5.*** "Let's turn to Relationship Care Handout 5, which introduces Two-Way-Street and One-Way-Street relationships. It is on page 204. It looks like this."

☆ *Teaching points.* "Sometimes we have Two-Way-Street relationships with people, which occurs when both people talk and listen to each other, taking turns. There is a balanced give-and-take between people. Each person cares about what the other person is thinking, feeling, and saying. A Two-Way-Street relationship can help people work together well. It takes two people to maintain a Two-Way-Street relationship. Even when we work very hard to keep a

Two-Way-Street relationship working, there are times when it gets out of balance. We may have to repair the relationship to fix the problem. Feeling cared for in a relationship and being able to give caring back adds to the quality of our lives.

"There are times when we try to have a Two-Way-Street relationship with someone, but it doesn't work out. Then it might be a One-Way-Street relationship. We may feel we are giving, but we do not feel heard or that the other person is giving back. If the other person is bothering us, we may decide that we do not want to have a Two-Way-Street relationship, and we stop having an equal give-and-take. It is important to notice when relationships are two-way or one-way streets. We use Clear Picture, On-Track Thinking, and On-Track Actions to make on-track relationship decisions in the moment."

➡ ***Orient to Learning Skills, Relationship Care Handout 6.*** "Good points. OK, there are times when we need to change off-track relationships. Since we have relationships with ourselves and other people, let's begin with learning how we get the relationship with ourselves back on-track when it is off-track. If you are ready, turn to Learning Skills, Relationship Care Handout 6 to learn more about how to do this. It is on page 206 of the *Skills System Workbook,* and it looks like this."

Note: The instructor goes through the points and has a brief discussion about the relevance of each. Additionally, the group talks about challenges related to making the changes from off-track to on-track.

➡ ***Orient to Learning Skills, Relationship Care Handout 7.*** "There are times even in great relationships that things go off-track. It is important to know how to repair relationships with other people. Finding Middle Ground and Steps of Responsibility help us get relationships back on-track. Let's go to Learning Skills, Relationship Care Handout 7 to learn more about Finding Middle Ground on page 209 of the *Skills System Workbook.*

☆ *Teaching points.* "There are times when relationships go off-track and we feel something isn't right between us and another person. Use of Finding Middle Ground can help us talk to someone to work out differences. We use all of our Calm-Only skills in Finding Middle Ground, so we have to be sure we are at or below a Level 3 feeling when we are doing it.

"When we notice a relationship problem, it is helpful to start with Problem Solving. We think about the issues and get a clear sense of the problem. If we check our options and decide Plan A is to try to work it out together, we decide how we are going to use Expressing Myself. Talking in person, on the phone, in letters, in email, and texting all work differently. We think about whether we are in the Right Mind, when is the Right Time and Place, and what are the Right Tone and the Right Words.

"We plan out whether we want to use Sugar and how we are going to Explain our concerns and side of the relationship story. In Finding Middle Ground, we want to know both sides of the story, so we ask questions to understand the other person's side of the story. If there is something I want from the person, maybe for him to act differently, I ask for it.

"Sometimes one or both people get upset. Feelings levels can go up when people are blaming each other. Using 'I statements,' such as 'I was hurt by how you said that,' can be more helpful than insulting someone by saying something like 'You are rude.' Continuing to talk and listen so both sides understand each other better can lead to win–win solutions. When two people work together to get a relationship back on track, they are Finding Middle Ground. Every situation is different, and that is why we may have to use many skills to repair relationships. We may have to use a 1236789 skills chain!"

➡ ***Orient to Learning Skills, Relationship Care Handout 8.*** "OK, let's turn now to Relationship Care Handout 8 on page 212."

☆ *Teaching points.* "When we have made a mistake that hurts another person, it is helpful to do the Steps of Responsibility. Doing these steps can help us keep self-respect and the respect of other people. First, I admit the problem; I tell the person what I did. I try to explain what I did and how I may have harmed the person. This is really difficult, because I may feel ashamed.

"Next, I apologize for what I did that I feel was a problem. I have to think about what exactly I wish I had done differently and what I wish I had not done. Then, I commit to changing my behavior in the future. I let the person know that I am going to try not to do it again. I finish doing the Steps of Responsibility, then do an On-Track Action that shows the person I mean what I am saying. Doing the Steps of Responsibility helps me regain self-trust and trust with the other people I have harmed. Completing Learning Skills, Relationship Care Worksheet 4 (p. 211) can help teach the Steps of Responsibility.

"There are times when a relationship ends. Sometimes we end a relationship, and other times, the other person ends the relationship. Relationships naturally change and end. People move in different directions and to different locations, or people die. We have to use all of our skills to manage the situation when people leave us before we are ready. It is important to get skills coaching in situations when we feel overwhelmed with sadness and hurt.

"Sometimes, we choose to end relationships. If a relationship is off-track and we can't fix it, we may want to end it. We might tell the person we are moving on, or we may just stop paying attention to the relationship, so that it just drifts apart. We have to use Clear Picture to know how we feel about our relationships and On-Track Thinking to make sure we do what fits for us. Problem Solving can help us figure out how to fix relationship problems. We are taking good care of ourselves when we keep our relationships in balance and change Off-Track Relationships."

➡ ***Orient to the end of the Encoding Phase.*** "Relationships are complicated! We have to use all of our skills to be able to do Relationship Care. We are going to talk more about different relationships so that we can learn how to handle all the different, changing relationships in our lives."

E-Spiral Phase 3. Elaboration: Practice and Linking

➡ ***Orient to the elaboration activity.*** "Please turn to Learning Skills, Relationship Care Worked Example 2 (p. 210) and Relationship Care Worksheet 4, the Finding Middle Ground Plan (p. 211). We will first go through the worked example; it looks like this. Let's read through this example to see how we might try to fix a relationship problem."

Instructions for the practice exercise. "Great, now we are going to make a Finding Middle Ground Plan using a relationship problem of someone in the group. We are also going to do a role play after we make the plan. Would anyone like to share a relationship problem that you would like to fix?"

Note: The instructor and group discuss the options and pick one that will work well. The answers are written on the board as the group members discuss each part of the plan. If no one volunteers, the instructor can invent a relevant scenario.

Disclosure question. "What did you learn from this exercise?"

➡ ***Orient to discussion.*** "Let's talk a little more about how we have used Relationship Care in the past, OK?"

Linking questions. "What is it like to use Relationship Care in Wise Mind?"; "This is a 1236789 skills chain; what does that mean?"

Disclosure question. "Have you ever tried to fix a relationship problem in the past?"

Expansion question. "Do you think you could try Finding Middle Ground with anyone in your life?"

➡ ***Orient to the end of the Elaboration Phase.*** "Are we ready to do a Finding Middle Ground role play?"

E-Spiral Phase 4. Efficacy: Bridge to Real Life

➡ ***Orient to efficacy activities.*** "OK, let's role-play the situation from Worked Example 2 about Pat and Cindy. This role play will help us practice Finding Middle Ground.

Note: The instructor asks for participants to play the roles of Pat and Cindy. Pat practices Finding Middle Ground with Cindy. The instructor supports Pat and Cindy and engages the rest of the group to explore the process.

Disclosure questions. "What was that exercise like for you?"; "What did you learn about Relationship Care?"

➡ ***Orient to discussion.*** "Before we finish for this week, I would like to ask a few more questions about some of the challenges in using Relationship Care."

Barrier questions. "What is difficult about doing Relationship Care with yourself?"; "What is difficult about doing Relationship Care with other people?"

Wisdom questions. "Is it important for you to do Relationship Care with yourself?"; "With other people?"

Commitment questions. "What Relationship Care will you do with yourself?"; "What Relationship Care will you do with other people?"

Coaching questions. "How can you coach yourself to do Relationship Care with yourself?"; "How can you coach yourself to do Relationship Care with other people?"

➡ ***Orient to home study.*** "This week we are going to practice using Relationship Care with ourselves and other people. Does that sound good? Also, if you want to study skills at home, review all the handouts we have gone over so far. You can also do Learning Skills, Relationship Care Worksheets 1–5."

➡ ***Orient to group ending.*** "As you know, we ring the bell six times at the end of group. We do one ring for each of the Clear Picture Do's. It is a chance to notice what is happening inside and outside of us right now. We take a moment to get a Clear Picture as we go back to our activities. Who would like to ring the bell today?"

Relationship Care Handouts to Review in Future Cycles or for Home Study

✓ Learning Skills, Relationship Care Summary Sheet (pp. 197–198).

☆ *Teaching points.* The summary sheet can be used during the encoding phase to explain concepts as teaching points. It may be too boring to read in group, but having different group members read different sections can break it up. Summary sheets are helpful for home study and for teaching skills to skills coaches.

✓ Learning Skills, Relationship Care Worksheet 1 (p. 201)

☆ *Teaching points.* This worksheet asks the individual to list things that will help her build on-track relationships with herself and others.

✓ Learning Skills, Relationship Care Worksheet 2 (p. 205)

☆ *Teaching points.* This worksheet asks the individual to list things that will help him have Two-Way-Street and One-Way-Street relationships with others.

✓ Learning Skills, Relationship Care Worked Example 1 (p. 207)

☆ *Teaching points.* This worked example shows how the individual can evaluate the status of a relationship and generate ways to make adjustments to increase balance in the relationship.

✓ Learning Skills, Relationship Care Worksheet 3 (p. 208)

☆ *Teaching points.* This worksheet helps the individual evaluate the status of a relationship and generate ways to make adjustments to increase balance in the relationship.

✓ Learning Skills, Relationship Care Worked Example 2 (p. 210)

☆ *Teaching points.* This worked example shows how a person plans to do Finding Middle Group with another person to resolve relationship conflicts.

✓ Learning Skills, Relationship Care Worked Example 3 (p. 213)

☆ *Teaching points.* This worked example is a sample of how a person can take the Steps of Responsibility after making a mistake in a relationship.

✓ Learning Skills, Relationship Care Worksheet 5 (p. 214)

☆ *Teaching points.* This worksheet offers the individual an opportunity to plan how she can admit a problem, apologize, commit to change, and take On-Track Actions to take responsibility for her actions.

WEEK 12: USING SKILLS IN MY LIFE

Preparing for Group

Handouts Needed

✓ Learning Skills, Using Skills in My Life, Skills Certificate (p. 225)

E-Spiral Phase 1. Exploring Existing Knowledge Base (Review)

➡ ***Welcome group.*** "Hello, everyone! We have made it to Week 12! How are you all doing today? Ready for the ringing of the bell?"

➡ ***Orient to the mindfulness activity: passing the bell and getting a Clear Picture.*** "We have to be able to get a Clear Picture in stressful situations, so we can use the rest of our skills. So, during this exercise, I am going to ask you to do more and continue to stay focused. When we use skills we can stay focused even in a crisis."

Instructions for the mindfulness exercise. "We are going to make things a little harder! We will choose six people to ring the bell and to say one of the Clear Picture Do's. The first person will say, 'Notice the Breath,' then ring the bell. When the sound has finished, the task will pass to the next person. That person will say, 'Notice Surroundings,' and ring the bell. When the sound is gone, the bell is passed. The next person says, 'Do a Body Check,' and rings the bell. When the bell sound is finished, then the bell is passed. The next person says, 'Label and Rate Feelings,' and rings the bell. When the sound is gone, the next person gets the bell. That person says, 'Notice Thoughts,' and rings the bell. When the sound of the bell has disappeared, the bell is passed to the last person, who says, 'Notice Urges,' and rings the bell. While all this is happening, we focus on doing the Clear Picture Do that is being stated at that moment. If you get lost or your mind begins to drift, gently bring your mind back to the bell and the instructions we are being given. We can do this! Any questions?"

Describe questions. "How did that exercise go for you?"; "Were you able to stay focused?"; "Were you able to bring your mind back?"

➡ ***Orient to Skills System review.*** "Ready to review our skills?"

Note: The skills instructor can choose a Basic Review Exercise from Week 1 (pp. 134–135), an Advanced Review Activity from Week 3 (p. 146), or create a new one.

➡ ***Orient to skills practice.*** "We are really learning our skills well! OK, it is time to go over our skills practice. Our homework this week was to practice Relationship Care. Who would like to start?"

Disclosure questions. "Who can share about Relationship Care that you did with yourself?"; "Who can tell us about Relationship Care that you did with other people?"

➡ ***Orient to new skills topic.*** "Good job. Today is a review of all of our skills. We are going to talk for a few minutes about how you are doing learning your skills. OK?"

Discuss existing knowledge about the new topic.

Assessment questions. "Which skills do you use the most?"; "For which skills do you need more practice?"

Note: Writing the answers on the board may be helpful.

Relevant context questions. "What is easy about learning skills?"; "What is hard about learning skills?"

Clarifying questions. "How is life different when people use skills?"; "How is life when we don't use skills?"

➡ ***Orient to relevant context of the new topic.*** "It is hard to remember all of our skills, especially when we are upset. We have to practice our skills a lot to learn them. As we get to know our skills better, we learn how to put them together to handle tough life situations."

E-Spiral Phase 2. Encoding: New Learning

➡ ***Orient to new learning.*** "Today we are going to fill out the Skills Quiz on page 217 in the Learning Skills, Using Skills in My Life section of the *Skills System Workbook.* None of us loves quizzes. This will help us find out the skills we understand and those with which we need more help. We will pass in the quizzes and go over the answers when we get done. I brought in sodas and cookies today to celebrate us finishing our 12 weeks. I am very proud of you all. Are we ready to get started?"

Note: The instructor can choose to do the quiz as a group or individually. The primary goal is to reflect on the past 12 weeks of learning and celebrate any gains. A secondary goal is to evaluate progress.

Instructions for the encoding activity. "If you have a hard time reading and writing, either I or your staff can help you. Let's take a few minutes to make a plan about how we can fill out this sheet. If you do not know the answer, you can guess or leave it blank. The good news is that once you hand in your quiz, you get a soda and cookies. Any questions?" (The answers are provided on the Skills Quiz Answer Sheet, p. 218.)

➡ ***Orient to the end of the Encoding Phase.*** "Great job! I think I saw a lot of people doing On-Track Actions here today."

E-Spiral Phase 3. Elaboration: Practice and Linking

➡ ***Orient to the elaboration activity.*** "OK, let's go over the quiz together."

Instructions for the practice exercise. "I will ask the group the questions, and let's come up with the right answers together."

Disclosure questions. "How do you think you did on the quiz?"; "How do you think you are doing learning your skills?"

➡ ***Orient to discussion.*** "We are going to talk a little more about how we are doing learning skills."

Linking question. "Has it been hard for you to learn to control yourself in the past?"

Disclosure questions. "What are you doing now that works?"; "What are you doing that does not work as well?"

Expansion question. "What do you need to do to make skills work better for you?"

➡ ***Orient to the end of the Elaboration Phase.*** "Great awareness. How about we talk more about how we use our skills together to handle tough situations?"

E-Spiral Phase 4. Efficacy: Bridge to Real Life

➡ ***Orient to efficacy activities: skills review activity.*** "Let's talk together about the situations in our lives that are really hard to deal with. We can work together to see how our skills can help us in those situations."

Instructions for the efficacy activity. "We are going to begin by listing difficult situations that you have faced in the last few months. We are going to make a list of these stressful situations on the board. Then we are going to look at making a skills plan for each of the situations. When we make a skills plan today, we are going to use the number of the skill to show what the plan is. For example, if the situation is one where we think there is risk, we might use 1. Clear Picture, 2. On-Track Thinking, 3. On-Track Action, 4. Safety Plan, and 5. New-Me Activity. So, that skills chain is a 12345. If we were bored and wanted to go watch TV, the skills chain would be a 1235: Clear Picture, On-Track Thinking, On-Track Action, and New-Me Activity. We talked last week about Relationship Care—Finding Middle Ground skills chains that need to include seven skills, 1236789, to solve relationship problems. Who would like to share a situation they handled using skills? We will all help you figure out the skills chain you used. Any questions?"

Disclosure questions. "How was it using the numbers to label skill chains?"; "Did it help you understand it better, or was it more confusing?"

➡ ***Orient to discussion.*** "Before we end for the day, let's talk about some of the challenges that we face when we are learning skills. OK?"

Barrier question. "What is difficult about learning skills?"

Wisdom questions. "Do you think it is important for you to learn skills?"; "Why?"

Commitment question. "What are you going to do to keep practicing skills?"

Coaching question. "How can you coach yourself to practice your skills?"

➡ ***Orient to home study.*** "This group has done an amazing job. I would like to hand out your certificates now. [The template for the Skills Certificate is on p. 225 of the *Skills System Workbook*.] I will announce your name and the number of cycles you have completed in the Skills System. This is like getting different belts in karate. The more cycles we get, the more skills we are able to use. Fantastic, I am so happy that you are all here and have worked so hard. It is our favorite part: homework! Please practice putting your skills together in skills chains this week. If you want to study skills at home, review all the handouts we have gone over so far. You can also do any worksheet that you have not completed yet. Thank you all!"

➡ ***Orient to group ending.*** "As you know, we ring the bell six times at the end of group. We do one ring for each of the Clear Picture Do's. It is a chance to notice what is happening inside and outside of us right now. We take a moment to get a Clear Picture as we go back to our activities. Who would like to ring the bell today?"

Note: Instructors may want to develop a graduation ceremony process for individuals who have completed a certain number of cycles through the Skills System curriculum. Creating a diploma, inviting friends/family members, providing refreshments, and having individuals share about how they integrated the skills are meaningful transitional activities.

Using Skills in My Life Handouts to Review in Future Cycles or for Home Study

✓ Learning Skills, System Tools Review Questions (p. 47)

☆ *Teaching points.* Instructors can use these questions to review skills in the beginning of group.

✓ Learning Skills, Using Skills in My Life Skills Quiz (p. 217)

☆ *Teaching points.* Instructors can use the quiz as a group activity or ask an individual to complete it. The individual can write the answers on the sheet or another person can write for them.

✓ Learning Skills, Using Skills in My Life Skills Quiz Answer Sheet (p. 218)

☆ *Teaching points.* The group or individual can review the answers to the quiz and clarify concepts.

✓ Learning Skills, Using Skills in My Life Skills Plan Map (p. 219)

☆ *Teaching points.* The Skills Plan Map has all of the skills and subskills on it. It offers a skills track for when the individual is at Level 0–3 feelings that include the All-the-Time and Calm-Only skills. The map also has the All-the-time skills for when the individual is a Level 4–5 feeling.

✓ Learning Skills, Using Skills In My Life Worksheet 1 (pp. 220–222)

☆ *Teaching points.* Worksheet 1 helps the individual create a Skills Plan when she is at or between a Level 0 and 3 feeling. It includes both All-the-Time and Calm-Only skills.

✓ Learning Skills, Using Skills In My Life Worksheet 2 (pp. 223–224)

☆ *Teaching points.* Worksheet 2 can be used to help an individual make a Skills Plan for when he is experiencing Level 4–5 feelings. This worksheet only includes All-the-Time skills.

✓ Learning Skills, Using Skills in My Life Skills Certificate (p. 225)

☆ *Teaching points.* The instructor can choose to use the certificate at the end of cycles through the 12-week curriculum.

SUBSEQUENT CYCLES THROUGH THE SKILLS SYSTEM CURRICULUM

Once the group members complete a 12-week cycle through the skills curriculum, they have a much better understanding of the skills concepts. For example, the group will have done 12 different mindfulness activities. During each group session, prior learning is reviewed, new learning is introduced, and new learning is linked to all the previous skills that were addressed. Due to the variable strengths of participants, each group member will have integrated different amounts of information.

The skills instructors juggle many things at the same time. Instructors have to teach the group while individualizing interventions for the diverse levels of skills integration and cognitive abilities of each group member. Although certain group members may be able to generalize all nine skills, others may struggle to remember even three names of the skills. Skills instructors must make the group an effective learning experience for each participant or find an alternative group for a client who is significantly ahead or behind the rest of the group.

Throughout each cycle of the group, there are opportunities to return to fundamental Skills System concepts and basic commitment to learning and utilizing skills. In general, teaching progresses in the following ways through multiple cycles of the Skills System curriculum:

- Teaching moves from being more general to more specific. For example, as the individual learns about breathing, she learns to focus awareness specifically on the nose or belly.
- Teaching integrates more detailed information as the knowledge base increases. For

example, as the individual understands On-Track Thinking, more of the steps of On-Track Thinking are integrated into the individual's behavior. Initially the person may take a second to think about a decision, while after repetition the client may Check It, Turn It, Cheerlead, and make a Skills Plan.

- Exercises become more realistic to replicate real-life forces in the participant's environment. For example, skills instructors may create distractions during a mindfulness breathing exercise so that the group learns to focus attention while experiencing interfering forces.
- The individual becomes more able to share helpful personal awareness and information related to skills discussions. For example, initially the participant may be hesitant to disclose that he has ever had difficulties related to overwhelming thoughts or feelings. As the individual gains competence managing feelings, he reduces his emotional vulnerabilities and increases his abilities to participate fully.
- Discussions become increasingly dialectical as the group progresses through the curriculum. During preliminary cycles, the group focuses heavily on integrating concrete skill information. As a group develops a skills knowledge base, discussions become more lively and expansive. As capacities increase, alternative views are encouraged and managed in group.
- Discussions related to barriers for skills use become increasingly personal and detailed. As skills instructors become familiar with each participant and as group members get to know each other, barriers to integrating skills are clearer. For example, initially the leader may not know that a participant lives with an abusive housemate. Throughout the group experience, individual challenges become evident. It is crucial that group leaders understand the forces that impede generalization of skills in each participant's life. Skills instructors coach participants to manage challenging situations throughout the cycles of the Skills System curriculum.

Skills System group members learn crucial information from both the teaching and social aspects of the curriculum. The participant cycles through the program, building skills that enhance self-awareness, self-acceptance, self-value, and self-trust. As these factors increase, the individual improves her ability to manage relationships effectively. The Skills System helps the individual navigate the human experience skillfully. Participants gain knowledge that allows them to create fulfilling lives that include freedom and joy.

TRANSITION TO CHAPTER 8

Chapter 8 presents skills coaching techniques that can be used by support providers, family members, and/or other people in participants' lives to help them generalize skills in the natural environment. The chapter explores how extrinsic emotion regulation supports can help individuals manage even challenging feelings and situations. Having a skills coach who understands the Skills System and the skills coaching techniques can help participants reach personal goals in their lives.

CHAPTER 8

Skills Coaching Techniques

Skills coaches are people who know the Skills System and skills coaching techniques who assist the individual to use her adaptive emotion regulation strategies in her natural environments. Skills coaches offer scaffolding that helps the individual build on her existing competencies to expand her abilities. Without adequate scaffolding, individuals may be less able to generalize adaptive strategies.

In addition to providing supports, coaches are part of the individual's environment. The individual and the coach are in a relationship of some kind that can be a one-way or two-way street. Coaches have opportunities to assist both through explicit coaching techniques and implicitly though their relationship with the individual. It is important to understand that it is possible for the coach to destabilize an individual, facilitating dysregulation. A coach's own emotion regulation actions affect the individual and vice versa. Therefore, Skills System coaching strategies involve the individual, the coach, and the interaction between them.

Throughout this chapter, the individual receiving coaching will be referred to as Person A or "the individual." The skills coach is called Person B or "the coach." By using skills, Person A and Person B each self-regulate. Additionally, when Person B engages with Person A using coaching strategies, the hope is that co-regulation is possible.

The first section of this chapter explains interpersonal emotion regulation and co-regulation to establish a theoretical basis for the skills coaching relationship. Next, the A + B = C Skills Coaching framework is described, including strategies for real-life situations when Person A discloses off-track thoughts/urges, is at a Level 4 or 5, and is less engaged in a skills coaching conversation.

EMOTION REGULATION AND SKILLS COACHING

The core tenet of DBT, dialectics, is relevant in skills coaching in multiple ways. Linehan (1993a) explains that validation strategies, delivered as extrinsic emotion regulation strategies by a therapist, can help the client decrease self-invalidation that undermines adaptive actions. This acceptance-based intervention is paired with change strategies that are designed to foster effective behaviors. In DBT, acceptance and change strategies are used to promote "the reconciliation of opposites in a continual process of synthesis" (Linehan, 1993a, p. 19). The combination of acceptance and change strategies provides key ingredients of growth.

Support staff members using the Skills System are encouraged to use both acceptance strategies (validation) and change strategies (skills coaching). Intertwining these strategies helps the individual both to co-regulate in the moment and experience longer-term intrapersonal development.

Interpersonal Emotion Regulation

Zaki and Williams (2013) explain that interpersonal emotion regulation happens within social interactions. The presence of other people in stressful situations serves to help an individual modulate negative affect (Beckes & Coan, 2011). In addition to this implicit benefit, relationships can serve a more active role in the emotion regulation process.

Intrinsic interpersonal emotion regulation occurs when the individual can seek out support to regulate an emotion (Zaki & Williams, 2013). The individual engages in interactions to help her up- or down-regulate emotions, depending on her goal in the situation. Extrinsic emotion regulation is not the individual (Person A) enacting strategies, but rather an external person (B) engaging in interpersonal behaviors that regulate the emotions of Person A. A skills coach engages in extrinsic emotion regulation strategies when he attempts to help someone regulate her emotions.

Within these two forms of interpersonal emotion regulation (intrinsic and extrinsic), there are two classes, "response-independent" and "response-dependent" (Zaki & Williams, 2013, p. 804). There are times when Person A can gain regulatory benefit just through an interaction regardless of Person B's responses (intrinsic response-independent). For example, when Person A labels a feeling during a conversation with Person B, it can serve as an emotion regulation function regardless of Person B's responses. Conversely, Person A's reactions can be response-dependent and impacted by Person B's responses during the same conversation. Response-dependent reactions can be risky, because if Person A seeks solace from Person B and he is unsupportive, Person A may feel worse.

Ideally, intrinsic interpersonal emotion regulation can make Person A feel safer (less alone in times of stress). It offers Person A an opportunity for combining psychological resources (A + B). When Person A shares an experience (i.e., being on the same page) with Person B it can communicate a sense of affiliation that can be rewarding for Person A. If Person A has an opportunity to label feelings and assess the causes of the feeling, there are emotion regulation benefits (Lieberman et al., 2011; Zaki & Williams, 2013).

Co-Regulation

Humans are equipped with a mirror neuron system (Plata-Bello et al., 2023). Our brains are built so that when people around us have experiences, we react with a simulated version of their experience. For example, if we see someone smiling, we have a simulated experience of happiness. Alternatively, if we see someone angry, it simulates experiences of anger for us. Therefore, we are all connected and all influence each other, whether we intend to or not.

These connections provide us with opportunities to help people. Person B's ability to manage her own feelings, thoughts, and urges can serve as a mirror for Person A. The opposite is also true. Coaches have the power to destabilize the individuals around them. If the coach is dysregulated, those within the environment will simulate that. It may be more difficult for Person A to be on-track when Person B is off-track.

Butler and Randell (2013) define co-regulation as the "bidirectional linkage of oscillating emotional channels (subjective experience, expressive behavior, and autonomic physiology) between partners, which contributes to emotional and physiological stability for both partners in a close relationship" (p. 202). This means that Person A and B are co-regulating when they are working together to manage feelings, maintain balance, and move toward personal goals. Therefore, if one or both engage effective skills and offer scaffolding to the other, the likelihood of their feelings being regulated is higher. Conversely, if one or both are not engaging in adaptive emotion regulation processes, feelings are likely to escalate and possibly last longer.

Coaching Conversations

Not all conversations are coaching conversations. Sometimes we are just talking, chatting, and interacting, one person to another. Other times, though, we are trying to help an individual deal with the situation they are experiencing, whether he is a friend, a person we are employed to support, our child, or a parent. Coaches help the individual reflect and take actions to reach their goals and live aligned with their values.

Coaching strategies are not one-size-fits-all. In Relationship Care, we discussed the different types of relationships. We have to adjust our coaching strategies to work within the boundaries of these different relationships. For example, parents serve a different role than friends; direct support professionals have a different role than therapists; and treating a 16-year-old like a 6-year-old is not going to work.

The coach who is sensitive to factors such as the individual's culture, ethnicity, age, developmental stage, physical and mental health issues, setting, and situation is often able to make the strongest coaching connection. A coach serves a different role in different peoples' lives, so it is necessary to make adjustments to address the unique needs of both the coach and the individual. Whether we are interacting with people we work with, family, or friends, we use our 123 Wise Mind to know when to offer skills coaching and how much coaching and/or what type is optimal for each individual and circumstance.

De-Escalation and Emergency Procedures

A + B = C is primarily used when individuals are between feelings Levels 0 and 3. Over a Level 3, people have difficulty processing information and it is important not to engage in interactions that increase cognitive load. All-the-Time skills may be used when over a Level 3, but the A + B = C model, because it relies on verbal processing, is not recommended when the individual is over a Level 3. Skills System concepts may be integrated into de-escalation strategies when the individual is above a Level 3 (e.g., Safety Plans, New-Me Activities), but A + B = C should not be the framework guiding the interactions.

Most models that include crisis interventions involve verbal de-escalation and nonviolent emergency strategies (e.g., Crisis Prevention Institute, Safety Care). Generally speaking, verbal de-escalation and environmental adjustments are used when the individual is at a Level 4 and emergency procedures are used when he is at a Level 5.

A + B = C SKILLS COACHING MODEL (0–3 FEELINGS)

In the "real world," the people supporting an individual who experiences emotion regulation challenges are often vulnerable, stressed, and have limited interest in delving into complex theory. The emotion regulation strategies must be built in to the lives of the coach and the individual in ways that minimize cognitive load and maximize supports. To that end, the A + B = C Skills Coaching model is a simple, user-friendly set of strategies that a coach can learn and practice.

A skills coaching conversation is not a regular dialogue between people. The coach is functioning to strategically help Person A effectively regulate feelings and reach her personal goals. The coach (Person B) may be a parent, support staff, or a partner who is attempting to help the individual make mindful decisions for herself. The coach is not controlling Person A in the relationship, he is helping her reach her unique potential.

A coaching conversation can range from a relaxed chat to a more complicated interaction when Person A or B are experiencing stress. It is important that the skills coach have a simple framework to guide strategies due to the potentially high cognitive load demands that can accompany complex situations.

The A + B = C framework is a simple way to conceptualize how to structure interpersonal emotion regulation interventions. Column "A" represents effort made first to clarify the individual's perspectives. In this first phase (A), the focus is on awareness and acceptance. The coach is hearing the individual without adding commentary.

Column "B" represents the perceptions of the coach (Person B). The Column B strategies help the coach know how and when to add his perspectives to the coaching conversation.

Column "C" represents a collaboration between Person A and Person B to create a Skills Plan that will help the individual manage the situation. There are times when Person A wants to function autonomously, and others when she requests collaboration. Column C strategies help balance coaching supports to optimize Person A's long- and short-term skills competency. Figure 8.1 presents an overview of the A + B = C concepts.

A: PERSON A'S PERSPECTIVE

Either Person A or Person B can initiate a coaching conversation. If Person A feels like she needs support, she may reach out to talk to Person B. Conversely, Person B may notice Person A's levels of feelings going up and/or behaviors changing and approach to offer skills coaching. In these circumstances, getting on the same page is an important first step. Person B asks questions and validates to help Person A with the goal of helping her get a Clear Picture of her internal and

A	+	B	=	C
Person A's Perspective		Person B's Perspective		Both People Work Together

A. Person A's perspective—getting on her page:

Person B tries to get a Clear Picture of Person A's situation. Person B asks questions *and* uses validation strategies. The focus is Person A's awareness and acceptance. If Person A is at a 0–3 feeling, Person B can get more details about the situation.

Getting a Clear Picture of Person A:

- Ask a general question about what is going on to **find out the cause of the emotion**. (*"What's going on?"*)
- Elicit a **label and rating** for the emotion. (*"How are you feeling? What level?"*)
- Ask about the **breath**. (*"What do you notice about your breath?"*)
- Ask about the **urge**. (*"What do you want to do?"*)
- Expand awareness to other Clear Picture Do's, if possible. (*"Surroundings?"; " Body sensations?"*)

Explore her On-Track Thinking:

- Ask about her plan of action. (*"So, what is your plan?"*)
- Ask about the goal. (*"What is your goal in this situation?"*)
- Help Person A assess the plan with Check It. (*"Do you think that will help you get to your goal?"*)

Executing On-Track Actions:

- Review the plan. (*"So, your plan is to . . . ?"*) Confirm the first On-Track Action. (*"Your On-Track Action will be . . . ?"*)

B. Person B's perspective—Person B offers his two cents:

Person B asks Person A if she would like to hear Person B's thoughts about the situation. (*"Would you like to hear what I am thinking?"*)

Person B waits for consent:

- If Person A says "no," Person B explains that he will be available at a later time. (*"No problem; if you want to chat later, I will be around."*)
- If Person A says "yes," Person B asks if she is comfortable in that location. (*"Is here OK or do you want to move to a different place to talk?"*)
- Once settled, Person B offers an opinion about whether Person A's plan will effectively reach her stated goal.

(*cont.*)

FIGURE 8.1. A + B = C Skills Coaching model.

Assessment to On-Track Action:

- If Person B thinks it is an on-track plan to the expressed goal, he supports it and tries to promote Person A taking an On-Track Action. (*"I think that plan will work; what will be your On-Track Action? . . . Great job!"*)
- If Person B thinks the plan will not reach Person A's goal, he explains the problem. (*"I am concerned that if you . . . it might . . . , which is not your goal."*)
- Person B offers skills coaching support. (*"Do you want to take a few minutes to talk about options?"*)

C. Both people work together—plan skills chains together:

If "yes," Persons A and B chat about the situation and what skills may be helpful to link together.

- Remember the Categories of Skills (*0–3 feeling = all nine skills/4–5 = All-the-Time skills, not Calm-Only skills*).
- Be sure to use enough skills (*Recipe for Skills*)!

Skills options:

- ***On-Track Thinking:*** Check It, Turn It, Cheerleading, and Make a Skills Plan.
- ***On-Track Actions:*** Take a Step to Your Goal, Switch Tracks, On-Track Action Plan, Accept the Situation, Turn the Page (All-the-Time skill).
- ***Safety Plans help in risky situations:*** Focus on a New-Me Activity, Move Away, and Leave (All-the-Time skill).
- ***New-Me Activities:*** Focus, Feel Good, Distraction, and Fun (All-the-Time skill).
- ***Problem Solving:*** Small problems—Quick Fix worksheet; medium and large problems—Clear Picture of the Problem, Check Options, Make Plans A, B, and C (Calm-Only skill).
- ***Expressing Myself:*** Communicating needs/concerns, etc; Expressing Myself Worksheet (Calm-Only skill).
- ***Getting It Right:*** Getting what he wants; Getting It Right Worksheet (Calm-Only skill).
- ***Relationship Care:*** Core Self; One- and Two-Way-Street relationships; Finding Middle Ground Worksheet; Steps of Responsibility Worksheet (Calm-Only skill).

Executing On-Track Actions:

- Review the plan. (*"So, your plan is to . . . ?"*)
- Confirm and support the first On-Track Action. (*"Your On-Track Action will be . . . ? Good job!"*)

FIGURE 8.1 *(cont.)*

external experiences in the moment. Figure 8.2 offers an overview of Column A tasks that can help Person B assist Person A to use skills. The focus and scope of coaching questions and validation strategies change depending on Person A's level of feeling.

For example, if the individual is well-regulated and experiencing relatively low levels of feeling (0–3), the coach can inquire about the details of the situation. At these levels, it is possible to have an in-depth conversation with Person A about a complex situation, discussing details about content, reflecting on short- and long-term goals, and brainstorming about skills options (including Calm-Only skills).

Whether the individual approaches the coach or vice versa, the coach may choose to begin by eliciting information about the situation. A general inquiry, such as "How are you doing?", "What's up?", "Are you doing OK?", or "What is bothering you?" offers Person A an opportunity to share her narrative. The coach needs to understand Person A's "perceived state of the world and [her] desired state of the world" (Gross, 2015, p. 10). Without going into depth, the coach asks Person A about (1) her situation and (2) how she wants it to be. When Person A is at a Level 3 feeling or below, the conversation can meander in an exploratory way following a natural cadence. Refer to the section later in this chapter that shares strategies that can help when the individual escalates to a Level 4 (p. 223).

An easy transition question to On-Track Thinking is "What is your plan?" This implicitly communicates that (1) a plan is necessary, (2) the urge and the plan are different, and (3) intentional behavior that executes the plan will follow. Referring to the generic word "plan" highlights Person A's freedom to choose a course of action. Person B's role as a coach is to help Person A activate On-Track Actions. In this situation, there is no need for the coach to add his "two cents"; the individual was effective and self-reliant. This is a positive interaction for both Person A and Person B.

Finding a Mutually Agreed-Upon Location

One of the first tasks for the coach is to be sure that Person A and B are in an area where they can communicate well. Being in a loud or public place may be less conducive for coaching conversations. The coach will also want to protect Person A's privacy. The skills coach may want to make it clear to the individual that moving to another, perhaps more private, area to talk may be an option. Discussing the best location for the conversation is an important process.

Discussing options for where the pair can go to talk can be a process that reflects the coach's commitment to having a two-way-street relationship. If the coach dictates where the conversation happens, it may disempower Person A, creating a one-way street. When the coach

- Make a general inquiry to start the coaching conversation
- Facilitate the dyad speaking in a suitable location
- Rate her own feelings level and estimate that of Person A
- Use validation strategies
- Invite Person A to get a Clear Picture
- Guide Person A through On-Track Thinking
- Assess Person A's plan-goal alignment
- Clarify Person A's On-Track Action
- Summarize Person A's Skills Plan
- Reduce barriers with practice and troubleshooting
- Elicit Cheerleading statements from Person A
- Offer Person A positive reinforcement

FIGURE 8.2. Overview of the coach's Column A tasks.

collaborates with the individual to find a mutually agreed-upon location, it not only facilitates the pair finding the best location to talk but also establishes a strong relationship connection that may sustain an effective skills coaching session and promote future collaboration.

Person B Gets a Clear Picture

Not only does the coach monitor the feelings rating of Person A, but he also self-monitors and makes necessary adjustments throughout the experience. The coach uses the Skills System guidelines to manage the immediate coaching situation that includes him as part of the transactional equation. For example, if the coach is at a Level 4 feeling, he may need to Switch Tracks and do a Safety Plan—Move Away, rather than doing an in-depth coaching session at that time. At a Level 4 feeling, the coach will have difficulty managing effective Two-Way-Street relationship behaviors. If it is not possible due to logistical constraints to withdraw from a coaching situation at that time, doing basic skills coaching of All-the-Time skills is preferred.

Estimating Person A's Feelings Level

Since it is impossible for a coach to know exactly what an individual's level of feeling is, coaches estimate Person A's level of feeling throughout a coaching conversation. The coach reflects on whether Person A is communicating in a two-way-street fashion. She assesses whether she feels like Person A is talking and listening. If the person's voice is raised or he is noncommunicative, the coach may estimate that Person A is at a Level 4 feeling. If the individual is not usually able to talk and listen due to communication issues, the coach assesses whether Person A is at his baseline or less able to communicate than usual.

If Person A tends to overregulate feelings, he may appear to be at a lower feelings level than he seems. For example, the individual could be talking calmly, yet be emotionally, cognitively, and behaviorally dysregulated without the coach being aware. If the coach is experiencing a two-way-street conversation with this person (suspecting he is at a Level 3), she could ask another follow-up question: "I am feeling like we are talking and listening to each other right now. Do you feel like you and I are talking and listening to each other?" Conversely, it is possible that Person A could overrate his feelings level, reporting at a higher level that he is. For example, Person A may say that he is at a Level 5 feeling even though he is talking calmly to the coach. When the coach suspects overrating (Person A appears not to be at a Level 5), she may want to ask Person A, "Are you hurting yourself, others, or property?" These simple questions can help Person A and B to get on the same page and develop a Skills Plans that accurately reflects Person A's current level of feeling.

Once Person B has a reasonable estimate of Person A's feelings level, Person B uses the Quick Step Assessment to adjust coaching strategies to accommodate Person A's level of affective arousal and cognitive regulation. For example, if the individual is over a Level 3 feeling, she is experiencing higher cognitive load. In that case, the coach focuses the coaching conversation on emotion regulation processes (All-the-Time skills) versus the content of the situation (Calm-Only skills). If Person A is at a Level 4 feeling, he may be experiencing stronger urges to use Calm-Only skills. To preserve the coaching connection, Person B uses care to shift the focus of the conversation from content (e.g., why he is angry at someone) to how he is going to manage his anger (the final two sections of this chapter offer strategies for handling this type of situation).

Validate!

As introduced in Chapter 5, coaches weave validation strategies throughout coaching conversations (Linehan, 2025a, pp. 88–90). Validation strategies offer the individual opportunities to experience external validation that they then internalize, often leading to self-validation—this is money in the self-regulation bank! Increasing Person A's abilities for self-validation reduces the corrosive effects of self-invalidation that erode her efforts to change and grow. The coach wants to (1) empower Person A's Core Self and (2) assist her to use adaptive skills in the situation. Validation builds long-term core capacity that increases Person A's competency to manage feelings independently.

Person B continually mines the conversation for opportunities to validate Person A. Generally, if Person A is at 0–3, all levels of validation are available, but if the individual is at a 4–5, the coach may want to avoid lengthy conversations that require verbal processing. Additionally, coaches should be mindful not to be more validating when Person A is at a Level 4–5 then when they are at 0–3, to avoid intermittently reinforcing her emotional escalation.

Invite Person A to Get a Clear Picture

The coach, Person B, uses the Quick Step to decide how to approach helping Person A get a Clear Picture. If Person A has experience with the Skills System, it may be best to ask her using Skills System terms, "Can you help me get a Clear Picture of your situation?" and/or "Could we go through the Clear Picture Do's together, so I really understand what is going on with you?" This approach will tap into Person A's knowledge base and create a bridge of understanding between Person A and Person B. If the individual has the ability, the coach may witness and reinforce Person A as she recalls the six Clear Picture Do's. If Person A struggles to recall all six of the Do's, the coach may want to either verbally support her to remember or use a visual aid to scaffold the Clear Picture process. For example, the coach may ask:

- "Where do you notice your breath?"; "What does it feel like?"
- "What do you notice in your surroundings?"; "What do you see, hear, smell, taste, and touch?"
- "What body sensations do you notice?"
- "What feeling do you notice?"; "What Level, 0-1-2-3-4-5, is it?"; "Do you feel like you can talk and listen with me?"
- "What thoughts are you noticing?"
- "What urge are you noticing?"; "What do you feel like doing?"

If the individual is not familiar with Skills System terms, the coach can still help Person A get a Clear Picture. Eliciting Person A's awareness of her breath, surroundings, body sensations, feeling, rating of the feeling, thoughts, and urges facilitates late-stage, second-phase processing.

When Person A shares her Clear Picture with the coach, it helps her have clarity of the situation and helps her and Person B to get on the same page.

Guide Person A through On-Track Thinking: Ask about the Plan and Goal

When Person A is at or between a Level 0 and 3 feeling and has a Clear Picture, the coach asks questions that guide Person A to do On-Track Thinking. In particular, the coach needs to understand what Person A's goal and plan are. At this phase of the process, the coach is still not offering personal commentary, so the questions he asks to illuminate the plan and goal must be asked without judgment or influence.

To help Person A clarify her goal, Person B may try asking simple questions like, "What do you want to happen here?"; "How do you want this to turn out?"; "Do you want your feelings to go up or down?"; "Do you want to feel better or worse?" Expressing both a plan and a goal helps Person A elaborate her appraisal process.

Once the goal and plan have been established, the coach and Person A have an opportunity to reflect on whether the plan will get Person A effectively to her goal. Person B does not comment on what Person A should or should not do; he evaluates how the plan will function to get her to the stated outcome. The coach may want to prompt the individual to Check It by asking, "Do you think your plan will get you to your goal?" Coaching strategies that expand Person A's awareness of the situation, attention, and appraisal increase the likelihood that she will remain on-track to her goals. If the coach assesses that Person A's plan is on-track to her expressed goal, he supports the plan: "I think this plan will work to get you to your goal," or "It seems like a good plan." More personal disclosure could be more reinforcing, such as, "I really like your plan," or "That is exactly what I was thinking."

Clarify Person A's On-Track Action

Once there is a Skills Plan, then the coach can ask what action Person A is going to take first: "What is your On-Track Action going to be?" If Person A describes vague steps, the coach helps guide him to set a clear course of simple, step-by-step actions. For example, if the individual states that he is going to do a New-Me Activity, the coach will ask what steps he is going to take to do the activity. The On-Track Actions may include leaving the living room, going to his bedroom, putting on some music, and working on his coloring book.

If the individual experiences executive functioning challenges or high cognitive load, it may be difficult for Person A to recall his skills plan. The coach may want to ask the individual to restate his plan so the coach can assess whether he remembers what to do. If Person A has difficulty recalling the strategies and tactics he will use, the coach may want to design some scaffolding to support Person A. The coach can suggest creative ways (e.g., visual aids, technology, people to remind him) to help remind Person A about the skills he will use.

Practicing, Troubleshooting, and Cheerleading

It is important that Person A have the ability to complete the strategies that are part of his skills plan. Optimally, Person A and B practice strategies prior to challenging situations, so the actions are familiar and within his repertoire of skills. To increase effective generalization, the coach and Person A may want to do troubleshooting before ending a coaching conversation to clarify any potential barriers and adjustments that could help him stay on-track. The coach may want to ask Person A to share a few Cheerleading statements that will remind Person A about his goals and abilities to prime encouragement and efficacy.

Reinforce Skillful Behaviors

Person A will demonstrate some skillful *responses* and strategies during a coaching conversation. As she displays skills and/or verbalizes skills concepts, the coach reinforces Person A's competency. If Person A demonstrates a skill, the coach may ask her to label the skill, asking "What skill was that you just did?" If Person A can't label the skill, the coach can tell her what skill it was.

A coach can reinforce skills most powerfully when he targets specific skills and terms to reinforce. For example, if Person A's plan is to go to her room and listen to music, the coach may ask, "What skill is it when you move away like that?" and/or "What skill is it when you listen to music?" If Person A does not know sufficient skills language to answer "Safety Plan" and "New-Me Activity," the coach may want to highlight the term and function of the skill: "Moving away from risk by going to your room is a Safety Plan," and "Listening to music is a Feel Good New-Me Activity." Labeling and reinforcing skills language in context can facilitate learning and generalization.

+ B: PERSON B'S PERSPECTIVE

There are times when Person B will have the urge to offer his opinion and other times not. Perhaps he has information that could help the individual. Perhaps he believes that Person A's plan will not likely reach the intended goal. Perhaps Person B wants to offer positive feedback to Person A. Alternatively, Person B may believe Person A is on-track and just needs to move in the direction of his plan; in this case Person B may want to simply offer positive feedback or orientation that she is available for coaching. Person B does 123 Wise Mind to be sure she is helping Person A move in the direction of his goals.

At this point, the coach may want to offer his perspective, although it is not necessary. If Person A is on-track, has a strong plan, and intends to execute a series of On-Track Actions, the coach may choose to say, "Great job, I am here if you need me." It is important that the coach not push Person A into a coaching conversation. If Person A says she does not want to hear Person B's opinions, it is fine. The coach can orient Person A to his availability at a later time, if coaching assistance is required. If Person A says "yes" about wanting to hear an opinion, then Person B can share. If Person A and Person B agree that the coach will share his perspective, there are a series of Column B tasks that can be followed (Figure 8.3).

Person B Asks for Consent to Share Perspectives

There are times when Person B feels it would be either on-track Relationship Care or effective skills coaching to offer a personal perspective to Person A. If the comments are going to highlight a different perspective from Person A's, it can be helpful to ask permission first. Getting

Ask whether Person A is willing to hear the coach's perspectives

- Wait for consent to offer perspectives
- Listen to Person A's responses to the coach's perspective
- Return to the Column A tasks: Clarify Person A's plan and assess the alignment
- Ask whether Person A wants to collaborate

FIGURE 8.3. Overview of the coach's Column B tasks.

informed consent (e.g., "Would you like to hear my thoughts?" or "Can I share my ideas about this with you?") establishes Person A as a viable, in-control entity. This simple strategy helps Person A experience a sense of identity and an even playing field. Person B's request for permission allows for reciprocity, collaboration, and respect, while simultaneously allowing for self-determination and independence of both parties. The partners can be together and separate at the same time, creating a dialectical synthesis that promotes personal and relationship growth. It is important for Person B to remember to wait for consent to share his thoughts. It is Person A's decision whether she wants to hear the coach's perspectives, so the coach must wait for consent prior to giving his "two cents."

For example, if the coach does not think the individual's skills plan will help her reach her goal, he may want to voice his concern. First, the coach asks for consent to share his opinion: "I have a few thoughts. Could I share them with you?" If Person A agrees, the coach may share his insights about the plan and goal alignment (e.g., "I am concerned that if you confront Jim in the break room, it might not work out well"). It is also possible to encourage Person A to understand Person B's perspective by asking questions that help her get a Clear Picture (e.g., "If you confronted Jim in the break room, could there be any negative consequences?"). If Person A is unable to foresee problems, the coach can highlight his concerns (e.g., "I think it will drive Jim's and your own feelings up at work. You said your goal was to keep this job. I am worried that he or you will go over a Level 3, start yelling, and get in trouble with your supervisor").

Return to the Column A Tasks: Clarify Person A's Plan and Assess the Alignment

After waiting for consent and sharing his perspectives, the coach gives Person A time to think and then listens to Person A's responses. If Person A's plan appears to have changed at all, the coach asks again what the plan is. The coach maintains a nonjudgmental stance and continues to assess the alignment of Person A's plan and goal throughout the coaching conversation. If the plan seems to be aligned, the coach continues with the Column A tasks:

- Clarifies Person A's On-Track Action
- Summarizes Person A's plan
- Reduces barriers with practice and troubleshooting

- Elicits Cheerleading statements from Person A
- Offers Person A positive reinforcement

Ask for Consent to Collaborate

If the coach assesses that Person A is having difficulty generating a Skills Plan that will align with her stated goal, he may want to offer to collaborate with the individual to create one together. The coach offers to brainstorm with Person A, exploring other options. Continuing with the work example, the coach might help Person A manage the relationship problem and keep her job. Person B could say, "I know Jim is a problem, but we may want to figure out a way to deal with it that doesn't put your job at risk. You getting fired is not going to help. Can we talk about other options?" The coach waits for consent at every decision point, not assuming that Person A wants to continue the process. If Person A declines the offer to reevaluate the plan and look at other skills options, the coach can orient Person A to his availability at a later time.

C: COLLABORATING ON A SKILLS PLAN

Collaborating is foundational for co-regulating. When Person A and Person B work together, both using skills, diverse entities connect in a dialectical synthesis process. They come together to do more than coexist, they connect in ways that benefit both parties. Once Person A consents to hear Person B's perspectives and Person A is ready to make a skills plan, there are a series of Column C tasks that can facilitate this process (Figure 8.4).

Plan Skills Chains Together

If Person A wants the coach's support in developing a Skills Plan that better aligns with her goals, the pair explores options. It is important to outline clearly which skills are available for Person A to use. If she is over a Level 3, only All-the-Time skills are available. If she is at or below a Level 3, all nine skills are accessible. Reviewing the Recipe for Skills can help as well. To this point, Person A has done Clear Picture and On-Track Thinking, so the pair can figure out together how many and which additional skills will facilitate Person A in reaching her personal goal.

Explore Skills Options

To find effective skills options, it may make sense to review each possible skill to discuss its applicability. There are various Skills System resources that can support this process. In the

Plan skills chains together
- Explore skills options
- Execute On-Track Actions

FIGURE 8.4. Overview of Column C: Collaborating.

Skills System Workbook, Learning Skills, Skills List Handout 2 (p. 24) highlights the functions of each skill. This can help the pair decide which skills may be effective in a given situation. Learning Skills, Using Skills in My Life Worksheets 1 and 2 (pp. 220–222, 223–224) can be used to create a Skills Plan. These worksheets can guide Person A and B through a coaching conversation once Person A has agreed to collaborate. Using Skills in My Life Worksheet 1 is appropriate when Person A is at a Level 3 or below, whereas Using Skills in My Life Worksheet 2 is appropriate when she is above a Level 3. Additionally, Table 8.1 highlights an assortment of common goals in situations and potential skills chains.

Complex situations may require addressing multiple goals; therefore, combined skills chains are necessary. For example, if the person tends to escalate to Level 5 feelings, the Skills Plan will have to include multiple On-Track Actions and/or New-Me Activities due to the requirement of using at least six skills (Recipe for Skills). When an individual is at or below a Level 3, integrating Calm-Only skills is often effective. For example, solving a problem may require the individual to use Expressing Myself and/or Getting It Right as part of the solution. This skills chain would be 123678.

Execute On-Track Actions

Once Person A has a plan that fits the situation, the coach helps her clarify it and take an On-Track Action. The plan may include several On-Track Actions; the coach focuses on the one that is a step toward the goal. To increase the likelihood of executing multiskill plans, the coach asks Person A to summarize the plan and offers her scaffolding to remember the skills. In addition, the coach supports Person A to take the first On-Track Action to get the plan started. For example, if Person A plans to go do a Focus New-Me Activity, getting the deck of cards to play solitaire may be the first On-Track Action.

The contextual application of skills is more complex than just collaborating on the creation of a Skills Plan during a coaching conversation. Rehearsing any multistep skills can improve generalization. Troubleshooting barriers can prepare Person A to have more flexible responses during unexpected circumstances. Addressing any possible problems ahead of time will reduce cognitive load when issues arise. For example, if Person A is planning to play solitaire and can't find any cards in her room, the plan may increase her feelings level rather than helping reduce them. In addition, highlighting Cheerleading statements can promote motivation, self-efficacy, and skills-efficacy.

ADJUSTING COACHING STRATEGIES

We all know that real life includes unexpected and often rapid changes. One moment a coaching conversation can be peaceful and the next, escalated. Because of the variable nature of human beings (Person A and Person B), it is important to know how to make adjustments in coaching strategies. This next section will explore three common situations that arise during coaching conversations and adjustments that might be helpful:

TABLE 8.1. Goals and Skills Chains

Factors	Skills chains: All-the-Time skills
Be aware of a situation.	1 (Clear Picture)
Make an on-track decision.	12 (On-Track Thinking)
Move toward my goal.	123 (On-Track Action—Take a Step toward My Goal)
Shift from off-track to on-track.	123 (On-Track Action—Switch Tracks to On-Track Action)
Keep my mind and body on-track.	123 (On-Track Action—On-Track Action Plans)
Tolerate a difficult situation.	123 (On-Track Action—Accepting the Situation)
Let go and move on from off-track TUFFs (Thoughts, Urges, Feelings, and Fantasies).	123 (On-Track Action—Turn the Page)
Manage inside and outside risks.	1234 (Safety Plan) and 12345 (Safety Plan and New-Me Activity)
Get more focused.	1235 (Focus New-Me Activity)
Be more comfortable.	1235 (Feel Good New-Me Activity)
Get my mind off of something that I can't change.	1235 (Distraction New-Me Activity: Distract My Mind and/or Distract My Body activities)
Increase positive emotions.	1235 (Fun New-Me Activity)
Solve small problems.	1236 (Problem Solving Worksheet—Quick Fix)
Solve medium and large problems.	1236 (Problem Solving Worksheets)
Share something that is on my mind and/or in my heart.	1237 (Expressing Myself Worksheets)
Get something I want or need from someone.	1238 (Getting It Right Plan Worksheet)
Improve my relationship with myself.	1239 (Relationship Care Core Self Handouts)
Improve relationships with others.	1239 (Relationship Care Handouts)
Understand how I should deal with different people in my life.	1239 (Relationship Care Handouts—Different Types of Relationships)

(*cont.*)

TABLE 8.1 *(cont.)*

Factors	Skills chains: All-the-Time skills
Get closer or further away from people in relationships.	1239 (Relationship Care Handout—Keeping Relationships On-Track)
Think about what type of relationship I have or want.	1239 (Relationship Care Handout—One-Way-and Two-Way-Street Relationships)
Change off-track personal habits.	1239 (Relationship Care Handout—Getting On-Track with Myself)
Fix relationship problems.	1236789 (Relationship Care Handout and Worksheets—Finding Middle Ground)
Repair a relationship.	1239 (Relationship Care Handout and Worksheet—Steps of Responsibility)

1. The individual discloses off-track thoughts or urges.
2. The individual escalates over a Level 3 feeling.
3. The individual is not engaged in the coaching conversation.

Person A Discloses "Off-Track" Thoughts or Urges

Sometimes in the midst of a coaching conversation, Person A will express off-track thoughts or urges. One of the (perhaps counterintuitive) ways to address this is to reinforce the individual's Clear Picture. For example, if Person A says, "He is a jerk," the coach may want to say, "Good Clear Picture of your thought." This is different than reinforcing the content of the thought by saying, "Great thought." If Person A says, "I want to punch him in the face," the coach may say, "Good Clear Picture of the urge," which is different than saying "Good idea." Reinforcing the separation of awareness (Clear Picture) and plan of action (On-Track Thinking and On-Track Action) is crucial.

If the coach jumps right to a change strategy—like responding to Person A saying, "I want to punch him in the face!" with "You can't do that, you will get arrested!"—it can prematurely derail Person A's late-stage processing. Alternatively, by using an acceptance strategy and saying, "Good Clear Picture of your urge," the coach may be able to avoid reinforcing patterns of dysregulation. In cases like this, it is very important that the coach clarify whether the off-track thought is Person A's urge or her plan (e.g., "Is that what you would like to do [punch him in the face] or what you are going to do?"). This helps the individual understand that (1) urges are not actions, and (2) just because she has an urge does not mean she has to act on it.

Coaches continually assess potential risks; if there is imminent risk to self or others, the coach shifts from A + B = C to de-escalation and/or emergency procedures. If Person A is merely expressing an urge, rather than a plan, and the coach reacts by highlighting potential consequences of her actions, Person A's learning process can be truncated. It is difficult, at times, for coaches to tolerate the uncertainty of Person A contemplating taking off-track actions, but this process may help her prepare and take On-Track Actions instead.

Person A Is at a Level 4 or Higher

When Person A begins to escalate to a Level 4 feeling, she becomes less able to process verbal information. It can be difficult to determine whether Person A is at a Level 3 (experiencing feelings and able to talk and listen) or is clearly at a Level 4 (unable to talk and listen and have a two-way-street interaction). In unclear situations, the coach will want to switch tracks from discussing details of content to focusing more on strategies that reduce arousal levels. For example, if the coach dives into hot topics at that time, asking "why" questions, and having lengthy conversations about the content of the situation, the likelihood of co-dysregulation rises. These missteps often increase Person A's cognitive load and feelings level, and reinforce the individual for using Calm-Only skills over a Level 3.

To determine the best coaching strategy, the coach should do the Quick Step and Targeting Strategy (Chapter 5) to evaluate the best path forward. Person B will want to determine whether it is time to shift to de-escalation strategies or if A + B = C will be best. In one situation, the coach may want to help the individual get a Clear Picture. If the individual's feelings level reduces, the coach may be able to resume doing the A + B = C coaching framework (Column A tasks).

In another situation the coach may evaluate and decide that reducing verbal interactions would be helpful. Instead of getting a Clear Picture, the coach may shift to suggesting Person A moves to a safe area (Safety Plan) and/or do one or more solo New-Me Activities.

If the individual appears to be escalating to a Level 5 behavior, it is important that safety be the priority. If Person A has a formal individual support plan and/or de-escalation procedures, it is important to use those protocols consistently. A lack of clarity about how and when to shift from A + B = C Skills Coaching to safety-oriented procedures may inadvertently intermittently reinforce the individual's escalation.

When Person A is at Level 4–5 feelings, it is more likely the coach will be at high levels, too. At a Level 4 feeling, the coach's abilities to process information, manage urges effectively, and take On-Track Actions are more difficult. The ability to co-regulate decreases when coaches are at a Level 4 feeling. The coach should use Clear Picture, On-Track Thinking, On-Track Action, Safety Plan, and New-Me Activities to manage his own feelings. It may be helpful for the coach to ask another person to step into the coaching role if the coach is over a Level 3 feeling. If the coach is at a Level 4 feeling and can't move away, he may be in a Safety Pickle. In Safety Pickles, the coach continues to get a Clear Picture, does lots of On-Track Thinking, Check the Urge, and Turn It, and does Cheerleading to stay on-track. There are a number of other strategies the coach can attempt to regulate their own feelings level, such as Accept the Situation, Written Safety Plans, or New-Me Activities, like breathing exercises, to help stay focused.

Person A Is Less Engaged

There are times when Person B notices that skills coaching would likely help Person A be on-track to her goals. While it is vital to respect Person A's autonomy, it is also important for Person

B to make efforts to reach across gaps in the relationship to see if co-regulation is possible. This section will present six coaching tactics that may help the coach engage Person A in a coaching conversation:

1. Give space and be available.
2. Validate and highlight the benefits of Clear Picture.
3. Validate and reflect on Categories of Skills.
4. Validate and reflect on the emotion regulation goal.
5. Validate and Switch Tracks to New-Me Activities.
6. Focus on Safety Planning.

Give Space and Be Available

If the coach assesses there is not an imminent safety risk, she can give Person A some time and space to deal with his situation. It may be helpful for the coach to communicate that she is available and explain how the individual can access coaching support—for example: "I would like to help if I can. I will be in the living room. Text me if you would like to chat." Person A may be independently doing Clear Picture, On-Track Thinking, On-Track Action, and a Thinking Safety Plan, and giving space may be the best way to support the individual to apply his skills autonomously in his life context.

Validate and Highlight the Benefits of Clear Picture

If the individual is not interested in engaging in the coaching conversations, the coach may want to validate the individual and highlight the benefits of Clear Picture. For example, the coach can validate the individual's current strategies: "Taking some time for ourselves can be helpful." The coach could make a radically genuine statement that communicates nonjudgment, understanding, and willingness to help: "I am here to help, if you need it." The coach can ask consent to share her two cents: "Could I share a thought I am having?" If permission is granted, the coach can highlight that getting a Clear Picture might help the individual feel better. For example, "I know it doesn't seem like it right now but getting a Clear Picture can help us feel better. When we have a fuzzy picture, it can make us feel worse. Would you like to try to get a Clear Picture with me? I can lead us through it if you would like." Person A may be experiencing high cognitive load, so the coach may want to use visual aids to support Person A through the Clear Picture Do's.

Validate and Reflect on Categories of Skills

If the individual is engaging in Calm-Only skills when over a Level 3 feeling, the coach may want to validate Person A's urge to use skills without validating their actions: "When we have strong feelings, most of us have urges to fix the situation." At that point the coach can also ask to share her two cents—"Can I tell you what I am thinking?"—and, when Person A has given consent, the coach can highlight concepts related to the Categories of Skills. Coaches use the Quick Step to determine how to describe the concepts. For example, the coach may choose to speak conceptually by saying, "When we are really upset, it is often best to wait to solve problems when we are calmer," or the coach may want to use Skills System terms like, "When we are over a 3, doing Problem Solving can make things worse for us. Doing some All-the-Time skills, like New-Me Activities could help you stay on-track. Do you want to chat about some ideas?" The coach could then ask if Person A wants to brainstorm about alternatives, or the individual may Switch Tracks on his own.

Validate and Reflect on the Emotion Regulation Goal

If the coach assesses that the individual's current strategies are making her uncomfortable feelings increase, the coach may want to ask about the individual's emotion regulation goal. The emotion regulation goal is associated with Person A's hopes about the current feeling and whether she wants it to increase or decrease in intensity and/or duration. Knowing what Person A's emotion regulation goal is helps the coach and Person A have clarity, which is foundational for co-regulation.

To elicit Person A's emotion regulation goal, it may be best to begin with validation, like a radically genuine statement, "I am a little confused right now," or a normalizing statement, "Life can get a little confusing sometimes." Once again, the coach gets consent to ask questions or tell his perspective. If Person A is open to a dialogue, the coach can ask about Person A's emotion regulation goal: "So I understand and have a Clear Picture, would you like this feeling to go up or down?" or "Would you like to feel better?" If the individual says she would like her feelings to be different than they are, the coach may want to offer to collaborate to make a Skills Plan. The coach could say, "That is possible. Would you like to chat about how you could do that?" If Person A consents again, the dyad moves into collaboration.

Validate and Switch Tracks to New-Me Activities

If the individual appears to be escalating over a Level 3, interacting verbally may increase levels of feelings. Engaging in Solo New-Me Activities may help Person A minimize escalation caused by verbal interactions. Additionally, a New-Me Activity may reduce feelings levels via the emotion regulation properties of the activity.

The coach uses the Targeting Strategy proactively to determine which New-Me Activity to suggest. The coach reflects about what type of New-Me Activity best serves the situation:

- If Person A is unfocused and confused, a Focus New-Me Activity may help improve cognitive processing that facilitates On-Track Thinking, leading to more On-Track Actions.
- If Person A is mentally, emotionally, or physically uncomfortable, doing a Feel Good New-Me Activity can soothe Person A's distress, allowing him to Switch Tracks from reacting to pain to an on-track Skills Plan.
- If Person A is overwhelmed by the current situation, it may be helpful for the coach to suggest a Distraction New-Me Activity. If Person A has done all he can in a situation and just needs to get his mind off the circumstances, choosing a form of distraction can help him get distance from the stressors and reduce arousal levels.

- If Person A is down-regulating to the point where he is increasing uncomfortable feelings, the coach may suggest doing a Solo Fun New-Me Activity. Fun New-Me Activities often serve the other functions of focus, self-soothing, and distraction as well.

From a behavioral perspective, it is important not to provide certain New-Me Activities only at high levels of feeling to mollify Person A. For example, if Person A only has access to a favorite video game when he is upset (Level 4), it can increase the likelihood of Level 4 behavior to elicit access to the video game. Therefore, if the coach wants to avoid intermittently reinforcing escalating behaviors, suggesting a high-reinforcing activity at a Level 4–5 may be counterproductive.

In addition to targeting, the coach uses the Quick Step to determine how best to facilitate the Solo New-Me Activity. For example, a lower-cognitive-load option would be for the coach to suggest a Solo New-Me Activity that Person A is familiar with, likes, and has immediate access to. A high-load option would be to present many options for Person A to choose from. The highest load would be to engage Person A in a brainstorming conversation about multiple alternatives, possible functions of each, and making choices from different possibilities.

Once the coach is ready to progress, she will want to use some kind of validation that requires minimal verbal interaction, such as "It seems like you might be feeling . . . (label a feeling that there is evidence of)?" or "This is a hard situation," or "I'm sorry you are going through this," or "I can see why you are feeling this way." Before sharing ideas, the coach asks if she can offer her two cents: "Could I make a suggestion?" or "I think there are some New-Me Activities that could help you. Do you want to hear about them?" If Person A agrees, the coach can suggest one or more Solo New-Me Activities. At a Level 4, doing Partnership New-Me Activities involves Relationship Care, which is a Calm-Only skill and is recommended when all involved are between 0 and 3 level feelings.

Once Person A gives permission, the coach may suggest one or more New-Me Activities that could help the individual in the moment. For example, a lower load suggestion might be, "Would you like to do your coloring or your puzzle?" A higher load suggestion would be, "Is there a Solo New-Me Activity that would help you right now?" The coach may want to offer positive reinforcement of On-Track Actions that Person A demonstrated to help increase both self- and skill efficacy.

Focus on Safety Planning

If the coach believes the individual is experiencing risk that requires addressing, she needs to intervene to reduce risk. The coach:

- Follows any de-escalation and/or nonviolent crisis intervention models that are in place (e.g., Crisis Prevention Institute, Safety Care, Mandt system).
- Follows written Safety Plans that have been created.
- Accesses additional supports to manage risks (e.g., other staff, emergency services).
- Addresses environmental factors to increase safety and reduce potential harm (e.g., removing risks from Person A's proximity, removing others from risks).

At Level 5 behaviors, the coach's goal is to minimize damage and create opportunities that are likely to support safety and de-escalation. Once Person A returns to a Level 4, the coach's goal is often to support Person A to manage the feeling in ways that continue to align with his goals. It is difficult to predict how long Person A will be at a Level 4. Person A may still feel uncomfortable for quite some time, but he can stay on-track by being in 123 Wise Mind. The coach uses the Quick Step to determine how and when to engage Person A using the A + B = C model and the other coaching strategies addressed in this chapter.

TRANSITION TO CHAPTER 9

Chapter 9 introduces strategies associated with conducting targeted instruction. Participating in targeted instruction helps the individual create skills plans, reflect on progress, highlight areas of need, and apply additional skills to reach his personal goals within the context of his life. Targeted instruction deepens skills competency and enhances generalization.

CHAPTER 9

Targeted Instruction

This chapter explains how to conduct targeted instruction. Targeted instruction is teaching that builds emotion regulation process competencies that help the individual reach specific goals. Previous chapters focus primarily on individuals' learning skills, but this chapter explains pre-learning activities and techniques designed to help the individual in reaching goals. Pre-learning, which happens prior to learning skills, is an important step that creates a foundation for learning and developing competency. The Reaching Goals strategies target specific skills gaps and improve skill use in those situations during the individual's daily life.

There are many steps required to reach goals. There are actions and patterns of behavior that align with goals and those that do not. For example, if the individual has a goal of maintaining a full-time job, getting up early and getting to work on time would be goal-aligned behavior. Conversely, sleeping in and being late 2 days per week might get her fired and is therefore not aligned with her goal. By increasing actions that are goal-aligned (On-Track Actions) and reducing behaviors that tend to be barriers (off-track actions), the individual is more likely to make progress toward reaching her goals.

Targets are specific things that the individual can identify and work on to increase goal-aligned actions and reduce barriers to her goals. For example, if the individual has a problem with oversleeping and being late for work, one of her targets may be to get up earlier. Other targets could include getting to work on time or going to bed earlier. Each of these patterns of behaviors are different and have multiple, unique microprocesses within each chain, so changing the behavior requires adjusting the processes that are within or support the behavior. When the individual changes key processes, she can change behavior. Not adjusting enough or the correct microprocesses likely sustains default behaviors.

Targeted instruction helps the individual change specific behaviors (microprocesses) within a situation. The instructor and the individual explore the situation in depth so that the individual has clarity about her on-track and off-track patterns of behavior. Since behavior patterns are often challenging to change, a series of "trial and error," or plan-and-replan activities are necessary to create an on-track habit. For example, if the individual has a long-standing, reinforced pattern of oversleeping and she wants to change that behavior, targeted instruction would help her:

- Create a Skills Plan of specific skill-related actions that would support her getting up an hour earlier.
- Execute that Skills Plan in real life.
- Monitor progress related to getting up earlier on workdays.
- Meet with the instructor to review progress related to getting up earlier on workdays.
- Examine specific behaviors she took that were (1) goal-aligned or (2) barriers (Back-Track).
- Explore ways she could have bolstered On-Track Actions and reduced off-track functioning in that situation (Re-Track).
- Create a new Skills Plan to reach the goal and address the target.

Targeted instruction is usually done by an individual therapist who is a Skills System instructor. Nontherapists, like behavior analysts (who are skills instructors), may also do targeted instruction. Targeted instruction activities often happen during a 1-hour weekly/biweekly, one-on-one session with the individual and instructor. Ideally the individual participates in both standard instruction and targeted instruction to expand her skills application and competency.

This chapter explores how to go about targeted instruction. The first section reviews pre-learning activities that create a foundation for targeted instruction. During the process of learning skills, we use "reaching goals" strategies to target instruction. Reaching goals begins with creating a Skills Plan using the My Skills Plan worksheet (Reaching Goals Worksheet 1 on p. 230 of the *Skills System Workbook*). The chapter then addresses monitoring progress using a Diary Card or other methods (Reaching Goals, Worksheet 2) and the My Progress worksheet (Reaching Goals Worksheet 3). Finally, we explain how the instructor can Back-Track—understand the specific chains of behavior that the individual engaged in (Reaching Goals Worksheet 4)—and Re-Track—adjust and enhance skills components (Reaching Goals Worksheet 5)—to improve future functioning.

LAYING THE FOUNDATION: PRE-LEARNING

The information about pre-instruction sessions provided in Chapter 6 of this book will help prepare an instructor to do targeted instruction. There are six worked examples and worksheets in the Pre-Learning section of the *Skills System Workbook* that may be useful to complete during pre-instruction sessions when beginning targeted instruction. Below are the names of the worksheets and functions within targeted instruction. The worksheets help the individual, as well as the instructor, to clarify important information that supports learning and collaboration. Each worksheet is preceded by a corresponding worked example that illustrates how the worksheet can be completed.

- Pre-Learning Worksheet 1: Getting to Know Me (p. 6)
    - Function: This worksheet helps the individual describe her strengths, supports, spirituality, challenges, and successes. It is important to understand and expand adaptive resources and begin to clarify barriers to reaching goals.

- Pre-Learning Worksheet 2: Getting to Know My Feelings (p. 7)
  - Function: This worksheet helps the individual better understand whether she experiences emotional dysregulation. When the individual understands that her feelings are in the driver's seat more often than necessary and to her detriment, it can increase her motivation to learn skills. The instructor frames learning skills as a way to get the individual navigating her life, rather than her feelings.
- Pre-Learning Worksheet 3: My New-Me and My Old-Me (p. 10)
  - Function: This worksheet helps the individual further clarify her goals, values, and vision for who she wants to be and how she wants to live (i.e., New-Me) and what she wants to leave behind (i.e., Old-Me). Many people (and the teams that support them) who have long histories of challenging behaviors can lose track of the individual's potential, which is vital to mobilize during targeted instruction. Additionally, exploring Old-Me starts the process of highlighting elements that need addressing.
- Pre-Learning Worksheet 4: My Goals (p. 12)
  - Function: This worksheet asks the individual to list her goals to get a broad sense of what she is working on. Additionally, the individual rates the level of priority of the goals. The priority helps the instructor and the individual throughout the targeted instruction process to ensure the dyad is targeting the highest priority goals.
- Pre-Learning Worksheet 5: Exploring My Goals (p. 14)
  - Function: This worksheet helps the instructor and individual clarify a specific goal and barriers to the goal. The individual would likely complete this process for multiple goals that will be address during targeted instruction.
- Pre-Learning Worksheet 6: Exploring Targets to Reach My Goals (p. 16)
  - Function: This worksheet helps the individual highlight what she needs to do more of and less of to reach a specific goal. These actions are the targets of instruction in that the individual works on learning how to do more adaptive strategies and less actions that are barriers to a specific goal.

CYCLES OF TARGETED INSTRUCTION

Once the Pre-Learning activities have been completed, the instructor and individual begin the cycle of targeted instruction. This process is a series of steps, repeated over time, that create, practice, monitor, and adjust Skills Plans. This cycle of instruction creates specific learning experiences that fill skills gaps and develop skills competency.

During targeted instruction sessions, the instructor rotates through tasks that:

- Clarify behaviors the individual has recently demonstrated
- Determine whether the actions taken were effective
- Examine possible adjustments
- Create a new Skills Plan for the immediate future

When the new Skills Plan is created, the individual and instructor then:

- Review progress related to the plan
- Do a detailed review of one situation (Back-Track)
- Fill gaps that were present (Re-Track)
- Create a new, fortified Skills Plan

Figure 9.1 diagrams how these processes work together, session after session, to help the individual reach his personal goals.

Making and Executing a Skills Plan

During a targeted instruction session, the individual and the instructor discuss how things are going in the individual's daily life, including his progress with behaviors he is trying to increase and behaviors he wants to decrease. The instructor uses the Targeting Strategy to move the conversation toward making a Skills Plan for the coming week (or time in between instruction sessions).

When making a Skills Plan, the instructor and the individual work together to brainstorm options and discuss the benefits and costs of different choices. The instructor's role is to help consolidate and capture the ideas and create a visual aid that will assist the individual to execute the plan. To maintain a Two-Way-Street relationship and optimize autonomy, the instructor continues to use A + B = C Skills Coaching strategies (see Chapter 8). For example, when the instructor wants to add her perspective, make a suggestion, or offer instruction, she asks permission to share her insights.

A Skills Plan is a process or document that helps the individual remember what skills to use within the context of his life. An instructor uses the Quick Step to proactively and reactively create Skills Plans. Using the Quick Step, the instructor assesses preexisting and current condi-

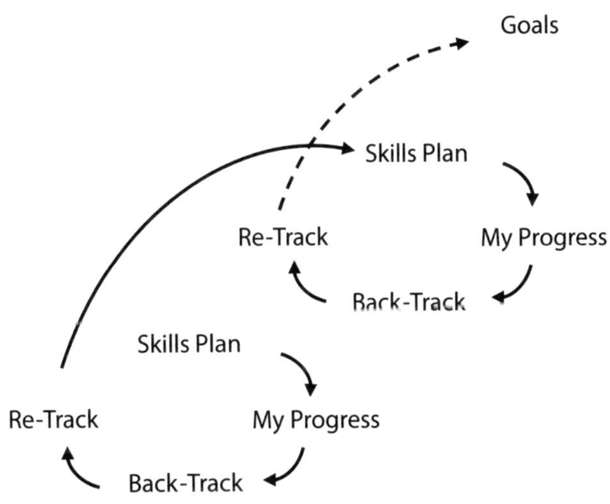

FIGURE 9.1. Targeted instruction cycle.

tions to determine how best to remind the individual about (1) salient issues and (2) what skill tactics to apply within the context. For example, if the individual is trying not to oversleep, the Skills Plan may involve going to bed early, setting an alarm, not hitting the snooze button in the morning, and asking someone to wake them if all else fails. Skills Plans are not general, they are specific, so the individual clearly understands what actions to take.

The form of the Skills Plan is dictated by the individual's abilities to understand and execute the plan. If an individual experiences high cognitive load, the instructor may want to simplify the plan and use pictures instead of making a text-heavy document. For example, Skills Plans can consist of a few pictures of desired actions, places the individual should go, or people he should talk to. Similarly, creating a simple written list or checklist of skills to use can provide important scaffolding for the individual. The instructor individualizes Skills Plans as much as possible so the individual knows what to do and when to do it in the target situation.

If the individual is a reader, it may be helpful to use the My Skills Plan worked example and worksheet in the Reaching Goals section of the *Skills System Workbook* (pp. 229 and 230). The instructor does the Quick Step to determine who should do the writing. For example, if the individual can read, but does not have clear handwriting, the instructor may want to fill out the Skills Plan. Alternatively, the instructor may assess that it is important for the individual to complete the plan himself. Either way, it is important that the individual understands the Skills Plan and can do the tasks that are listed.

Reaching Goals Worksheet 1 (My Skills Plan) asks the individual to list his goal (e.g., I want to keep my job) and the target (e.g., I want to go to work on time) that he will be addressing in the upcoming time frame (between targeted instructions sessions). The individual is asked to check off skills that will help him in the specific situation and to consider whether he'll need All-the-Time skills, Calm-Only skills, or a mix of the two, keeping in mind that he can only use Calm-Only skills when between 0 and 3 level feelings.

Once the individual has a Skills Plan, the instructor works with him to increase the likelihood that the individual will do the Skills Plan. For example, the instructor may ask the individual to practice specific elements of the plan, or it may be helpful to do troubleshooting about environmental factors that could disrupt the individual's efforts.

Diary Card

The dyad also discusses how the individual will monitor his progress during the week. Unlike DBT, Skills System targeted instruction does not require a formal document or Diary Card. The instructor uses the Quick Step to develop a way for the individual and instructor to monitor progress. For example, if the individual lives in a residential setting, he may bring documentation from his program to share with the instructor. The instructor can make a simple weekly checklist or ask the individual to document skills use, off-track urges, and off-track actions that happen during the week. While not required, it is possible that the dyad will decide that it would be best to track progress on targets using a Diary Card. A Diary Card Worksheet and Worked Example are provided in the Reaching Goals section of the *Skills System Workbook* (Reaching Goals Worked Example 2 and Worksheet 2 on pp. 231 and 232).

Many individuals with learning challenges have difficulty reading and writing, so using a Diary Card is optional. If a Diary Card is not possible, it can be helpful to verbally recall the previous events. It may be helpful to read any documentation that is available that describes the individual's on-track and off-track behaviors. When providing targeted instruction for individuals who have executive functioning challenges, using some forms of written record, either self-report or program documentation can facilitate the process of getting clarity about time frames and events.

Progress Review

When the individual returns to the next targeted instruction session, the instructor asks him about his progress related to his goals and targets. If the individual completed a Diary Card, the dyad reviews it at the beginning of the session. It is helpful to ask specifically about On-Track Actions, off-track urges, and off-track actions as they relate to both general functioning and specific goals and targets on the Skills Plan. The purpose of this progress review is for the instructor to determine what chains of behavior should be looked at in more depth (Back-Track).

When considering both on-track and off-track functioning, it is helpful to establish a timeline of when (days and times) particular events happened. For example, if the individual reports waking up on time on Monday and not on Wednesday, the instructor will want to clarify the factors associated with both. Perhaps he went to bed at 10 P.M. on Sunday and was well rested for work on Monday. Perhaps he played video games until 3 A.M. on Tuesday morning and was unprepared to wake up and go to work on Wednesday. The dyad explores the individual's experiences during the week that contribute to both on-track to off-track behavior.

The progress review may cause the individual to have high feelings that increase cognitive load (e.g., shame, disappointment, anger). If the individual has a preexisting executive functioning issue, the progress review, even before the increased emotion levels, may affect his abilities to recall time frames and sequencing; his abilities may reduce further as emotions increase. It is important that the instructor use the Quick Step and validation strategies throughout the progress review process.

Reaching Goals Worked Example 3 and Worksheet 3 in the *Skills System Workbook* (pp. 233 and 234) are used by the instructor to organize the individual's self-report about his progress. During progress review the instructor:

- Confirms the goal and target that the individual worked on
- Asks the individual to describe On-Track Actions he took in relation to his goals and targets
- Asks the individual to describe off-track urges the individual experienced
- Asks the individual to describe off-track actions demonstrated

Back-Track

Doing a Back-Track means getting a Clear Picture of each level of feeling in a situation in order to provide clarity to the individual and instructor. Reaching Goals Worked Example 4 and Worksheet 4 in the *Skills System Workbook* (pp. 235 and 236) can be used to guide the Back-Track process. The worksheet can support the examination of the behavior chain; additional information can be added on the back of the page or on a separate paper if necessary. Figure 9.2

shows a streamlined version of the Back-Track process, using an incident when the individual overslept and did not go to work. This chain highlights several microtransitions within a brief time frame where the instructor and individual could intervene to change the outcome of the situation. The instructor may have chosen this situation because she assessed that it was an opportunity for the individual to Switch Tracks. A different response to the alarm, for example, may have led to the individual getting up and going to work. The Back-Track gives the dyad clarity on the escalation pattern.

It is important that the instructor have a positive, nonjudgmental attitude about Back-Tracking. Challenging behaviors are not personal failures, the end of the world, or impossible to fix; they are skills issues that can be easily corrected. Back-Tracking can be like doing an escape room together: looking for clues and ideas about how to reach goals. This type of attitude helps the individual accept that doing Back-Tracks are an important aspect of learning skills.

Throughout the process, the instructor makes adjustments to illuminate the most relevant factors that led to off-track actions. The more the instructor knows about the individual's patterns and environment, the more she can explore factors the individual doesn't mention. For example, the instructor may know enough to ask about situations that occurred at other times that may have increased the individual's vulnerability (e.g., playing video games until 3 A.M. the night before). Similarly, the instructor may get more information about the events that followed this situation that might include factors that contribute to the escalation (e.g., meeting a new supervisor at work).

Various factors affect the individual's ability to self-report accurately. It is possible the individual is experiencing barriers to recalling and/or communicating the urges they experienced. For example, the individual may be cognitively overloaded, lack self-awareness, have memory problems, have strong shame responses, not trust the therapist, or she may be avoiding. If doing a Back-Track is not possible, it may be necessary for the instructor to help the individual shape her

Level	Breath	Surrounding	Body	Feelings	Thoughts	Urges	Action
5							
4	Tense	Covers over my head—7:10	Stomachache	Shame 4	I'm not going in.	Roll over and go to sleep.	Stayed in bed and blew off work.
3	Heavy	Rolling around the bed.	Tight muscles.	Frustrated 3	I can't deal with work today.	Turn off the alarm.	Turned off the alarm; did not get up.
2	Shallow	Lying in bed—7:05	Groggy	Annoyed 2	I don't want to work.	Hit the snooze button.	Hit the snooze button.
1	Quick	In bed and alarm goes off—7 am	Startled and Sleepy	Anxious 1	I don't feel right.	Throw the alarm.	Laid in bed.

FIGURE 9.2. Sample of a Back-Track.

ability to participate in this process over time. For example, the Back-Track may need to focus on "cooler" versus "hotter" situations. The Back-Track could also be shortened or eliminate details related to high-feelings processes. During this shaping process, it is important that the instructor be mindful of not reinforcing the individual's avoiding by not doing the Back-Track at all.

Targeting for Back-Track

Once the progress review is complete, the instructor must do the Quick Step to assess the individual's preexisting and current cognitive load. As in the Targeting Strategy, the instructor needs to determine whether a lower load approach is necessary, or if a high-load tactic is possible. The following list highlights some guidelines for the instructor when she is determining what events to Back-Track:

- If the individual is not cognitively overloaded, do a Back-Track of a high-risk, off-track behavior.
- If the individual is overloaded, consider doing the Back-Track of the high-risk situation at a later time.
- If there are no high-risk situations, do a Back-Track of a situation when the individual did off-track actions.
- If there are no off-track actions, do a Back-Track of a situation when the individual had off-track urges.
- If there are no off-track actions or off-track urges, do a Back-Track of a situation that included the most actions that are barriers to the individual reaching his goal.
- If there are no off-track actions or off-track urges, it may also be helpful to do a Back-Track of the individual's On-Track Actions to build self-awareness, skill awareness, self-efficacy, and skill efficacy.
- If there are off-track actions and/or off-track urges, but the individual's cognitive load is too high, consider (1) doing a New-Me Activity to help decrease the feelings and increase focus or (2) doing a Back-Track of a situation when the individual demonstrated On-Track Actions.

How to Back-Track

There is no prescribed way to progress through a Back-Track. The instructor can ask questions in a structured way using Reaching Goals Worksheet 4 (p. 236 of the *Skills System Workbook*). Alternatively, the individual can describe a situation and the instructor can ask clarifying questions to get a Clear Picture of what happened. The instructor uses the Quick Step to design the optimal way to get ample information about what happened and what could be enhanced in the future. The following strategies may help the instructor elicit accurate information about a situation:

- Start by asking the individual about his highest level of feeling and what action he took, then clarify the Clear Picture Do's for that level—for example: "You mentioned you were at a Level 5, what did you do? Where were you? What was your breath like?"

- Once the highest level of feeling has been clarified, ask where he was when he was at the next level of feeling—for example: "Where were you when you were at a Level 4?" The instructor asks about the Clear Picture Do's for the Level 4 situation.
- Continue to move down the Feelings Rating Scale, getting a Clear Picture of each level.
- If the individual is having difficulty moving backward in time after clarifying the top level, the instructor can try to establish when the individual was at a Level 1 or baseline. From the baseline state, the instructor can move forward up the scale (Level 1, 2, 3,4, 5) again clarifying the actions, locations, and other Clear Picture Do's.
- An individual with executive functioning challenges likely has difficulty with sequencing, which will make the Back-Track more challenging. For example, the individual's description may not track level to level accurately, or the individual may disclose events from other days without the instructor being aware of the switch. Asking clarifying questions to confirm the individual and instructor are on the same page is helpful. Additionally, using diagrams and maps of areas can help the dyad create an accurate reflection of the situation.

There is utility in creating a visual depiction of the progression from Level 1 to the highest level of feeling, so the individual and instructor can see the chain. The instructor creates a 0-1-2-3-4-5 feelings-level diagram progression and asks the individual to describe what was happening at each level using the Clear Picture Do's as a guide. It can be helpful to establish where the individual was (Notice Surroundings) to clarify physical movements during a situation; linking locations to the feelings level can help the individual scaffold his recollections and improve accuracy.

Re-Track

Back-Tracking helps the individual and instructor get a Clear Picture of the situation. Re-Tracking helps the pair go through the steps of On-Track Thinking to determine what On-Track Actions could help in the future. A Re-Track is when the instructor reviews the information gleaned from a Back-Track, adjusting to improve the emotion regulation process for a similar situation in the future.

For each feelings level that is a part of the individual's Back-Track, the instructor helps him reflect on these questions:

- Was the thought at that level an on-track or off-track thought? Was the urge at that level an on-track or off-track urge (i.e., "Would acting on the thought or urge help you reach your goal?")?
- If it was an off-track thought or urge, what could a Turn It thought be?
- If it was an on-track thought or urge, what could Cheerleading statements be that would encourage you to take an On-Track Action?
- What could a Skills Plan be to manage that level of feeling in the future?

The Re-Track worked example and worksheet in the *Skills System Workbook* (Reaching Goals Worked Example 5 and Worksheet 5 on pp. 237 and 238) is used in conjunction with the Back-Track worksheet (Reaching Goals Worksheet 4, p. 236). The right column of the Back-

Track worksheet contains the action the individual took at each level of feeling. The left column of the Re-Track worksheet also lists the feelings levels, so the sheets align. Level 1 on the Back-Track flows into the Level 1 of the Re-Track, all the way to 5 at the top. Figure 9.3 shows how the Back-Track and Re-Track worksheets fit together.

How to Re-Track

Once the instructor helps the individual get a Clear Picture of the chain via the Back-Track, the instructor begins asking the Re-Track questions about the lowest level of feeling.

Check the Thought and Urge

The first task is to use Check It to check the thought and urge. For example, "When you were lying in bed you had the urge to throw the alarm. Was that an on-track or off-track urge?" If the instructor disagrees with the individual's assessment, she can ask permission to share her perspectives using the Column B tactics from the A + B = C coaching framework (Chapter 8). Both thoughts and urges can be checked. This can help the individual understand how thoughts can lead to urges and ultimately actions (as well as body sensations and feelings).

This tactic serves multiple functions for the instructor and individual. The instructor wants to help the individual improve self-awareness that will increase the individual's ability to recognize when skills are needed and where to intervene. As cognitive load allows, the instructor may

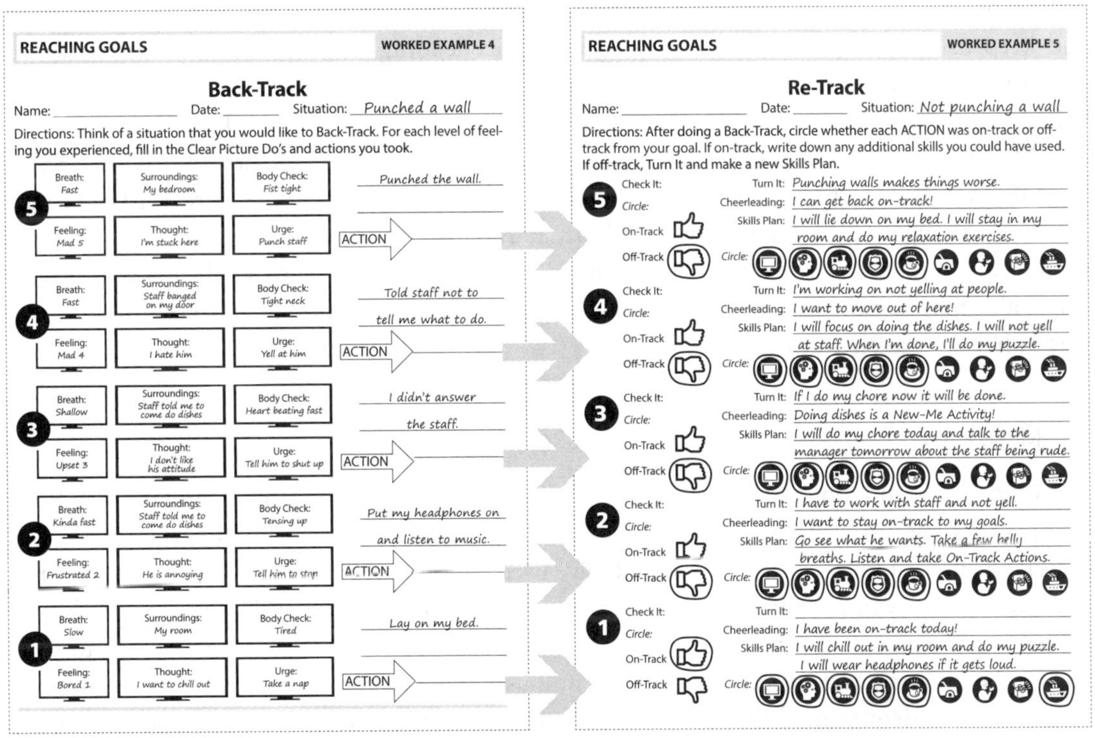

FIGURE 9.3. Images of the Back-Track and Re-Track worksheets fit together.

create learning experiences that increase the individual's awareness; this process also allows the instructor and individual to find effective intervention points for new skills and tactics.

Create a Turn It Thought

If the individual's thought and urge are deemed on-track, the instructor can skip this step and progress to the next one, eliciting Cheerleading statements to strengthen on-track functioning. If the individual's thoughts and/or urges are evaluated to be off-track from his goal, the instructor prompts him to generate a Turn It thought. For example, "You say the urge to hit the snooze button was off-track. What is a Turn It thought that might help you turn off the alarm, instead of hitting the snooze button?"

Turn It thoughts are immediate, targeted interventions that help change the individual's course of action from off- to on-track. The Turn It thought can highlight or bring to awareness (1) the positive consequences of being on-track to his goal and/or (2) the negative outcomes of remaining off-track. In addition to the Switch Tracks benefit, turned thoughts can lead to changes in breath, surroundings, body sensations, feelings, thoughts, and urges. The individual learns that through these skills, he can change the trajectory and intensity of his emotions, remaining on-track to his goal at all levels of feeling.

Elicit Cheerleading

If the individual was having on-track urges and/or has generated a Turn It thought, the instructor asks him to say a few Cheerleading statements to encourage himself to stay on-track and keep using skills. The instructor can elicit Cheerleading before making a Skills Plan to increase motivation and solidify connection to the goal. The instructor can also ask the individual to generate cheers after a Skills Plan is developed to boost self- and skill-efficacy.

Many individuals who experience emotion regulation problems tend toward being self-invalidating. The instructor may have to help the individual check and turn off-track, self-devaluing thoughts by overcorrecting with an abundance of Cheerleading. Both Turn It and Cheerleading statements may not be in the individual's repertoire, so explicit teaching and visual aids may be necessary to provide scaffolding to support the individual to use these strategies in her natural environments.

Make a Skills Plan

Once the foundational steps of getting a Clear Picture, Check It, Turn It, and doing Cheerleading are done (to whatever degree the Quick Step and time allow), the instructor asks the individual about additional skills he might have used at each level of feeling in the situation. For example, "When you were at a Level 2 annoyed, thinking about not wanting to go to work, and having urges to hit the snooze button, what skills could you have used to be on-track to your goal?" The instructor reviews the Back-Track and uses the Targeting Strategy (Chapter 5) when Re-Tracking to determine skills and tactics that can be added to the individual's Skills Plan. In the context of the example in Figure 9.2, Figure 9.4 lists a variety of skills that could have been used to help the individual stay on track.

Clear Picture:

- Practice getting a Clear Picture when he first awakens.
- Use a visual aid to remember what the Clear Picture Do's are.
- Create a recording on his phone that helps him go through the six Clear Picture Do's.

On-Track Thinking:

- Check and turn off-track thoughts after getting a Clear Picture.
- Begin the day with positive affirmations (Learning Skills, On-Track Thinking Worksheet 5—Cheerleading: Blast It, p. 95).
- Cheer himself on to face any upcoming challenges.
- Use visual aids to recall his goals and on-track thoughts.

On-Track Action:

- Take On-Track Action—First Step to the Goal: List multiple On-Track Actions the individual can to that will move him from bed to work.
- Switch Tracks—Opposite to the Urge: Practice jumping out of bed with enthusiasm to seize the day!
- Practice moving from being comfortable (e.g., lying in bed) to being in a less comfortable position (e.g., doing some simple stretching and/or getting in the shower).
- On-Track Action Plan:
    - Go to bed by 10 P.M. the night before having to go to work.
    - Do laundry so there are clean clothes.
    - Have medication refilled and organized.
    - Do grocery shopping so there is food to eat.
- Secure reliable transportation to work.
- Accept the Situation: Accept that transitions are part of life and working is a necessity.
- Turn the Page: Focus on what he is grateful for rather than how horrible work is; focus on looking good today rather than lamenting not staying in bed.

Safety Plan:

- Set the alarm early enough to have ample time to get ready for the day.
- Have the alarm more than arms-length from the bed, forcing him to get out of bed.
- Set out clean clothes picked out to wear to work the next day.
- Have hygiene products available so there are no barriers to getting ready for work.
- Have a friend or family member call him to be sure he is up.
- Have something yummy available for breakfast.
- Ensure access to morning beverages.
- Check the weather so he can plan accordingly.
- Have enough money to meet the needs of the day.

(cont.)

FIGURE 9.4. Skills that could be used in the context of the Figure 9.2 example.

New-Me Activities:

- Take a shower.
- Do ample grooming to look and feel good.
- Wear clean clothes.
- Eat breakfast and/or drink a beverage.
- Take medications.
- Listen to music or a podcast.
- Watch TV while he gets ready.
- Read inspirational material.
- Have some time for quiet reflection.
- Call or text a friend or family member to say, "Good morning!" and perhaps that he loves them and hopes they have a good day.

FIGURE 9.4 *(cont.)*

Re-Tracking Helpful Hints

Use Foundational Strategies

The instructor uses validation strategies, the Quick Step, and the Targeting Strategy when doing a Re-Track. The goal is to broaden the individual's awareness of skills that he could use throughout the situation and focus on a few specific skills to get behavioral activation.

Find the On-Track to Off-Track Shift

It is important for the instructor and individual to find the point when the individual was on-track and then shifted off-track. This point can be a change in the individual's surroundings, body sensations, feelings, thoughts, and/or urges. The instructor focuses on exploration of that moment in time and targets additional skill options to support on-track functions, countering the off-track pressures.

Make Concepts Clear and Concrete

It is important to note that thoughts and urges can be abstract concepts for some individuals, making them difficult to understand and communicate. The instructor should clarify that the individual understands what thoughts and urges are before using the terms. Cognitive overload can degrade the individual's self-awareness, contextual understanding, and ability to communicate; the instructor uses validation and the Quick Step when Re-Tracking.

Adjust Questions to Maximize Participation

If the individual is experiencing low cognitive load, the instructor may want to ask open-ended questions about possible skills or brainstorm options with the individual. If the individual is experiencing high cognitive load, the instructor will want to progress slowly, going step-by-step, one skills concept at a time—for example: "Do you think that getting a Clear Picture at that point could be helpful?"

Create a New Skills Plan

Once the instructor has expanded skill options across the situation during the Re-Tracking process, the instructor and individual create a new Skills Plan. The Re-Track is an exploration process and the new Skills Plan filters the many possible options into a more organized skills to-do list (for more detail, see the previous section in this chapter about creating a Skills Plan). The targeted instruction process rotates through a Skills Plan, Back-Track, Re-Track, Skills Plan cycle (see Figure 9.1) to (1) develop skill competency and (2) reduce specific barriers to goals.

TARGETING INSTRUCTION

Throughout the targeted instruction cycle (but most likely after the Re-Track is complete), it may be helpful to provide instruction to the individual on topics that will facilitate on-track functioning. The instructor evaluates what is missing and fills the knowledge and competency gaps. For example, if the individual is experiencing a medium risk and needs to do a Talking Safety Plan, but does not know how, the instructor needs to be sure he learns before leaving the session. The instructor will have to use available teaching resources and activities (e.g., visual aids, demonstration, roleplay) to help the individual—as best she can in the available time—talk to someone in his environment about managing the risk.

The individual may have multiple gaps in capacities that present barriers for on-track functioning. The instructor can use the Targeting Strategy to target instruction (see Chapter 5). For example, if the individual has a medium-risk situation and takes immediate action on an urge, he may not be doing Clear Picture or On-Track Thinking. Without a Clear Picture of his surroundings, feelings, thoughts, and urges, he will not be able to do an effective Safety Plan. Similarly, if the individual does not Check It, Turn It, and make a Skills Plan, the chances of doing a Talking Safety Plan decrease.

The Targeting Strategy helps the instructor evaluate which is the best emotion regulation process to teach, given the individual's abilities in the moment. For example, the instructor could start by helping the individual do some of the Clear Picture Do's. This would support the individual's awareness of himself and the risk. From that base of awareness, he can be taught to use On-Track Thinking to take On-Track Actions. If the individual's cognitive load is high, it may be difficult to instruct him in doing a Talking Safety Plan. A Talking Safety Plan relies on another person, and depending on the relationship and the individual's training, the process of doing a Talking Safety Plan could increase the individual's level of feeling. A poorly executed Talking Safety Plan can also increase risk. The instructor remains flexible and relies on the Quick Step to determine how much teaching can happen and what the focus of that teaching should be. In this case, the instructor might want to choose a "cooler," lower-load skill option, like Safety Plan—Move Away or New-Me Activities to manage imminent risk. Suggesting a

Focus or Feel Good New-Me Activity in the individual's bedroom, for example, may serve as a de facto Safety Plan in addition to providing the benefits of the New-Me Activity.

Although 123 Wise Mind is optimal (because it builds emotion regulation competency across the span of an emotion), it takes time to build competencies in the six Clear Picture Do's and the four parts of On-Track Thinking to take On-Track Actions. Instructors must be realistic in each teaching interaction; the instructor may only be able to address one or two processes using an a-la-carte approach. Doing a Talking Safety Plan may be necessary in the long term for the individual, but the process of teaching that particular skill in that moment may have higher costs than benefits.

TRANSITION TO BEING AN INSTRUCTOR!

You have made it through the second edition of *The Emotion Regulation Skills System!* It's time to jump in and teach skills! There is no better way to learn how to teach skills than by starting a skills group or doing one-on-one skills instruction. In addition to the accompanying *Skills System Workbook,* additional online resources that can help expand your teaching tools can be found at *http://skillssystem.com.*

APPENDIX

Lesson Planning Worked Example and Worksheet

LESSON PLANNING WORKED EXAMPLE

Week number: *Week 3* Topic of group: *Clear Picture*

Element	Plan
Mindfulness activity How many minutes: *3*	*Notice our breath for one minute: Notice where we feel it and what it feels like.*
Skills review exercise/game How many minutes: *5*	*Ask the group quiz questions about the names, numbers, pictures and functions of the 9 core skills (Visual aid: Skills System Handout 2).*
Homework review activity How many minutes: *10*	*Ask the group, "Who used skills this week?" The group share examples.*
Discussion about relevant context and new teaching How many minutes: *5*	*Ask: "What is it like to have a fuzzy picture?" "What can happen when we have a fuzzy picture?"*
Teaching points How are you going to teach the main topic for the week? (If you are going to use handouts/worksheets, list which one/ones you will use) How many minutes: *10*	*The group looks at Clear Picture Handout 1. The instructor reads the description of each Clear Picture Do On the Summary Sheet.*
Practice exercise How many minutes: *10*	*The group practices each Clear Picture Do after the instructor reads the description.*
Activity: Role play How many minutes: *10*	*The instructor leads the group using the Clear Picture Handout 1 to get a Clear Picture.*
Efficacy: Troubleshooting and commitment discussion How many minutes: *5*	*Ask: When could you practice getting a Clear Picture this week? How could it help you?*
Cool down How many minutes: *2*	*Notice our breath for one minute.*

LESSON PLANNING WORKSHEET

Week number: ________________ Topic of group: ____

Element	Plan
Mindfulness activity How many minutes:	
Skills review exercise/game How many minutes:	
Homework review activity How many minutes:	
Discussion about relevant context and new teaching How many minutes:	
Teaching points How are you going to teach the main topic for the week? (If you are going to use handouts/worksheets, list which one/ones you will use) How many minutes:	
Practice exercise How many minutes:	
Activity: Role play How many minutes:	
Efficacy: Troubleshooting and commitment discussion How many minutes:	
Cool down How many minutes:	

References

American Psychological Association. (2007). *APA dictionary of psychology.* Washington, DC: Author.

Beckes, L., & Coan, J. (2011). Social baseline theory: The role of social proximity in emotion and economy of action. *Social and Personality Psychology Compass, 5,* 976–988.

Brown, J. F. (2019). Improving accessibility to dialectical behavior therapy for individuals with cognitive challenges. In M. Swales (Ed.), *The Oxford handbook of dialectical behaviour therapy* (769–795). London: Oxford University Press.

Brown, J. F., Brown, M. Z., & Dibiasio, P. (2013). Treating individuals with intellectual disabilities and challenging behaviors with adapted dialectical behavior therapy. *Journal of Mental Health Research in Intellectual Disabilities, 6*(4), 280–303.

Butler, E. A., & Randall, A. K. (2013). Emotion coregulation in close relationships. *Emotion Review, 5*(2), 202–210.

Denny, B. T. (2020). Getting better over time: A framework for examining the impact of emotion regulation training. *Emotion, 20*(1), 110–114.

Etkin, A., Buchel, C., & Gross, J. J. (2015). The neural bases of emotion regulation. *Nature Reviews, 16,* 693–700.

Ford, B. Q., Gross, J. J., & Gruber, J. (2019). Broadening our field of view: The role of emotion polyregulation. *Emotion Review, 11*(3), 197–208.

Gold, M. W. (1972). Stimulus factors in skills training of retarded adolescents on a complex assembly task: Acquisition, transfer, and retention. *American Journal on Mental Retardation, 76*(5), 517–526.

Gross, J. J. (Ed.). (2007). *Handbook of emotion regulation.* New York: Guilford Press.

Gross, J. J. (2013). Emotion regulation: Taking stock and moving forward. *Emotion, 13*(3), 359–365.

Gross, J. J. (2014a). Emotion regulation: Conceptual and empirical foundations. In J. J. Gross (Ed.), *Handbook of emotion regulation* (2nd ed., pp. 3–22). New York: Guilford Press.

Gross, J. J. (Ed.). (2014b). *Handbook of emotion regulation* (2nd ed.). New York: Guilford Press.

Gross, J. J. (2015). Emotion regulation: Current status and future prospects. *Psychological Inquiry, 26*(1), 1–26.

Gross, J. J. (2024). Conceptual foundations of emotion regulation. In J. J. Gross & B. Q. Ford (Eds.), *Handbook of emotion regulation* (3rd ed., pp. 3–13). New York: Guilford Press.

Gross, J. J., & Thompson, R. A. (2007). Emotion regulation: Conceptual foundations. In J. J. Gross (Ed.), *Handbook of emotion regulation* (pp. 3–26). New York: Guilford Press.

Haaven, J., Little, R., & Petre-Miller, D. (1989). *Treating intellectually disabled sex offenders: A model residential program.* Brandon, VT: Safer Society Press.

Hamid, A., & Darweesh, A.(2020). Cognitive impairment in psychiatric patients in the United Arab Emirates. *Applied Neuropsychology: Adult, 2*(1), 87–93.

Haq, I. U. (2013). Dialectical behavior therapy for challenging behavior in patients with learning disabilities. *Journal of Pakistan Psychiatric Society, 10*(1), 51–52.

Hartmann, S., Pruessner, L., & Barnow, S. (2024). Contextual variations in emotion regulation: How do regulatory goals shape the use and success of emotion regulation strategies in everyday life? *Emotion, 24*(3), 574–588.

Kalyuga, S. (2011). Cognitive load theory: How many types of load does it really need? *Educational Psychology Review, 23*(1), 1–19.

Kurban, F. (2024). Evolution of pre-service mathematics teachers' spatial visualization skills during a cognitive load theory-based education. *Problems of Education in the 21st Century, 82*(2), 202–220.

Laurinaitiene, K., & Steibliene, V. (2019). Young woman with confusion and cognitive impairment: A case report. *Biologne Psichiatrija ir Psichofarmakologia, 21*(2), 41–45.

Lieberman, M. D., Inagaki, T. K., Tabibnia, G., & Crockett, M. J. (2011). Subjective responses to emotional stimuli during labeling, reappraisal, and distraction. *Emotion, 11*(3), 468–480.

Linehan, M. M. (1993a). *Cognitive-behavioral treatment of borderline personality disorder.* New York: Guilford Press.

Linehan, M. M. (1993b). *Skills training manual for treating borderline personality disorder.* New York: Guilford Press.

Linehan, M. M. (2025a). *DBT skills training manual* (rev. ed.). New York: Guilford Press.

Linehan, M. M. (2025b). *DBT skills training handouts and worksheets* (rev. ed.). New York: Guilford Press.

McNair, L., Woodrow, C., & Hare, D. (2017). Dialectical behavioral therapy (DBT) with people with intellectual disabilities: A systematic review and narrative analysis. *Journal of Applied Research in Intellectual Disabilities, 30,* 787–804.

Mevissen, L., Lievegoed, R., Seubert, A., & De Jongh, A. (2011). Do persons with intellectual disability and limited verbal capacities respond to trauma treatment? *Journal of Intellectual and Developmental Disability, 36*(4), 278–283.

Miller, A. L., Rathus, J. H., & Linehan, M. M. (2007). *Dialectical behavior therapy with suicidal adolescents.* New York: Guilford Press.

Najjar, L. J. (1996). *The effects of multimedia and elaborative encoding on learning* (Technical Report G-IT-GUU-96-05). Atlanta: Georgia Institute of Technology.

Paas, F., & Sweller, J. (2012). An evolutionary upgrade of cognitive load theory: Using the human motor system and collaboration to support the learning of complex cognitive tasks. *Educational Psychology Review, 24*(1), 27–45.

Patterson, C., Williams, J., & Jones, R. (2020). DBT and intellectual disabilities: The relationship between treatment fidelity and therapeutic adaptation. *Advances in Mental Health and Intellectual Disability.* [Epub ahead of print]

Plata-Bello, J., Privato, N., Modroño, C., Pérez-Martín, Y., Borges, Á., & González-Mora, J. L. (2023). Empathy modulates the activity of the sensorimotor mirror neuron system during pain observation. *Behavioral Science, 13,* 947–962.

Preece, D. A., & Sikka, P. (2024). Alexithymia. In J. J. Gross & B. Q. Ford (Eds.), *Handbook of emotion regulation* (3rd ed., pp. 233–240). New York: Guilford Press.

Prochaska, J. O., DiClemente, C. C., & Norcross, J. C. (1992). In search of how people change: Applications to addictive behaviors. *American Psychologist, 47*(9), 1102–1114.

Rutherford, A. V., & Joormann, J. (2024). Depression. In J. J. Gross & B. Q. Ford (Eds.), *Handbook of emotion regulation* (3rd ed., pp. 338–343). New York: Guilford Press.

Sakdalan, J. A., & Collier, V. (2012). Piloting an evidence-based group treatment programme for high risk sex offenders with intellectual disability in the New Zealand setting. *New Zealand Journal of Psychology, 41*(3), 6–12.

Southward, M. W., Sauer-Zavaka, S., & Cheavens, J. S. (2021). Specifying the mechanisms and targets of emotion regulation: A translational framework from affective science to psychological treatment. *Clinical Psychology: Science and Practice, 26*(2), 168–182. [Epub ahead of print]

Stanoi, O. A., & Ochsner, K. N. (2024). Research methods in emotion regulation: Evolving questions and new approaches. In J. J. Gross & B. Q. Ford (Eds.), *Handbook of emotion regulation* (3rd ed., pp. 13–21). New York: Guilford Press.

Suri, G., Gross, J. J., & McClelland, J. L. (2020). Value-based decision making: An interactive perspective. *Psychological Review, 127*(2), 153–185.

Sweller, J. (1988). Cognitive load during problem solving: Effects on learning. *Cognitive Science, 12,* 257–285.

Sweller, J. (1989). Cognitive technology: Some procedures for facilitating learning and problem solving in mathematics and science. *Journal of Educational Psychology, 81*(4), 457–466.

Sweller, J. (2010). Element interactivity and intrinsic, extraneous, and germane cognitive load. *Educational Psychology Review, 22*(2), 123–138.

Sweller, J. (2022). The role of evolutionary psychology in our understanding of human cognition: Consequences for cognitive load theory and instructional procedures. *Educational Psychology Review, 34*(4), 2229–2241. [Epub ahead of print].

Sweller, J., van Merrienboer, J. J. G., & Paas, F. G. W. C. (1998). Cognitive architecture and instructional design. *Educational Psychology Review, 10*(3), 251–296.

Sweller, J., van Merrienboer, J. J. G., & Paas, F. (2019). Cognitive architecture and instructional design: 20 years later. *Educational Psychology Review, 31,* 261–292.

Tomasulo, D. (2005). The interactive–behavioral model of group counseling for people with mental retardation and chronic psychiatric illness. *NADD Bulletin, III*(6), Article 3.

van Gog, T., Paas, F., & Sweller, J. (2010). Cognitive load theory: Advances in research on worked examples, animations, and cognitive load measurement. *Educational Psychology Review, 22*(4), 375–378.

Vine, V., Bernstein, E. E., & Nolen-Hoeksema, S. (2019). Less is more: Effects of exhaustive vs. minimal emotion labeling on emotion regulation strategies planning. *Cognition and Emotion, 33*(4), 855–862.

Zaki, J., & Williams, W. C. (2013). Interpersonal emotion regulation. *Emotion, 13*(5), 803–810.

Index

Note. *f* or *t* following a page number indicates a figure or table.

D

E

H

Q

R

T

U

V

W